PROSTHETI
DEPT.
R.e.e.

The Child With a Limb Deficiency

Shriners Hospitals for Crippled Childen Symposium

Published by the

American Academy of
Orthopaedic Surgeons

The Child With a Limb Deficiency

Edited by
John A. Herring, MD
Chief of Staff
Texas Scottish Rite Hospital
Professor of Orthopaedic Surgery
University of Texas Southwestern Medical School
Dallas, Texas

John G. Birch, MD
Associate Chief of Staff
Texas Scottish Rite Hospital
Pediatric Orthopaedics
Dallas, Texas

Symposium
Dallas, Texas
April 14-15, 1997

Supported by the
Shriners Hospitals for Crippled Children

Published by the
American Academy of Orthopaedic Surgeons
6300 North River Road
Rosemont, IL 60018

The Child With a Limb Deficiency

American Academy of Orthopaedic Surgeons

First Edition
Copyright © 1998 by the
American Academy of Orthopaedic Surgeons

ISBN 0-89203-175-1

Library of Congress Cataloging-in-Publication Data
The child with a limb deficiency/edited by John A. Herring, John G. Birch. -- 1st ed.
p. cm.
"Symposium, Dallas, Texas, April 14-15, 1997, supported by the Shriners Hospitals for Crippled Children, in collaboration with the Pediatric Orthopaedic Society of North America."
Includes bibliographical references and index.
1. Extremities (Anatomy)--Abnormalities--Congresses.
2. Prosthesis--Congresses. 3. Pediatric orthopaedics--Congresses.
4. Physically handicapped children--Rehabilitation--Congresses.
I. Herring, John A. II. Birch, John G. III. Shriners Hospitals for Crippled Children. IV. Pediatric Orthopaedic Society of North America.
[DNLM: 1. Limb Deformities, Congenital--congresses. 2. Amputation--in infancy & childhood--congresses. 3. Prostheses and Implants--in infancy & childhood--congresses. 4. Rehabilitation--in infancy & childhood. WE 865 C536 1998]
RD775.C48 1998
618.92'09758--dc21
DNLM/DLC
for Library of Congress   98-11882 CIP

Contributors

William P. Adams, Jr, MD
Assistant Professor
Department of Plastic and
   Reconstructive Surgery
University of Texas, Southwestern
   Medical Center
Dallas, Texas

Todd F. Anderson, CP, BS
Prosthetic Manager
Shriners Hospitals, Twin Cities
Minneapolis, Minnesota

Diane J. Atkins, OTR
Coordinator, Amputee Program
The Institute for Rehabilitation and
   Research
Assistant Professor
Department of Physical Medicine
   and Rehabilitation
Baylor College of Medicine
Houston, Texas

James B. Bennett, MD
Consultant
Shriners Hospital for Children,
   Houston
Hand Surgeon
Texas Orthopedic Hospital
Houston, Texas

John G. Birch, MD
Assistant Chief of Staff
Texas Scottish Rite Hospital
Pediatric Orthopaedics
Dallas, Texas

Kenneth L.B. Brown, MD, MSc,
   FRCSC
Clinical Associate Professor
Department of Orthopaedic Surgery
University of British Columbia
British Columbia Childrens Hospital
Vancouver, BC, Canada

Maurizio A. Catagni, MD
Chief of the Ilizarov Unit
Department of Orthopaedics
Lecco General Hospital
Lecco, Italy

Frank M. Chang, MD
Director, Orthopaedic Surgery
The Children's Hospital, Denver
Associate Professor
University of Colorado Department
   of Orthopaedic Surgery
Denver, Colorado

Mary Williams Clark, MD
Chief, Division of Pediatric
   Orthopaedics
Department of Orthopaedic Surgery
Medical College of Ohio
Toledo, Ohio

Gregory Clines, BS
MSTP Student
McDermott Center
University of Texas, Southwestern
   Medical Center
Dallas, Texas

Colleen Coulter-O'Berry, MS, PT, PCS
Board Certified Pediatric Clinical
   Specialist
Team Leader Limb Deficiency and
   Seating/Mobility
Department of Orthotics and
   Prosthetics
Scottish Rite Children's Medical
   Center
Atlanta, Georgia

Donald R. Cummings, CP
Director of Prosthetics
Texas Scottish Rite Hospital for
   Children
Dallas, Texas

Jon R. Davids, MD
Director, Motion Analysis
  Laboratory
Shriners Hospital for Children
Greenville, South Carolina

Darin Davidson
Orthopaedic Research Fellow
Division of Pediatric Orthopaedics
Childrens Hospital, Eastern Ontario
Ottawa, Ontario, Canada

John P. Dormans, MD
Associate Professor of Orthopaedic
  Surgery
The University of Pennsylvania
Chief of Orthopaedic Surgery
The Children's Hospital of
  Philadelphia
Philadelphia, Pennsylvania

Marybeth Ezaki, MD
Director of Hand Surgery
Texas Scottish Rite Hospital for
  Children
Dallas, Texas

Eileen Fowler, PhD, PT
Assistant Professor
Department of Orthopaedic Surgery
University of California at Los
  Angeles
Los Angeles, California

Robert Gillespie, MB, ChB,
  FRCSC, FRCS(Ed)
Head, Department of Pediatric
  Orthopaedics
The Children's Hospital of Buffalo
Buffalo, New York

Francesco Guerreschi, MD
Orthopaedic Surgeon
Lecco General Hospital
Orthopaedic Department
Lecco, Italy

Nasreen F. Haideri, ME
Supervisor
Movement Science Lab
Texas Scottish Rite Hospital for
  Children
Dallas, Texas

John E. Hall, MD
Professor of Orthopaedic Surgery
Harvard Medical School
Children's Hospital
Boston, Massachusetts

James A. Harder, BSc, MD, FRCSC
Clinical Associate Professor
Division of Pediatric Orthopaedic
  Surgery
University of Calgary
Alberta Children's Hospital
Calgary, Alberta, Canada

Winfried Heim, CP(C)
Certified Prosthetist
Amputee Program, Myoelectric
  Services
Bloorview MacMillan Centre
Toronto, Ontario, Canada

John A. Herring, MD
Chief of Staff
Texas Scottish Rite Hospital
Professor of Orthopaedic Surgery
University of Texas Southwestern
  Medical School
Dallas, Texas

P. Craig Hobar, MD
Assistant Professor
Craniofacial Director
Department of Plastic and
  Reconstructive Surgery
University of Texas, Southwestern
  Medical Center
Dallas, Texas

Sheila A. Hubbard, PT, OT, BSc
Physical and Occupational
  Therapist
Clinical Coordinator, Amputee
  Program
Bloorview MacMillan Centre
Toronto, Ontario, Canada

Charles E. Johnston II, MD
Assistant Chief of Staff
Texas Scottish Rite Hospital
Dallas, Texas

J. Ivan Krajbich, MD, FRCSC
Director, Spinal Deformity and
  Tumor Programs
Shriners Hospital for Children,
  Portland Unit
Associate Professor, Department of
  Surgery
Oregon Health Science University
Portland, Oregon

Leon M. Kruger, MD
Chief of Staff Emeritus
Shriners Hospital for Children
Springfield, Massachusetts

Isaac Kurtz, MHSc, PEng
Electronics Coordinator
Rehabilitation Engineering Department
Bloorview MacMillan Centre
Toronto, Ontario, Canada

Merv Letts, MD, FRCSC
Head, Division of Pediatric
  Orthopaedics
Surgeon-in-Chief, Childrens
  Hospital, Eastern Ontario
University of Ottawa
Ottawa, Ontario, Canada

Todd L. Lincoln, MD
Assistant Professor of Orthopaedic
  Surgery
Division of Orthopaedic Surgery
Stanford University
Palo Alto, California

Randall T. Loder, MD
Associate Professor
Section of Orthopaedic Surgery
University of Michigan
Ann Arbor, Michigan

Michael Lovett, PhD
Associate Professor
McDermott Center
University of Texas, Southwestern
  Medical Center
Dallas, Texas

Philip William Mack, MD
Orthopaedic Surgery
Flagstaff Medical Center
Flagstaff, Arizona

Daniel Massey*
Quadrimelic Congenital Amputee
Dallas, Texas

Newton C. McCollough III, MD*
Director of Medical Affairs
Shriners Hospitals for Children
Tampa, Florida

Gert Montgomery, BScN, MSW, CSW
Social Worker
Bloorview MacMillan Centre
Toronto, Ontario, Canada

Anne A. Morton, PhD
Director of Psychology
Texas Scottish Rite Hospital for
  Children
Dallas, Texas

Kenneth J. Noonan, MD
Assistant Professor
Pediatric Orthopaedic Surgery
Riley Children's Hospital
Indianapolis, Indiana

William L. Oppenheim, MD
Professor and Head of Children's
  Orthopedics
UCLA School of Medicine
Department of Orthopaedic Surgery
University of California, Los
  Angeles
Los Angeles, California

Dror Paley, MD, FRCSC
Professor of Orthopaedics
Chief, Pediatric Orthopaedics
Co-Director, Maryland Center for
  Limb Lengthening
University of Maryland
Kernan Hospital
Baltimore, Maryland

Joanna G. Patton, BS, OTR
Clinical Occupational Therapist and
  Instructor
Child Amputee Prosthetics Project
Shriners Hospital for Children,
  Los Angeles
Los Angeles, California

Charles T. Price, MD
Surgeon in Chief
Nemours Childrens' Clinic, Orlando
Director, Pediatric Orthopaedics
Orlando Regional Healthcare
  System
Orlando, Florida

Sheri D. Pruitt, PhD
Assistant Professor
Department of Psychiatry
University of California, San Diego
  School of Medicine
San Diego, California

Daniel C. Riordan, MD
Emeritus Professor, Clinical
  Orthopaedics
Tulane University Medical School
New Orleans, Louisiana

Thomas W. Sadler, PhD
Professor
Director, UNC Birth Defects Center
Department of Cell Biology and
  Anatomy
University of North Carolina
Chapel Hill, North Carolina

Perry L. Schoenecker, MD
Professor of Orthopaedics
Washington University
Chief of Staff
St. Louis Shriners Hospital
St. Louis, Missouri

C. Michael Schuch, BA, CPO
Assistant Clinical Professor and
  Director
Department of Prosthetics and
  Orthotics
Duke University Medical Center
Durham, North Carolina

Michael Seid, PhD
Research Associate
Center for Child Health Outcomes
Children's Hospital, San Diego
San Diego, California

Yoshio Setoguchi, MD
Medical Director
Child Amputee Prosthetics Project
Shriners Hospital for Children
Los Angeles, California

Julie Shaperman, MSPH, OTR
Research Associate
Rehabilitation Engineering
  Program
Rancho Los Amigos Medical
  Center
Downey, California

Howard H. Steel, MD, PhD
Chief Surgeon, Emeritus
Shriners' Hospital for Children
Philadelphia, Pennsylvania

Jeanine R. Thomas, PT
Physical Therapy
Texas Scottish Rite Hospital
Dallas, Texas

James W. Varni, PhD
Professor of Psychiatry
University of California, San Diego
San Diego, California

Hugh G. Watts, MD
Clinical Professor, Orthopaedics
University of California, Los
    Angeles
Shriners Hospital
Los Angeles, California

David D. Weaver, MD
Professor and Director of Clinical
    Service
Department of Medical and
    Molecular Genetics
Indiana University School of
    Medicine
Indianapolis, Indiana

Golder N. Wilson, MD, PhD
Director, Division of Pediatric
    Genetics and Metabolism
Mary McDermott Cook
    Distinguished Professor of
    Pediatric Genetics
Department of Pediatrics
University of Texas Southwestern
    Medical Center
Dallas, Texas

Carol A. Wise, PhD
Research Scientist
Texas Scottish Rite Hospital
Dallas, Texas

* Participant in symposium

Contents

Foreword

This volume is the third in a series of pediatric orthopaedic symposia published by the American Academy of Orthopaedic Surgeons and made possible through sponsorship by Shriners Hospitals for Children. Beginning in 1990, Shriners Hospitals have provided the Academy with funds to support triennial symposia on selected topics in pediatric orthopaedics. The topics chosen are those for which treatment is difficult or controversial, and about which there is little available current literature to guide patient care.

The symposia are developed by the Committee on Pediatric Orthopaedics of the Academy in collaboration with the Pediatric Orthopaedic Society of North America. They are intended to define the current status of patient care, to develop consensus on controversial issues, and to identify research priorities. In order to have maximal impact on patient care, the Academy has agreed to publish these symposia, making the information widely available to those in the health care professions.

This symposium on the Child With a Limb Deficiency was organized and conducted under the very capable leadership of Dr. John A. Herring as chairman and Dr. John Birch as Vice Chairman. They selected an outstanding group of participants and contributors for the symposium who represented many disciplines. Further, they identified the most perplexing and difficult limb deficient conditions for in-depth consideration by these experts. Many controversies in approach to treatment were identified and discussed. Dr. Herring was extremely effective in driving the participants to consensus and in organizing the work product of the group.

Shriners Hospitals for Children alone have more than 6,000 active patients with limb deficiencies, who account for over 500 admissions for inpatient care annually to its 19 pediatric orthopaedic hospitals. These children pose unique challenges in functional and cosmetic restoration for the clinic team. Interdisciplinary assessment and communication is essential for an optimum result. It is hoped that the information contained in these pages will facilitate that communication to the ultimate benefit of limb deficient children and their families.

NEWTON C. MCCOLLOUGH III, MD
DIRECTOR OF MEDICAL AFFAIRS
SHRINERS HOSPITALS FOR CHILDREN
TAMPA, FLORIDA

Preface

For two days in April of 1997 some 38 people met in Dallas to educate one another, to agree upon some things and disagree on others having to do with children with limb deficiencies. This book is the visible result of that interaction. The invisible result was that each participant went home filled with new ideas and broadened perceptions about these important children and adolescents. It is our sincere hope that the multidisciplinary approach of this work will appeal to and educate all those involved in the care of such children.

This symposium occurred through the generosity of the Shrine Hospital system combined with the management skills of the American Academy of Orthopaedic Surgeons, and is the third such symposium. The book is directed toward any professional person dealing with children who have limb deficiencies. We also welcome parents and children as readers. Each author has written a state of the art chapter in an area of his or her expertise, in language understandable by most people in related fields. The consensus statements were forged by the entire group working together, and reflect either general agreement or the fact that at times agreement was not possible. These statements, in fact, reflect the similarities and differences in the state of the art as practiced in different centers in North America and Europe.

The basic science sections are extensive and worth reading by every person in the field. An example is the subclavian artery disruption sequence, an hypothetical sequence of events that may account for a number of seemingly unrelated congenital defects. While the actual mechanism may or may not exactly fit the hypothesis, understanding this piece of embryology may open productive new avenues of research and thought. The long-neglected genetic aspects of limb deficiency are now coming to the forefront as the genetic revolution gathers momentum. The related chapters emphasize that there are many more heritable limb abnormalities than we have previously recognized.

Another reason to publish the efforts of so many diverse workers is illustrated in the chapters by our psychologic colleagues. Dr. Varni admonishes us to measure the effects we glibly speak of while Dr. Morton lets us glimpse the world of difficulties a child enters when he or she undertakes a major surgical procedure for correction of deformity. The psychologic costs and benefits of any of our interventions must be carefully weighed when we contemplate treatment alternatives.

In several chapters many questions are asked and discussed regarding the classification and management of specific limb deficiencies. The proposed classifications are oriented toward helping with treatment decisions, and as such will evolve as our interventions evolve. These types of classification have their place just as anatomic classifications have theirs. The topics of rotationplasty, limb lengthening, and hip stabilization in children with femoral deficiency are thoroughly debated. There was hot debate about the appropriateness of multiple limb lengthening procedures in children with large discrepancies, and only time and experience will resolve the questions raised. We are making progress, but progress is difficult, and proposals that seem out of bounds today may be easily accomplished tomorrow. Others will fall by the wayside as better approaches become available. The management of fibular hemimelia is also thoroughly discussed, and the different chapters provide a balance between those who prefer amputation for moderately severe deficiencies and those who recommend limb lengthening. In the end, the choice remains for the reader to make.

Finally the topics of limb salvage, management of residual limbs, or "stumps" as Dr. Watts insists they be called, and prevention of amputation are important for all readers. Dr. Letts rightly admonishes those of us who treat children who have suffered traumatic amputations to become advocates at the forefront of the efforts to rid the world of land mines and other hazards to children.

The editors wish to thank the Shrine Hospitals for their support of this project, as well as the American Academy of Orthopaedic Surgeons without whose sponsorship this work would not have happened. Special thanks goes to the AAOS Publications Department who have tirelessly copy edited the book and prepared it for publication. Also much thanks to Louise Hamilton and Phyllis Cuesta of our office who spent a great deal of time organizing the symposium. We were amazed that so many individuals from so many different disciplines were able to work successfully together in the consensus process. We would also like to thank the authors for their timely manuscript completion. Finally a special word of thanks to Daniel Massey, a remarkably accomplished young man who joined all our deliberations and just happens to have congenital quadrimelic limb deficiency.

JOHN A. HERRING, MD
JOHN G. BIRCH, MD

Section 1
Embryology and Genetics of the Normal and Deficient Limb

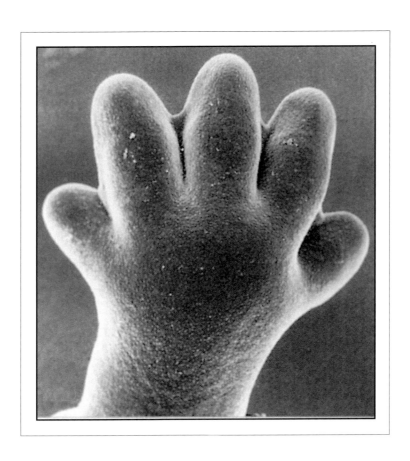

Chapter 1

Embryology and Gene Regulation of Limb Development

Thomas W. Sadler, PhD

Limb Morphogenesis

Limb development begins during the fourth week (postfertilization) along the flank of the embryo in predetermined regions opposite cervicothoracic and lumbosacral segments (Fig. 1). These limb fields are defined prior to limb outgrowth and appear to depend on signals from intermediate mesoderm of the mesonephric kidney and the somites.[1] Initiation of growth involves thickening of lateral plate mesoderm that, in turn, signals the overlying ectoderm to thicken and form a ridge over the tip of the limb bud (Fig. 2). This apical ectodermal ridge (AER) controls proximodistal limb growth by keeping the mesenchyme cells beneath it in a rapidly proliferating state, the progress zone. As mesoderm cells move away from this subectodermal progress zone, they cease proliferating and begin to differentiate. In this manner, the limb develops in a proximodistal direction from the limb girdle to the digits. Proximal bones of the limb girdle and the humerus/femur are patterned before differentiation of ridge ectoderm, while the formation of the remaining bones and digits depends on the AER.[2,3] Lateral plate mesoderm forms the bones and connective tissues of the limb, and muscles are derived from myotome regions of somitic mesoderm.

Growth of fore and hind limbs occurs by similar mechanisms, although lower limb development lags behind that of the upper limb by 1 to 2 days. As growth proceeds, three axes are established: (1) proximodistal, from flank to digit tip, controlled by the AER; (2) anteroposterior, from the radial (thumb) side to the ulna, controlled by the zone of polarizing activity (ZPA); and (3) dorsoventral, from the back of the hand to the palm, controlled by the dorsal ectoderm. By the sixth week, distal portions of the limbs flatten to form hand and footplates, while the first cartilage appears proximally. During the seventh week, the limbs rotate: the forelimb rotates laterally 90°, placing the thumb in a lateral position, while the hindlimb rotates medially 90°, placing the big toe in a medial position. Digital rays appear in the hand and footplates, and cell death occurs in the AER and the intervening spaces between each digit. Continued extension of each digit then depends on the cap of AER that remains at each tip. Final separation

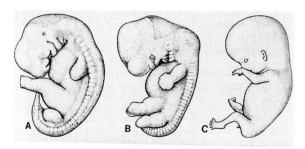

Fig. 1 *Growth of the limbs begins at the end of the fourth week postfertilization (**A**) with buds that form in mesoderm along the flank of the embryo. Growth of the forelimb precedes that of the hindlimb by 1 to 2 days. As the buds extend distally during the sixth week, the terminal portion flattens to form the hand and foot plates complete with digital rays (**B**). By 8 weeks, digits are present and the limbs have rotated to their normal position (**C**). Cartilage first appears in proximal segments and ossification centers are present in the long bones by the twelfth week. (Reproduced with permission from Sadler TW: Skeletal development, in* Langman's Medical Embryology, *ed 7. Baltimore, MD, Williams & Wilkins, 1995.)*

of the digits depends on additional cell death in the webbed area between each digit. By 8 weeks, the limbs are in their proper position and all segments are complete, including the digits. Ossification begins about this time, and by 12 weeks, ossification centers are present in all of the long bones.

Most limb defects occur early in the period of limb morphogenesis, when cells and tissues are rapidly proliferating and differentiating. This time is the limb's "sensitive period," which reaches a peak during the fifth and sixth weeks after fertilization. Unfortunately, this time is often prior to a woman's first prenatal visit, such that counseling for potential factors that cause birth defects is often too late to be effective.

Regulation of Limb Growth and Patterning

Factors regulating limb growth and patterning have been the subject of a great many studies and, in fact, limb morphogenesis is one of the most commonly investigated models of epithelial mesenchymal interactions and cell differentiation. Investigators have benefited from the accessibility of limb tissue in laboratory animals and from the fact that morphogenetic and genetic factors controlling limb development are highly conserved among different species. Early experiments relied on tissue transplants and morphologic analyses to establish the roles of various cells and tissues of the limb in induction and signaling. Now, with the advent of molecular biology, the genes and their products responsible for orchestrating limb development are being identified. In turn, their identification is providing potential candidate genes that may be involved in limb defects, either directly or through the actions of teratogens.

The Apical Ectodermal Ridge and Fibroblast Growth Factors

The role of the AER in regulating limb growth in a promodistal direction has been known for some time. Elegant experiments with chick embryos have demonstrated that removal of the ridge results in truncated limbs and that the earlier the AER is removed, the more severe the truncation.[3-6] The underlying mesenchyme induces and maintains the AER and, in turn, the AER keeps mesenchyme in the distal tip of the limb in an undifferentiated rapidly proliferating state (Fig. 2). Although the AER promotes limb outgrowth, the mesenchyme dictates the type of limb that will form. For example, mesenchyme from a hindlimb grafted beneath the AER of a forelimb or wing will form a hindlimb.[4,7] Thus, reciprocal signals are established between ectoderm and mesoderm. For years, investigators have searched for the signaling molecules and postulated theories about morphogen gradients to account for limb outgrowth and patterning.

Molecular biologists are now elucidating the factors involved in signaling and have shown that fibroblast growth factors (FGFs) play a pivotal role in limb outgrowth. Both FGF-4 and FGF-8[8,9] are present in the AER, and both can substitute for an intact ridge when applied exogenously to limb bud mesoderm.[10,11] Although both FGF-4 and FGF-8 may be important for a functional AER, evidence suggests that FGF-4 is present in the ectoderm only after an AER is induced,[12] whereas FGF-8 is present in pre-limb ectoderm before establishment of the AER.[9] Thus, FGF-8 may be involved in the initiation of limb outgrowth and, thereafter, both factors play roles in maintaining this growth. In this regard, both genes are also capable of maintaining genes expressed in the ZPA, which is important for anterior-posterior patterning (See below.)

Considering roles that FGFs might play in clinical dysmorphology of the limb, it is interesting to note that overexpression of FGF-8 in chick embryos resulted in truncations, deletions, extra digits, and other abnormalities.[9] In some cases, limb reductions were accompanied by shortening of all skeletal elements, producing a phenotype similar to that of achondroplasia. This form of dwarfism is caused by mutations in the FGF-3 receptor (FGFR-3), such that the receptor is hyperactive.[13,14] Thus, overexpression of FGF-8 may interfere with normal signaling by the FGFs and/or their receptors, which appear to be involved in a number of human skeletal dysmorphologies.[14] Interestingly, limb mesoderm cells express FGFR-1, whereas FGFR-2 is expressed in limb ectoderm[15] providing additional support for the hypothesis that these molecules are involved in signaling pathways important for limb development.

The Zone of Polarizing Activity and *Shh*

Like that of the AER, the functional role of the ZPA has been known for some time. This activity initially is localized in a small area of mesoderm along the posterior border of the limb near the body wall (Fig. 3). As the limb grows, this area moves outward, maintaining its posterior location close to the posterior border of the AER. Transplant studies in chick

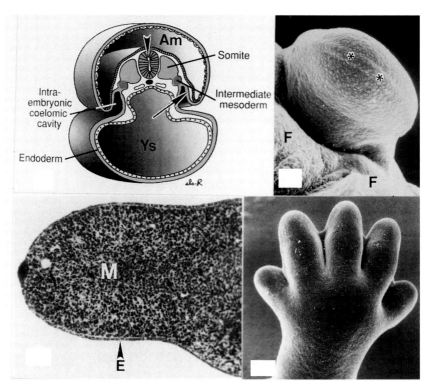

Fig. 2 Top left, *Cross section through an embryo showing the neural tube (arrowhead), somites, and intermediate mesoderm. This mesoderm signals lateral plate mesoderm (arrow) to initiate limb development. Am = amnion; Ys = yolk sac. (Reproduced with permission from Sadler TW: Skeletal development, in* Langman's Medical Embryology, *ed 7. Baltimore, MD, Williams & Wilkins, 1995.)* **Top right,** *As the limb grows out from the flank (F), the apical ectodermal ridge (AER; asterisks) forms at the limb tip and regulates proximodistal growth.* **Bottom left,** *Longitudinal section of a developing mouse limb bud showing the ectoderm (E) surrounding a core of undifferentiated meso-derm (M). At the limb tip, the ectoderm is thickened (arrows) to form the AER. (Reproduced with permission from Sadler TW: Skeletal development, in* Langman's Medical Embryology, *ed 7. Baltimore, MD, Williams & Wilkins, 1995.)* **Bottom right,** *Digits form following programmed cell death in the AER in the spaces between the dig-its. Each digit then continues to grow under the influence of its own AER. Tissue between the digits will also be removed by gene-regulated programmed cell death.*

embryos have shown that the ZPA is involved in anteroposterior patterning of the limb and digits. For example, transplanting an extra ZPA to the ante-rior region of a normal chick limb results in a mirror image duplication of the digits[16–18] (Fig. 3). Once again the hypothesis was raised that one or more morphogens were responsible for this activity and that a gradient was established, such that specific thresholds for the morphogen resulted in the induction of anterior to posterior structures.[19] In this model, the highest concentration of the proposed morphogen was at the posterior border of the

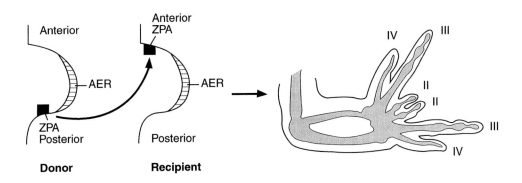

Fig. 3 *Regulation of the anteroposterior limb axis. A small block of mesoderm near the posterior border of the limb, the zone of polarizing activity (ZPA), regulates anteroposterior patterning of the limb, assuring, for example, that the digits appear in their proper order. If the ZPA is transplanted into the anterior margin of a normal recipient limb, then it will result in a mirror image duplication of the digits as shown in the caricature of a chick limb that would normally have 3 digits, with digit 2 on the radial side. In normal limbs, as the apical ectodermal ridge (AER) regulates distal growth, the ZPA is moved distally as well, maintaining close proximity to the posterior border of the AER. Signals from the AER support gene expression in the ZPA.*

limb, near the ZPA, while the lowest was at the anterior border, farthest from the ZPA.

Searches for the morphogen at first suggested that retinoic acid was the molecule, and studies showed that its exogenous application to the anterior border of a normal limb could mimic results from ZPA transplant studies and cause mirror image duplications.[20] However, it now appears that the action of the ZPA resides in the protein produced by the *sonic hedgehog* gene (*shh*),[21] and that the effect of retinoic acid, when placed in anterior limb mesoderm, is to induce expression of this gene, thereby creating a new ZPA.[22] Whether or not retinoic acid acts endogenously in a normal limb to induce a ZPA is not yet clear. Interestingly, however, retinoids as teratogens can mimic virtually every limb defect known clinically, thereby attesting to their powerful effects.[23,24]

Shh is a homologue of the *Drosophila* segment polarity gene *hh*. It is a secreted protein expressed by ZPA mesoderm and possesses all the activity of the ZPA. Thus, ectopic expression of the gene results in mirror image duplications like those the grafting experiments had produced.[21] Extrapolation of the role of *Shh* expression patterns to human limb abnormalities would suggest that a gradient is essential and that overexpression might result in duplications (polydactyly), whereas underexpression might lead to deletions. In this regard, it is interesting that *shh* concentration gradients depend on cholesterol, which serves as a transport molecule for *sonic* protein.[25,26] Children with Smith-Lemli-Opitz syndrome, who suffer from a cholesterol deficiency resulting from abnormalities in cholesterol biosynthesis,[27] exhibit a variety of birth defects, including limb anomalies, such as postaxial polydactyly, short fingers, and distal axial triradius. These observations suggest a link between a defect in a metabolic pathway and gene function and probably represent only one of many sites of gene-environment interactions leading to limb anomalies.

Dorsal Ectoderm, *Wnt-7a*, and Feedback Loops

Patterning along the dorsoventral axis from the back of the hand to the palm depends on signals from the dorsal ectoderm. If this ectoderm is reversed dorsoventrally from the mesoderm, the polarity of the skeletal pattern is reversed as well.[28,29] Recent evidence suggests that *Wnt-7a*, a proto-oncogene and secreted signaling molecule, is localized exclusively to the dorsal ectoderm[30,31] and is responsible for this patterning. Thus, mice lacking this gene after targeted mutagenesis show alterations in dosoventral polarity, such that ventral structures form on the dorsal side of the limb.[32] These mice also exhibit a decrease in *shh* expression and absence of posterior limb structures. Because the *Wnt* family members are homologues of the *Drosophila* gene *wingless*, which is essential for *hh* expression,[33,34] it is hypothesized that in vertebrates there is a similar signaling pathway, which involves *Wnt-7a* and *shh*, whereby maintenance of *shh* expression depends on *Wnt-7a*. Evidence for this hypothesis is derived from studies showing that removal of dorsal ectoderm from developing chick limbs results in loss of the ulna and most posterior digit and in a decrease in *shh* expression. Furthermore, providing a source of *shh* to ectoderm-denuded limbs restores formation of these structures.[35] Thus, dorsal ectoderm influences both dorsoventral (directly) and anteroposterior (through *shh*) patterning of the limb. In fact, signals for all three limb axes interact in feedback loops: FGFs in the AER activate *shh* in the ZPA while *Wnt-7a* maintains the *shh* signal.[35]

Downstream Regulators, the Hox Genes

Homeobox (Hox) genes contain a conserved 180 base pair DNA sequence called the homeodomain. These genes act as transcription factors and appear in all species. In the limb, genes of the *HoxA*[36] cluster may play a role in proximodistal patterning, whereas genes of the *HoxD* cluster appear to contribute to anteroposterior patterning.[37] Both clusters are regulated by signals from the ZPA and the AER.[38] For example, grafting studies of ZPA mesoderm that result in mirror image duplications of the digits, also result in mirror image duplication of *HoxD* gene expression.[39-41] Furthermore, this response of the *HoxD* genes depends on an intact AER.[40,41]

Expression of the *HoxD* gene cluster itself is intriguing and suggests that these genes play a patterning role. *HoxD* genes in this cluster include, *HoxD9, HoxD10, HoxD11, HoxD12,* and *HoxD13*. These genes are "nested" in overlapping expression patterns in the limb (Fig. 4), suggesting that their combined expression specifies digit identity.[38,42] In support of this hypothesis, misexpression of *HoxD11* across the entire limb bud results in transformation of digit 1 into digit 2.[43]

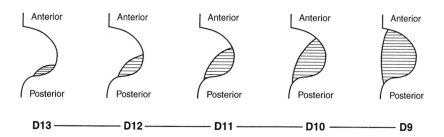

Fig. 4 *Homeobox gene expression in the limb. Expression of homeobox genes of the Hox D cluster are 'nested' in the limb bud in an overlapping pattern. Thus, D13 is expressed only in the most posterior border of the limb; D12 overlaps this expression pattern, but also extends over a slightly larger area and so on for each succeeding gene in the cluster. Because the homeobox genes are transcription factors that control gene expression, it is thought that this pattern is critical in specifying anteroposterior position across the limb.*

Mutant Mice Support a Role for Gene Interaction

Mice homozygous for mutations at the *limb deformity (ld)* locus exhibit shortened limbs, missing digits, and renal aplasia.[44] This locus encodes a group of protein isoforms termed *formins* that are normally expressed in the ureteric bud, AER, and other regions.[45-47] Mutations in the genes encoding these proteins result in a disorganized AER and improper gene signaling. For example, some mutants show expression of FGF-8, but no expression of FGF-4. Therefore, initiation of limb outgrowth occurs, but continued growth is disrupted by the absence of FGF-4 in the AER. Also, without an intact ridge and FGF-4, *shh* expression is downregulated and, consequently, anteroposterior patterning is disrupted. Finally, expression of the *HoxD* domains is delayed, either because of disruption of these signals and/or because of a lack of *ld* transcripts directly.[47-49] Tissue transplant experiments indicate that *ld* mesenchyme is unable to induce a normal AER, thereby accounting for signal disruption and, ultimately, limb abnormalities.[49]

Genes, Genes, Genes, and Teratogens

It is obvious that limb development is a complex process that involves the orchestration of a number of genes. Disruption of one player affects others that participate in the expression cascades that regulate cell phenomena responsible for limb development. It should not be surprising that loss or impairment of different genes may result in the same type of limb deformity, because these genes participate in interacting signaling pathways. It should also be noted that these same genes, such as *shh, Wnt, HoxD,* and so forth, are also found at other sites in the embryo where epithelial-mesenchymal interactions occur. For example, *Wnt* and *shh* both appear to be involved in craniofacial morphogenesis. Thus, multiple malformations may result from disruption of one of these genes, thereby forming a basis for some syndromes. Also, it should not be forgotten that teratogens and other factors, such as retinoic acid and low cholesterol, can inhibit normal gene expression or may act on cells and tissues directly, thereby producing phenocopies that appear to be genetic in origin, but are not.

References

1. Stephens TD, Spall R, Baker WC, et al: Axial and paraxial influences on limb morphogenesis. *J Morphol* 1991;208:367–379.

2. Saunders JW Jr: The proximo-distal sequence of origin of the parts of the chick wing and the role of the ectoderm. *J Exp Zool* 1948;108:363–403.

3. Summerbell D: A quantitative analysis of the effect of excision of the AER from the chick limb-bud. *J Embryol Exp Morphol* 1974;32:651–660.

4. Zwilling E: Ectoderm: Mesoderm relationship in the development of the chick embryo limb bud. *J Exp Zool* 1955;128:423–441.

5. Saunders JW Jr, Cairns JM, Gasseling MT: The role of the apical ridge of ectoderm in the differentiation of the morphological structure and inductive specificity of limb parts in the chick. *J Morphol* 1957;101:57–87.

6. Saunders JW Jr: Developmental control of three-dimensional polarity in the avian limb. *Ann NY Acad Sci* 1972;193:29–42.

7. Harrison RG: Experiments on the development of the fore limb of Amblystoma, a self-differentiating equipotential system. *J Exp Zool* 1918;25:413–461.

8. Heikinheimo M, Lawshé A, Shackleford GM, Wilson DB, MacArthur CA: FGF-8 expression in the post-gastrulation mouse suggests roles in the development of the face, limbs and central nervous system. *Mech Dev* 1994;48:129–138.

9. Vogel A, Rodriguez C, Izpisua-Belmonte JC: Involvement of FGF-8 in initiation, outgrowth and patterning of the vertebrate limb. *Development* 1996;122:1737–1750.

10. Niswander L, Martin GR: Fgf-4 and BMP-2 have opposite effects on limb growth. *Nature* 1993;361:68–71.

11. Mahmood R, Bresnick J, Hornbruch A, et al: A role for FGF-8 in the initiation and maintenance of vertebrate limb bud outgrowth. *Curr Biol* 1995;5:797–806.

12. Niswander L, Martin GR: Fgf-4 expression during gastrulation, myogenesis, limb, and tooth development in the mouse. *Development* 1992;114:755–768.

13. Rousseau F, Bonaventure J, Legeai-Mallet L, et al: Mutations in the gene encoding fibroblast growth factor receptor-3 in achondroplasia. *Nature* 1994;371:252–254.

14. Wilkie AO, Morriss-Kay GM, Jones EY, Heath JK: Functions of fibroblast growth factors and their receptors. *Curr Biol* 1995;5:500–507.

15. Orr-Urtreger A, Givol D, Yayon A, Yarden Y, Lonai P: Developmental expression of two murine fibroblast growth factor receptors flg and bek. *Development* 1991;113:1419–1434.

16. Saunders JW Jr, Gasseling MT: Ectodermal-mesenchymal interactions in the origin of limb symmetry, in Fleischmajer R, Billingham RE (eds): *Epithelial-Mesenchymal Interactions.* Baltimore, MD, Williams & Wilkins, 1968, pp 78–97.

17. Summerbell D: The zone of polarizing activity: Evidence for a role in normal chick limb morphogenesis. *J Embryol Exp Morphol* 1979;50:217–233.

18. Tickle C, Summerbell D, Wolpert L: Positional signalling and specification of digits in chick limb morphogenesis. *Nature* 1975;254:199–202.

19. Wolpert L: Positional information and the spatial pattern of cellular differentiation. *J Theor Biol* 1969;25:1–47.

20. Tickle C, Alberts B, Wolpert L, Lee J: Local application of retinoic acid to the limb bond mimics the action of the polarizing region. *Nature* 1982;296:564–566.

21. Riddle RD, Johnson RL, Laufer E, Tabin C: *Sonic hedgehog* mediates the polarizing activity of the ZPA. *Cell* 1993;75:1401–1416.

22. Wanek N, Gardiner DM, Muneoka K, Bryant SV: Conversion by retinoic acid of anterior cells into ZPA cells in the chick wing bud. *Nature* 1991;350:81–83.

23. Kochhar DM: Limb development in mouse embryos: I. Analysis of teratogenic effects of retinoic acid. *Teratology* 1973;7:289–295.

24. Kochhar DM: Cellular basis of congenital limb deformity induced in mice by vitamin A, in Bergsma D, Lenz W, Greene SC (eds): *Morphogenesis and Malformation of the Limb*. New York, NY, Alan R Liss, 1977, pp 111–154.

25. Porter JA, Ekker SC, Park WJ, et al: *Hedgehog* patterning activity: Role of a lipophilic modification mediated by the carboxy-terminal autoprocessing domain. *Cell* 1996;86:21–34.

26. Porter JA, Young EK, Beachy PA: Cholesterol modification of hedgehog signaling proteins in animal development. *Science* 1996;274:255–259.

27. Tint GS, Irons M, Elias ER, et al: Defective cholesterol biosynthesis associated with the Smith-Lemli-Opitz syndrome. *N Engl J Med* 1994;330:107–113.

28. MacCabe JA, Errick J, Saunders JW Jr: Ectodermal control of the dorsoventral axis in the leg bud of the chick embryo. *Dev Biol* 1974;39:69–82.

29. Pautou MP: Dorso-ventral axis determination of chick limb bud development, in Ede DA, Hinchliffe JR, Balls M (eds): *Vertebrate Limb and Somite Morphogenesis*. Cambridge, England, Cambridge University Press, 1977, pp 257–266.

30. Dealy CN, Roth A, Ferrari D, Brown AM, Kosher RA: Wnt-5a and Wnt-7a are expressed in the developing chick limb bud in a manner suggesting roles in pattern formation along the proximodistal and dorsoventral axes. *Mech Dev* 1993;43:175–186.

31. Parr BA, Shea MJ, Vassileva G, McMahon AP: Mouse Wnt genes exhibit discrete domains of expression in the early embryonic CNS and limb buds. *Development* 1993;119:247–261.

32. Parr BA, McMahon AP: Dorsalizing signal Wnt-7A required for normal polarity of D-V and A-P axes of mouse limb. *Nature* 1995;374:350–353.

33. Lee JJ, von Kessler DP, Parks S, Beachy PA: Secretion and localized transcription suggest a role in positional signaling for products of the segmentation gene hedgehog. *Cell* 1992;71:33-50.

34. Tabata T, Eaton S, Kornberg TB: The Drosophila hedgehog gene is expressed specifically in posterior compartment cells and is a target of engrailed regulation. *Genes Dev* 1992;6:2635–2645.

35. Yang Y, Niswander L: Interaction between the signaling molecules Wnt 7a and shh during vertebrate limb development: Dorsal signals regulate anteroposterior patterning. *Cell* 1995;80:939–947.

36. Yokouchi Y, Sasaki H, Kuroiwa A: Homeobox gene expression correlated with the bifurcation process of limb cartilage development. *Nature* 1991;353:443–445.

37. Dolle P, Izpisua-Belmonte JC, Falkenstein H, Renucci A, Duboule D: Coordinate expression of the murine Hox-5 complex homeobox-containing genes during limb pattern formation. *Nature* 1989;342:767–772.

38. Morgan BA, Tabin CJ: The role of homeobox genes in limb development. *Curr Opin Genet Dev* 1993;3:668–674.

39. Nohno T, Noji S, Koyama E, et al: Involvement of the Chox-4 chicken homeobox genes in determination of anterior posterior axial polarity during limb development. *Cell* 1991;64:1197–1205.

40. Izpisua-Belmonte JC, Tickle C, Dolle P, Wolpert L, Duboule D: Expression of the homeobox Hox-4 genes and the specification of position in chick wing development. *Nature* 1991;350:585–589.

41. Izpisua-Belmonte JC, Brown JM, Crawley A, Duboule D, Tickle C: Hox-4 gene expression in mouse/chicken heterospecific grafts of signalling regions to limb buds reveals similarities in patterning mechanisms. *Development* 1992;115:553–560.

42. Duboule D: How to make a limb? *Science* 1994;266:575–576.

43. Morgan BA, Izpisua-Belmonte JC, Duboule D, Tabin CJ: Targeted misexpression of Hox-4.6 in the avian limb bud causes apparent homeotic transformations. *Nature* 1992;358:236–239.

44. Kleinebrecht J, Selow J, Winkler W: The mouse mutant limb deformity (ld). *Anat Anz* 1982;152:313–324.

45. Woychik RP, Maas RL, Zeller R, Vogt TF, Leder P: 'Formins': Proteins deduced from the alternative transcripts of the limb deformity gene. *Nature* 1990;346:850–853.

46. Jackson-Grusby L, Kuo A, Leder P: A variant limb deformity transcript expressed in the embryonic mouse limb defines a novel formin. *Genes Dev* 1992;6:29–37.

47. Chan DC, Wynshaw-Boris A, Leder P: Formin isoforms are differentially expressed in the mouse embryo and are required for normal expression of Fgf-4 and shh in the limb bud. *Development* 1995;121:3151–3162.

48. Haramis AG, Brown JM, Zeller R: The limb deformity mutation disrupts the SHH/FGF-4 feedback loop and regulation of 5' Hox D genes during limb pattern formation. *Development* 1995;121:4237–4245.

49. Kuhlman J, Niswander L: Limb deformity proteins: Role in mesodermal induction of the apical ectodermal ridge. *Development* 1997;124:133–139.

Chapter 2
Genetic Control of Limb Development

Michael Lovett, PhD
Gregory Clines, BS
Carol A. Wise, PhD

Introduction

Our current understanding of the genetics of human limb development owes much to basic research conducted on three model organisms: the fruit fly, the mouse, and the chick. At first sight, vertebrate limb development, with the interplay of positional genetic cues, modeling, and growth signals, seems dauntingly complex. Despite this apparent complexity, it is becoming clear that many of the key genetic players fall into a series of discrete gene families. In the fruit fly, *Drosophila melanogastor*, these genes usually are present in only one or a very few copies. In mouse and man, these gene families, through the evolutionary process of duplication and divergence, exist in much larger numbers. In some cases, several members of a gene family have apparently overlapping functions; in most cases they are involved in several different developmental steps and act in several different tissues. One consequence of this is that disruptions of key controlling genes can have widespread deleterious effects that may not just involve limb abnormalities.

The developing limb has three axes: the anterior/posterior, the dorsal/ventral, and the proximal/distal (Fig. 1). Some of the important signals for initiating and maintaining these axes have now been worked out in detail (Fig. 1). Although it might seem easiest to describe the entire process of limb development with reference only to signals that control these three axes, the situation is not quite that simple. The genes that initiate and potentiate signals in different axes often interact and feed back, resulting in effects that are not confined to one direction of growth. Therefore, in the following sections we will describe the separate genes and gene families that are involved in this process and the signaling cascades that they participate in. The key genes involved in limb development are summarized in Table 1.

The past 5 years have seen a revolution in the understanding of limb development. Despite all this progress, it is nevertheless important to realize that large gaps still exist in this knowledge, especially in the steps that occur between the early inductive signals in limb bud differentiation and the final formation of the specialized tissues in the fully developed vertebrate limb.

Fibroblast Growth Factors

Retinoic acid, acting via a specific set of receptors, can function as a potent inducer of limb bud development.[1] In addition, specific homeobox genes

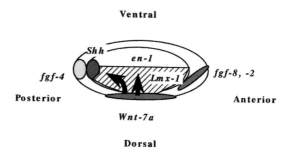

The dorsal/ventral boundary, as specifed by *lmx-1* and particularly *engrailed 1 (en-1)*, is where *radical fringe* is expressed to form the AER.

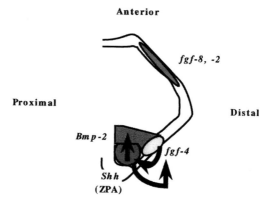

Fig. 1 The three axes of limb development and signaling molecules that are important in their specification. Key signaling molecules are shown according to where they are expressed. Arrows indicate either an inductive signal (eg, Shh turning on Bmp-2) or a feedback loop (eg, the feedback loop between Shh and fgr-4).

play a role in positioning where a limb bud will occur.[2] However, in a remarkable series of recent experiments[3–5] it has been shown that fibroblast growth factors *(Fgfs)* alone are sufficient to induce the complete development of additional limbs when applied to the flank of chick embryos. In support of this, an *Fgf-4* coated bead placed next to a limb bud from which the apical ectodermal ridge has been removed is able to maintain mouse limb bud outgrowth.[6,7] *Fgfs* are made by at least eight related genes and act through specific membrane bound receptors *(Fgfrs)* to send their signals. Any one of *Ffgfs 1, 2, 4, 6,* or *8* is sufficient to induce the signaling cascades that lead to the development of a complete limb.

The early limb bud consists of a layer of ectoderm overlaying a bud of mesenchyme. At the tip of the limb bud, running anteroposteriorly as a rim

Table 1 Key genes involved in limb development

Name of gene/gene family	Examples	Activity
Fibroblast growth factors	*FGFs -4, -6, -8*	Growth factors mostly in apical ectodermal ridge (AER)
Hedgehog genes	*Shh*	Membrane-bound signal for anteroposterior axes in zone of polarizing activity
Patched	*Ptc*	Receptor for hedgehog (*hh*) proteins
Smoothened	*Smo*	Bound to *Ptc* and released when *hh* proteins bind
Bone morphogenetic proteins (BMPs)	*Bmp-2, Bmp-7*	Switched on in mesenchyme *Shh* via pathway
Gli genes	*Gli-1, Gli-2, Gli-3*	Transcription factors turned on via *Shh* pathaway
Wnt genes	*Wnt-7a*	Dorsalizing signal, turns on *Lmx-1*; repressed by *engrailed-1*
Fringe genes	*Radical fringe*	Proximal/distal signal, turns on *Ser-2* and induces AER formation
Homeobox genes	*Hox-b8*	Transcription factors. Confer positional identity. Act both early and late in limb development
T-box genes	*Tbx-3, Tbx-5*	Transcription factors that may be turned on by BMPs or *Wnt* gene products

of taller epithelia, is a cluster of cells called the apical ectodermal ridge (AER). The signals that induce this ridge will be discussed further. *Fgf-8* is turned on very early in the ectoderm[8] and may induce the expression of other inductive signals such as *Sonic hedgehog*. *Fgf-2 is* present in both the ectoderm and the mesoderm[9] and *Fgf-4* is present in the ectoderm at the posterior margin of the ectodermal ridge.[10] This posterior area is very close to where the gene *Sonic hedgehog (Shh)* is expressed and the continued expression of *Fgf-4* is maintained by *Shh*.[11,12] In a sort of molecular quid pro quo, *Fgf-4*, in turn, feeds back to maintain *Shh* expression. To date, the *Fgf* genes, although having dramatic effects upon limb development, have not been associated with inherited genetic diseases in humans. However, mutations in the genes encoding three FGF receptors (FGFR1, 2, and 3) cause a number of human craniofacial developmental disorders[13] and other mutations in FGFR3 cause the dwarfing disorder achondroplasia.[14]

Sonic Hedgehog

The zone of polarizing activity (ZPA) in the developing limb bud is an area of posterior mesenchyme that lies below the ectoderm (the area where *Fgf-4* is expressed). The ZPA sets up a gradient of activity that defines the posterior/anterior axis of the limb. When the ZPA of one limb bud is transplanted to the anterior margin of another, a duplicate set of digits is formed in the reverse orientation; thus, the ZPA exhibits polarizing activity.[15] This implies that a morphogen present within the ZPA produces an anterior/posterior gradient within the limb bud; posterior digits form at high morphogen concentrations and anterior digits form at lower concentrations. Retinoic acid was an early candidate for this morphogen. It is well known that high doses of retinoid-containing drugs are associated with the development of limb abnormalities in mice and humans.[16] Furthermore, implantation of a retinoic acid-soaked bead to the anterior limb bud margin has the same digit-duplication effect as ZPA transplantation and acts in a dose-dependent manner.[17] However, the presence of endogenous retinoic acid within the limb bud is still controversial, and exogenous retinoic acid may only incidentally activate ZPA-associated genes. Recently, it has become clear that the ZPA inductive signal is in fact encoded by the *Shh* gene, which is expressed in the ZPA.[18] *Hedgehog* genes were originally described in *Drosophila* and are a multigene family with diverse signaling functions in higher vertebrates.[19] *Shh* acts as an inductive signal in the development of several tissues, but in the limb bud it is first seen in the ZPA.

Shh expression is sufficient to maintain ZPA activity, and therefore, it was thought to encode a diffusible signaling molecule that was in highest concentration at the ZPA and gradually decreased in concentration at greater distances from the ZPA. This does not appear to be the case. The *Shh* protein precursor is cleaved into two pieces, one diffusible and the other membrane bound, but it is the membrane bound, N-terminal piece that encodes the inductive activity.[20] *Shh* protein is bound to the membrane via cholesterol, and the presence of this membrane link is important for *Shh* signaling.[21] *Shh* expression may originally be induced in the ZPA by the action of *Fgfs* and/or homeobox genes. *Shh* induces the expression of a cascade of downstream genes, and it does this by binding to its specific receptor, which is called *Patched*. The downstream genes include bone morphogenetic proteins, *Wnt* genes, *Gli* transcription factors, and homeobox genes.[22] Levels of *Shh* in the ZPA can be experimentally reduced or eliminated in transgenic animals (animals into which a segment of DNA has been experimentally introduced).[23] Decreases in *Shh* protein lead to the loss of the ulna and posterior digits. Complete elimination of *Shh* activity leads to absence of distal limb structures. In humans, mutations in *Shh* cause the pleiotropic genetic disorder holoprosencephaly,[24] reflecting the many developmental steps in which this gene is involved.

Other *hedgehog* genes play decisive roles during later stages of limb development.[19] Among these is the *Indian hedgehog (Ihh)* gene which regulates the rate of cartilage differentiation.[25] This gene also binds to the receptor *Patched* and induces *Gli* transcription factors.

Patched and *Smoothened*

The *Patched (Ptc)* gene was first discovered in *Drosophila melanogaster*. In humans it appears to consist of only one gene that encodes a receptor for all the *hedgehog* proteins. It normally acts to repress the expression of genes such as bone morphogenetic proteins *(Bmps)*, homeobox genes, and *Gli* transcription factors.[20,26] When *Shh* binds to *Ptc* this repression is lifted and expression of these genes is induced. *Ptc* is associated in the cell membrane with the product of the *Smo* gene and appears to hold *Smo* in check. The structure of *Smoothened (Smo)* indicates that it encodes a seven transmembrane domain, G-coupled receptor. When *Shh* binds to *Ptc, Smo* is released and is free to transduce a signal to downstream genes. This is not the complete story of signal transduction from *Shh* to its downstream genes, because there appear to be at least two nonepistatic pathways leading from the *Shh-Ptc-Smo* interaction to the activation/repression of downstream genes. In humans, PTC acts as a tumor suppressor,[26] presumably because it normally keeps several potent growth control genes in check. When PTC function is completely lost, this leads to an increased incidence of basal cell nevus carcinoma, and mutations in PTC have also been found in some sporadic cases of basal cell carcinoma.

Bone Morphogenetic Proteins

Bmps were discovered by their ability to form ectopic bone when implanted under the skin or muscles of rats.[27,28] The products of these genes are related to the transforming growth factor-beta (TGF-ß) family of proteins and participate in fracture healing and in the developmental specification of joint placement.[29] Three BMP genes *(Bmp-2, Bmp-4,* and *Bmp-7)* are expressed within the mesenchyme and AER of developing limb buds.[12,30,31] Two of these, *Bmp-2* and *Bmp-7,* are expressed in response to *Shh* but do not cooperate with *Shh* as anteroposterior polarizers.[12] Interestingly, the *Drosophila* homolog of these genes is *decapentaplegic,* which is also a member of the TGF-ß superfamily and is also expressed as a consequence of *Drosophila hedgehog* expression. The function of the BMPs in very early limb bud formation is not clear, but they do appear to have a role in subsequent digit formation. For example, *Bmp-7* gene knockout mice have additional anterior digits.[32] However, BMPs by themselves do not appear to be sufficient to induce digit formation.[30,31] The expression of *Bmp-2, Bmp-4,* and *Bmp-7* in chicks is correlated with the programmed cell death (apoptosis) of interdigital tissue that is involved in the formation of the future digits.[33,34] Additional demonstration of the role of BMPs in digitation is the report that functional inactivation of a BMP receptor results in incomplete interdigital cell death, and chickens that have webbed feet.[34]

The continual extension of the limb bud removes mesenchymal cells in a proximal to distal progression from the undifferentiating effects of the apical ridge. Mesenchymal cells, in turn, form high cell densities called condensations at positions corresponding to future skeletal elements.[35] In-situ hybridization studies detected *Bmp-2* and *Bmp-5* within these cartilaginous condensations[36,37] consistent with findings that endogenous injection of these BMPs leads to identical cellular aggregations.[38] Under the instruction of a BMP or other unidentified factor, the mesenchymal condensations then differentiate into chondroblasts, which secrete the cartilage matrix.

Gli Transcription Factors

One downstream effect of the hedgehog signaling pathway is the activation of a family of three *Gli* genes that encode transcription factors. The proteins made by these genes then continue the cascade of gene expression by firing genes further downstream. *Gli*s are the mammalian homologs of the *Drosophila cubitus interruptus (cu)* gene.[39] Like *cu* they are members of the zinc finger-containing *Kruppel* family of transcription factors. Altering the expression of *Gli* genes can have profound deleterious consequences. In humans, GLI genes have been found to be amplified in glioblastomas and disruption of the GLI3 gene results in the autosomal dominant disorder Greig cephalopolysyndactyly.[40]

Wnt Genes

The *Wnt* signaling cascade is a highly conserved signaling pathway through-out the animal kingdom, and the gene family that encodes these diffusible molecules has been implicated in early developmental decision making in vertebrates and flies.[41] There are ten *Wnt* genes in mouse and man. Two of these, *Wnt-5a* and *Wnt-7a,* are expressed in specific areas of the developing limb bud. However, it is *Wnt-7a* expression that specifies the dorsoventral polarity in the limb bud. *Wnt-7a* transcripts are localized to the dorsal limb bud ectoderm [42,43] and if the mouse *Wnt-7a* gene is knocked out, the result-ing mice have paws with a double ventral pattern.[44] In the chick, the dorsal-izing effects of *Wnt-7a* are mediated by the homeobox gene *Lmx-1* expressed in the underlying dorsal mesenchyme of the limb bud.[45,46] *Lmx-1* is a LIM homeodomain transcription factor that is sufficient to specify dor-sal cell fate in the limb bud. In *Drosophila* the *wingless* gene is necessary for proper dorsal ventral patterning of the wing and leads to the expression of the LIM homeodomain transcription factor *apterous.*[47] Like *Lmx-1* in verte-brates, *apterous* specifies dorsal cell fate in the *Drosophila* wing. The *apter-ous* gene, in turn, controls the expression of the secreted protein *fringe.* By contrast, another homeodomain transcription factor *Engrailed-1 is* expressed in the ventral limb bud ectoderm, and targeted inactivation of this gene in mice results in dorsal transformation of the limb.[48] *Engrailed-1* appears to function by repressing the actions of *Wnt-7a* and also represses the action of *fringe* genes.

As was mentioned above, *Shh* in the ZPA and *Fgf-4* in the posterior mar-gin of the AER coactivate each other, forming a positive feedback loop, and thus maintain the polarizing potential of the ZPA.[11,12] *Wnt-7a* also partici-pates in this activiation; the continued expression of *Wnt-7a* in the dorsal epithelia acts to maintain *Shh* expression.[20] Thus, *Wnt-7a,* the dorsalizing signal for limb bud differentiation in the dorsal ventral axis, potentiates the expression of *Shh,* which encodes the signal for polarization in the anterior posterior axis.

Radical Fringe and *Ser-2*

The AER appears to control the proximal/distal patterning of the limb bud and maintains the high proliferative rate of the mesenchymal cells immediately beneath it, called the progress zone.[49] As the limb bud elongates, proximal limb mesenchyme loses the rapid proliferative signals of the AER and begins a process of differentiation. The importance of the AER has been known since 1948 when it was reported that its removal in chick resulted in limb truncation and that the earlier the removal the more extreme the truncation.[50] Recently, some of the specific molecular signals involved in inducing this ridge have been elucidated. Yet again, these molecules have homologs with well-conserved functional properties in the fruit fly. In *Drosophila* a specialized group of cells arranged in a dorsal ventral border along the wing margin express the *fringe* gene.[47] The boundary between those cells that do, or do not, express *fringe* becomes the wing edge. *Fringe* in turn induces the *serrate* gene, which then turns on downstream genes. In vertebrates, a homolog of *fringe* called *Radical fringe* appears to specifiy the same type of positional cue within the AER.[51,52] *Radical fringe* is expressed in the dorsal parts of the limb ectoderm before the AER forms. A *Radical fringe* boundary is required to form the AER, and at this boundary a homolog of *serrate* called *Ser-2 is* expressed. Support for the inductive effects of *Radical fringe* comes from the observation that ectopic application of the *Radical fringe* protein to a ventral surface results in the formation of an additional AER.[52]

Homeobox Genes

Homeobox genes were originally discovered in fruit flies and are responsible for conferring positional information on many different cell types. Disruptions of these genes can lead to homeotic transformations in which, for example, a leg primordia develops into an antenna. There are 39 homeobox genes (HOX genes) in humans arranged in four gene clusters. In addition to these, there are many other genes that share conserved structural elements with the *Hox* genes but are distributed elsewhere in the genome. The *Hox* genes encode transcription factors that all share a conserved homeodomain of 61 amino acids. In fruit flies, *hox* genes are activated in a stepwise manner and, to some extent, this is conserved in vertebrates.[53] It is beyond the scope of this review to attempt to summarize the complex pattern of *Hox* gene expression that occurs in the developing limb. However, some examples serve to illustrate the important roles these genes play in specifying positional information. Some *Hox* genes are turned on early in limb development. Among these, *Hox-b8* appears to play a role in specifying where the ZPA will arise. This gene is normally expressed within a segmental boundary that lies adjacent to where the ZPA of the forelimb will arise. If the *Hox-b8* zone of expression is experimentally engineered to lie more anteriorly, then two ZPAs are induced, resulting in mirror image forelimbs growing out of one limb bud.[54]

The three-dimensional differential expression of *Shh, Fgfs,* and *Wnt-7a* result in the expression of specific *Hox* genes also within a three-dimensional space.[11,12] The differential expression of *Hox* genes then activates other downstream effectors to instruct the mesenchymal cells as to their position and future cell type. Of the four *Hox* complexes, *Hoxa* and *Hoxd* genes are reported to be the major players and form a series of overlapping domains in the distal tip of the limb bud.[55–57] Mouse gene knockouts have been constructed for several *Hox* genes, and these mutants show specific defects with a close relationship between the affected skeletal elements and the expression domains of the respective *Hox* genes. Mouse *Hoxd-13* homozygous deletions result in the delay of overall limb development in addition to abnormal morphology of the wrist bones, metacarpals, and phalanges.[58] It appears that vertebrate *Hox* genes have some overlap and redundancy of function, and double gene knockouts in the mouse have been useful in determining these overlaps and interactions.[57] Nevertheless, two heritable human disorders that affect limb development have recently been found to be caused by mutations in discrete HOX genes. Mutations in HOX-D13 cause synpolydactyly,[59] and mutations in HOX-A13 cause hand-foot-genital syndrome,[60] a disorder in which there are reduced anterior and posterior digits.

T-Box Genes

T-box genes were first described in mice where the *T*-locus encodes a mutant T-box gene that results in mice with shortened tails and vertebral defects.[61] Mice homozygous for the *T* mutation die very early in embryogenesis. There are eight T-box genes in humans and mice (*T, Tbr-1, Tbx-1* through *Tbx-6*). These encode transcription factors that share a common T-box binding domain. Of these, *Tbx-2, -3, -4,* and *-5* are expressed during limb development and may be turned on by *Bmps -2,* or *-4* or by *Wnt.*[62,63]

Their significance in human limb development was recently demonstrated when mutations in human TBX-5 were shown to cause the heart-hand genetic disorder Holt-Oram syndrome,[62,63] in which phocomelia is one phenotype. Subsequently, another genetic disorder, ulnar-mammary syndrome, which also involves limb malformations, was found to be caused by mutations in the TBX-3 gene,[64] which is located close to the TBX-5 on human chromosome 12.

Conclusion and Future Prospects

The pattern that emerges from all of these genes and interactions is that a relatively small set of genes and gene families appear to control the early steps in limb devlopment. Although the develomental programs are different at the morphologic level, there is a remarkable molecular conservation of the pathways from flies to men.[65] In general, humans have more genes in a particular gene family, and these are used, in sometimes overlapping pathways, to play variations on a common theme; but the important point is that the molecular theme is conserved. Studies in *Drosophila* and especially in transgenic mice will doubtless continue to shed light on this complex and intriguing process. However, it will also be interesting and important to discover the differences between various species. Of particular interest in this regard will be the molecular dissection of limb regeneration in uredele amphibians.[66] Despite the insights derived from lower organisms, new control genes (eg, the TBX genes) are still being found in man, and the correlation between these genes, human biology, and human disease is still in its infancy. Technologic advances in the positional cloning of human genetic disease genes and the Human Genome Project promise to yield an explosion of correlations between heritable disorders of limb growth/patterning and specific defective genes. These, in turn, should aid the understanding of the more frequent sporadic cases and eventually lead to therapeutic interventions that are based upon a true understanding of the molecular genetics of human limb development.

References

1. Cash DE, Bock CB, Schughart K, Linney E, Underhill TM: Retinoic acid receptor alpha function in vertebrate limb skeletogenesis: A modulator of chondrogenesis. *J Cell Biol* 1997;136:445–457.

2. Cohn MJ, Patel K, Krumlauf R, Wilkinson DG, Clarke JD, Tickle C: Hox 9 genes and vertebrate limb specification. *Nature* 1997;387:97–101.

3. Cohn MJ, Izpisua-Belmonte JC, Abud H, Heath JK, Tickle C: Fibroblast growth factors induce additional limb development from the flank of chick embryos. *Cell* 1995;80:739–746.

4. Ohuchi H, Nakagawa T, Yamauchi M, et al: An additional limb can be induced from the flank of the chick embryo by FGF4. *Biochem Biophys Res Commun* 1995;209:809–816.

5. Crossley PH, Minowada G, MacArthur CA, Martin GR: Roles for FGF8 in the induction, initiation, and maintenance of chick limb development. *Cell* 1996;84: 127–136.

6. Miswander L, Martin GR: FGF-4 and BMP-2 have opposite effects on limb growth. *Nature* 1993;361:68–71.

7. Niswander L, Tickle C, Vogel A, Booth I, Martin GR: FGF-4 replaces the apical ectodermal ridge and directs outgrowth and patterning of the limb. *Cell* 1993;75:579–587.

8. Vogel A, Rodriguez C, Izpisua-Belmonte JC: Involvement of FGF-8 in initiation, outgrowth and patterning of the vertebrate limb. *Development* 1996;122: 1737–1750.

9. Fallon JF, Lopez A, Ros MA, Savage MP, Olwin BB, Simandl BK: FGF-2: Apical ectodermal ridge growth signal for chick limb development. *Science* 1994;264: 104–107.

10. Niswander L, Martin GR: Fgf-4 expression during gastrulation, myogenesis, limb and tooth development in the mouse. *Development* 1992;114:755–768.

11. Niswander L, Jeffrey S, Martin GR, Tickle C: A positive feedback loop coordinates growth and patterning in the vertebrate limb. *Nature* 1994;371:609–612.

12. Laufer E, Nelson CE, Johnson RL, Morgan BA, Tabin C: Sonic Hedgehog and Fgf-4 act through a signaling cascade and feedback loop to integrate growth and patterning of the developing limb bud. *Cell* 1994;79:993–1003.

13. Muenke M, Schell U: Fibroblast-growth-factor receptor mutations in human skeletal disorders. *Trends Genet* 1995;11:308–313.

14. Shiang R, Thompson LM, Zhu YZ, et al: Mutations in the transmembrane domain of FGFR3 cause the most common genetic form of dwarfism, achondroplasia. *Cell* 1994;78:335–342.

15. Saunders JW Jr, Gasseling MT: Ectodermal-mesenchymal interactions in the origin of limb symmetry, in Fleischmajer R, Billingham RE (eds): *Epithelial-Mesenchymal Interactions.* Baltimore, MD, Williams & Wilkins, 1968, pp 78–97.

16. Rizzo R, Lammer EJ, Parano E, Pavone L, Argyle JC: Limb reduction defects in humans associated with prenatal isotretinoin exposure. *Teratology* 1991;44: 599–604.

17. Summerbell D: The effect of local application of retinoic acid to the anterior margin of the developing chick limb. *J Embryol Exp Morphol* 1983;78:269–289.

18. Riddle RD, Johnson RL, Laufer E, Tabin C: Sonic hedgehog mediates the polarizing activity of the ZPA. *Cell* 1993;75:1401–1416.

19. Hammerschmidt M, Brook A, McMahon AP: The world according to hedgehog. *Trends Genet* 1997;13:14–21.

20. Yang Y, Niswander L: Interaction between the signaling molecules WNT7a and SHH during vertebrate limb development: Dorsal signals regulate anteroposterior patterning. *Cell* 1995;80:939–947.

21. Porter JA, Young KE, Beachy PA: Cholesterol modification of hedgehog signaling proteins in animal development. *Science* 1996;274:255–259.

22. Roberts DJ, Johnson RL, Burke AC, Nelson CE, Morgan BA, Tabin C: Sonic hedgehog is an endodermal signal inducing Bmp-4 and Hox genes during induction and regionalization of the chick hindgut. *Development* 1995;121:3163–3174.

23. Chiang C, Litingtung Y, Lee E, et al: Cyclopia and defective axial patterning in mice lacking Sonic hedgehog gene function. *Nature* 1996;383:407–413.

24. Roessler E, Belloni E, Gaudenz K, et al: Mutations in the human Sonic Hedgehog gene cause holoprosencephaly. *Nat Genet* 1996;14:357–360.

25. Vortkamp A, Lee K, Lanske B, Segre GV, Kronenberg HM, Tabin CJ: Regulation of rate of cartilage differentiation by Indian hedgehog and PTH-related protein. *Science* 1996;273:613–622.

26. Stone DM, Hynes M, Armanini M, et al: The tumour-suppressor gene patched encodes a candidate receptor for Sonic hedgehog. *Nature* 1996;384:129–134.

27. Wang EA, Rosen V, D'Alessandro JS, et al: Recombinant human bone morphogenetic protein induces bone formation. *Proc Natl Acad Sci USA* 1990;87: 2220–2224.

28. Hogan BL: Bone morphogenetic proteins in development. *Curr Opin Genet Dev* 1996;6:432–438.

29. Storm EE, Kingsley DM: Joint patterning defects caused by single and double mutations in members of the bone morphogenetic protein (BMP) family. *Development* 1996;122:3969–3979.

30. Francis PH, Richardson MK, Brickell PM, Tickle C: Bone morphogenetic proteins and a signalling pathway that controls patterning in the developing chick limb. *Development* 1994;120:209–218.

31. Francis-West PH, Robertson KE, Ede DA, et al: Expression of genes encoding bone morphogenetic proteins and sonic hedgehog in talpid (ta3) limb buds: Their relationships in the signalling cascade involved in limb patterning. *Dev Dyn* 1995;203:187–197.

32. Jena N, Martin-Seisdedos C: McCue P, Croce CM: BMP7 null mutation in mice: Developmental defects in skeleton, kidney, and eye. *Exp Cell Res* 1997;230:28–37.

33. Ganan Y, Macias D, Duterque-Coquillaud M, Ros MA, Hurle JM: Role of TGF beta s and BMPs as signals controlling the position of the digits and the areas of interdigital cell death in the developing chick limb autopod. *Development* 1996;122:2349–2357.

34. Zou H, Niswander L: Requirement for BMP signaling in interdigital apoptosis and scale formation. *Science* 1996;272:738–741.

35. Ede DA, Flint OP, Wilby OK, Coquhoun P: The development of pre-cartilage condensations in limb bud mesenchyme in vivo and in vitro. *Symp Br Soc Devel Biol* 1977;3:161–179.

36. Lyons KM, Pelton RW, Hogan BL: Patterns of expression of murine Vgr-1 and BMP-2a RNA suggest that transforming growth factor-beta-like genes coordinately regulate aspects of embryonic development. *Genes Dev* 1989;3:1657–1668.

37. Wozney JM, Capparella J, Rosen V: The bone morphogenetic proteins in cartilage and bone development, in Bernfield M (ed): *Molecular Basis of Morphogenesis*. New York, NY, Wiley-Liss, 1993, pp 221–230.

38. Wozney JM, Rosen V, Celeste AJ, et al: Novel regulators of bone formation: Molecular clones and activities. *Science* 1988;242:1528–1534.

39. Alexandre C, Jacinto A, Ingham PW: Transcriptional activation of hedgehog target genes in Drosophila is mediated directly by the cubitus interruptus protein, a member of the GLI family of zinc finger DNA-binding proteins. *Genes Dev* 1996;10:2003–2013.

40. Vortkamp A, Gessler M, Grzeschik KH: GLI3 zinc-finger gene interrupted by translocations in Greig syndrome families. *Nature* 1991;352:539–540.

41. Serrano N, O'Farrell PH: Limb morphogenesis: connections between patterning and growth. *Curr Biol* 1997;7:R186–R195.

42. Dealy CN, Roth A, Ferrari D, Brown AM, Kosher RA: Wnt-5a and Wnt-7a are expressed in the developing chick limb bud in a manner suggesting roles in pattern formation along the proximodistal and dorsoventral axes. *Mech Dev* 1993;43:175–186.

43. Parr BA, Shea MJ, Vassileva G, McMahon AP: Mouse Wnt genes exhibit discrete domains of expression in the early embryonic CNS and limb buds. *Development* 1993;119:247–261.

44. Parr BA, McMahon AP: Dorsalizing signal Wnt-7a required for normal polarity of D-V and A-P axes of mouse limb. *Nature* 1995;374:350–353.

45. Riddle RD, Ensini M, Nelson C, Tsuchida T, Jessell TM, Tabin C: Induction of the LIM homeobox gene Lmx1 by Wnt7a establishes dorsoventral pattern in the vertebrate limb. *Cell* 1995;83:631–640.

46. Vogel A, Rodriguez C, Warnken W, Izpisua-Belmonte JC: Dorsal cell fate specified by chick Lmx1 during vertebrate limb development. *Nature* 1995;378:716–720.

47. Irvine KD, Wieschaus E: Fringe,a Boundary-specific signaling molecule, mediates interactions between dorsal and ventral cells during Drosophila wing development. *Cell* 1994;79:595–606.

48. Loomis CA, Harris E, Michaud J, Wurst W, Hanks M, Joyner AL: The mouse Engrailed-1 gene and ventral limb patterning. *Nature* 1996;382:360–363.

49. Summerbell D, Lewis JH, Wolpert L: Positional information in chick limb morphogenesis. *Nature* 1973;244:492–496.

50. Saunders JW Jr: The proximo-distal sequence of origin of the parts of the chick wing and the role of the ectoderm. *J Exp Zool* 1948;108:363–403.

51. Rodriguez-Esteban C, Schwabe JW, De La Pena J, Foys B, Eshelman B, Belmonte JC: Radical fringe positions the apical ectodermal ridge at the dorsoventral boundary of the vertebrate limb. *Nature* 1997;386:360–366.

52. Laufer E, Dahn R, Orozco OE, et al: Expression of Radical fringe in limb-bud ectoderm regulates apical ectodermal ridge formation. *Nature* 1997;386:366–373.

53 Morgan BA, Tabin CJ: The role of Hox genes in limb development. *Prog Clin Biol Res* 1993;383A:1–9.

54. Charite J, de Graaff W, Shen S, Deschamps J: Ectopic expression of Hoxb-8 causes duplication of the ZPA in the forelimb and homeotic transformation of axial structures. *Cell* 1994;78:589–601.

55. Izpisua-Belmonte JC, Tickle C, Dolle P, Wolpert L, Duboule D: Expression of the homeobox Hox-4 genes and the specification of position in chick wing development. *Nature* 1991;350:585–589.

56. Yokouchi Y, Sasaki H, Kuroiwa A: Homeobox gene expression correlated with the bifurcation process of limb cartilage development. *Nature* 1991;353:443–445.

57. Fromental-Ramain C, Warot X, Messadecq N, LeMeur M, Dolle P, Chambon P: Hoxa-13 and Hoxd-13 play a crucial role in the patterning of the limb autopod. *Development* 1996;122:2997–3011.

58. Dolle P, Dierich A, LeMeur M, et al: Disruption of the Hoxd-13 gene induces localized heterochrony leading to mice with neotenic limbs. *Cell* 1993;75: 431–441.

59. Muragaki Y, Mundlos S, Upton J, Olsen BR: Altered growth and branching patterns in synpolydactyly caused by mutations in HOXD13. *Science* 1996;272: 548–551.

60. Mortlock DP, Innis JW: Mutation of HOXA13 in hand-foot-genital syndrome. *Nat Genet* 1997;15:179–180.

61. Herrmann BG, Labeit S, Poustka A, King TR, Lehrach H: Cloning of the T gene required in mesoderm formation in the mouse. *Nature* 1990;343:617–622.

62. Li QY, Newbury-Ecob RA, Terrett JA, et al: Holt-Oram syndrome is caused by mutations in TBX5, a member of the Brachyury (T) gene family. *Nat Genet* 1997;15:21–29.

63. Basson CT, Bachinsky DR, Lin RC, et al: Mutations in human TBX5 cause limb and cardiac malformation in Holt-Oram syndrome. *Nat Genet* 1997;15:30–35.

64. Bamshad M, Lin RC, Law DJ, et al: Mutations in human TBX3 alter limb, apocrine and genital development in ulnar-mammary syndrome. *Nat Genet* 1997;16:311–315.

65. Shubin N, Tabin C, Carroll S: Fossils, genes and the evolution of animal limbs. *Nature* 1997;388:639–648.

66. Brockes JP: Amphibian limb regeneration: Rebuilding a complex structure. *Science* 1997;276:81–87.

Chapter 3

Vascular Etiology of Limb Defects: The Subclavian Artery Supply Disruption Sequence

David D. Weaver, MD

Introduction

A vascular pathogenesis of certain birth defects generally is accepted.[1-5] In most cases, however, the specific vascular insult leading to the development of a particular defect is not identified. In this chapter, I will review the evidence supporting a vascular etiology for birth defects, discuss several conditions thought to result from vascular disruption, and review some of the proposed mechanisms leading to vascular-induced defects, with emphasis on the subclavian artery supply disruption sequence.

Definitions

In this chapter, vascular refers to any component of the circulatory system, including the heart, arteries, veins, and capillaries. A disruption is a prenatal interference with an originally normal developmental process, or an abnormal loss of an organ, part of an organ, or a larger region of the body. Vascular disruption is a prenatal disruptive defect of vascular origin.

Characteristics of Vascular Disruptions

In general, the type and severity of a vascular disruption depends on the gestational timing, the location of the involved vessel, the degree of tissue damage, and the adherence between tissues or organs.[1] Less severe effects generally are seen when the abnormal vascular event occurs during the fetal period. During the fetal period, the lesions tend to be more confined, and the degree of tissue loss is minimized because, for the most part, anastomoses have developed.[1] When the disruptive event occurs early in development, it frequently is impossible, based on physical grounds alone, to distinguish a malformation from a vascular disruption.[1] Most vascular disruptions are not inherited, and thus, the recurrence risk for subsequent siblings is probably less than 1%. Some conditions presumed to have a vascular etiology are listed in Outline 1.

Outline 1 Conditions with implied vascular disruption pathogenesis[1]

Adams-Oliver syndrome

Amniotic band disruption sequence

Fetal brain disruption sequence

Gastroschisis

Hypoglossia-hypodactyly syndrome

Klippel-Feil syndrome

Limb-body wall complex

Möbius' syndrome

Oculoauriculovertebral spectrum

Poland's syndrome

Porencephalic cysts/hydranencephaly

Sirenomelia

Splenogonadol fusion sequence

Terminal transverse limb defects, isolated

Thrombocytopenia-absent radii syndrome

Twin reversal arterial perfusion sequence

Evidence for the Existence of Vascular Disruptions

Support for the occurrence of vascular disruptions comes from several sources. For instance, twins studies have shown that monozygotic twins have a 50% higher rate of birth defects than do single births.[1] Many of these defects are known to be or believed to be secondary to vascular mechanisms. One example is the twin reversed arterial profusion sequence.[6] In this condition, there is an artery-to-artery anastomosis at the placental or umbilical cord level of monozygotic twins. Subsequent to the establishment of the anastomosis and for reasons that are not entirely clear, the heart stops in one twin and the other twin begins pumping blood in a reverse direction through the umbilical artery of the first twin. As a result, the perfused twin becomes hypotensive and experiences hypoxemia. These factors, in turn, lead to interference in normal morphology and a variety of disruptive defects. The consequence of this process is often a very bizarre twin with various combinations of defects including acephaly, acardia, and amelia.[6]

Animal experimentation also has provided evidence for the presence of vascular disruptions. Noted among these studies is the work of Webster and associates[7] who have demonstrated that hemorrhage and tissue necrosis in the extremities of fetal rats may result from a number of factors, including temporary unilateral clamping of uterine blood vessels, handling the uterus, and stretching of the uterine blood vessels. The result of such manipulation apparently is fetal hypoperfusion and ischemia, the consequence of which is hypoplasia of digits, most commonly, terminal transverse limb defects.

Clinical data also support the presence of vascular disruptions. Until a few years ago, chorionic villus sampling (CVS) in humans was done between 8 and 14 weeks from the last menstrual period (LMP). Evidence since has been published that early CVS (done before 10 weeks post LMP) is associated with an increased incidence of limb defects.[8,9] If these data are correct, then the etiology of the limb defects most likely is secondary to a vascular disruptive event.

Other disorders that lend credence to the concept of a vascular etiology of birth defects are hydranencephaly, porencephalic cysts, the fetal brain disruption sequence, and amniotic bands. Hydranencephaly is believed to occur as a result of the obstruction of one or both internal carotid arteries during fetal development. The obstruction leads to partial or complete infarction of the cerebrum. A porencephalic cyst is a nonmembrane-lined brain cyst that, in most cases, appears to have arisen from localized necrosis of brain tissue, which probably was caused by an interrupted blood supply to the affected region. Therefore, in many cases, the pathogenesis of porencephalic cysts is similar to that of hydranencephaly, except that it is on a more localized basis.[10] Fetal brain disruption sequence is a form of hydranencephaly[10] that begins with necrosis of a sizable portion of the fetal brain during the last half of the pregnancy. Evidence indicates that this necrosis occurs both from vascular disruption and from infections of the brain.[10] Fetal brain disruption sequence differs from hydranencephaly in that the fetal skull collapses causing severe microcephaly, overlapping of the cranial sutures, and rugation of the scalp. Because excessive brain matter is lost, the prognosis for intellectual function in a child with this disorder is poor. Amniotic bands, strands of amnion that appear to result from amnionic rupture, have a tendency to wrap around an extremity and/or to be swallowed by the fetus. As the involved body part grows, the band does not. The result is compression of the tissues, venous and arterial occlusion, and eventually, necrosis and amputation of the distal or involved parts.

Mechanisms Producing Vascular Disruptions

Cohen[1] has summarized the methods by which vascular disruptions are believed to occur. These mechanisms include emboli of placental origin or depletion of thromboplastin, both resulting from death of a co-twin; transient hypertension or hypotension; and hypo- or hyperperfusion. Other possible mechanisms are described by Van Allen[3,5] and by Bavinck and Weaver.[11]

Embryology of the Vascular System

The vascular system is the first organ system to develop and become functional in the embryo. Actual circulation in the embryo begins by the end of the third week of development (postfertilization time). The vascular system is critical to the developing embryo, which rapidly outgrows the ability of oxygen and nutrients to diffuse from the outside to the inside. In addition to its early function, the vascular system must adapt to the changing needs and structures of the embryo and, eventually, must develop into the adult systems without interruption of function or loss of integrity. Therefore, new vessels

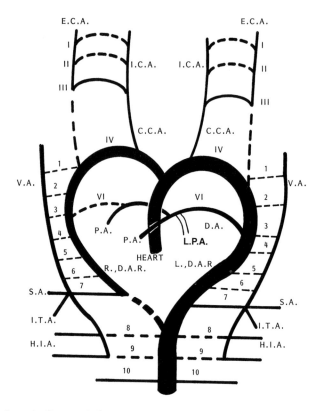

Fig. 1 *Schematic diagram indicating various components of the aortic arch complex, and subclavian arteries and its branches. The vascular components that do not normally persist in the adult are indicated by broken lines: I, II, III, IV, and VI aortic arches; 1, 2, 3, 4, 5, and 6 cervical intersegmental arteries; 8, 9, and 10 thoracic intersegmental arteries; C.C.A. = common carotid arteries; E.C.A. = external carotid arteries; D.A. = ductus arteriosus; H.I.A. = superior intercostal arteries; I.C.A. = internal carotid arteries; I.T.A. = internal thoracic arteries; L.D.A.R. = left dorsal aortic root; L.P.A. = left pulmonary artery; P.T. = pulmonary trunk; R.D.A.R. = right dorsal aortic root; R.P.A. = right pulmonary artery; S.A. = subclavian arteries; S.I.C.A. = superior intercostal arteries; V.A. = vertebral arteries; V.A.R. = ventral aortic root. (Reproduced with permission from Bavinck JN, Weaver DD: Subclavian artery supply disruption sequence: Hypothesis of a vascular etiology for Poland, Klippel-Feil, and Mobius anomalies. Am J Med Genet 1986;23:903–918. Reprinted by permission of Wiley-Liss, Inc., a subsidiary of John Wiley & Sons, Inc.)*

appear, others enlarge and take on increased functions, and still others regress and completely disappear.

Beginning at about day 20 of development, six aortic arches develop. Most of these arches regress or are incorporated into other vessels[11] (Fig. 1). The left fourth aortic arch, however, persists as the arch of the aorta, while the right proximal fourth arch becomes the proximal portion of the right subclavian artery. By about day 29, the embryo has some 30 pairs of dorsal

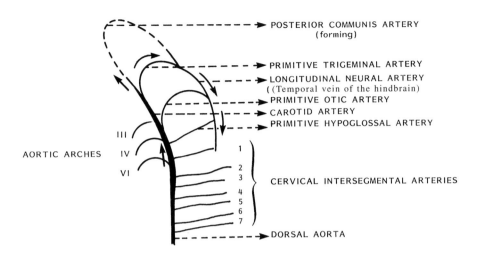

POSTERIOR COMMUNIS ARTERY
(forming)

PRIMITIVE TRIGEMINAL ARTERY

LONGITUDINAL NEURAL ARTERY
((Temporal vein of the hindbrain)

PRIMITIVE OTIC ARTERY

CAROTID ARTERY

PRIMITIVE HYPOGLOSSAL ARTERY

AORTIC ARCHES

III
IV
VI

1
2
3
4
5
6
7

CERVICAL INTERSEGMENTAL ARTERIES

DORSAL AORTA

Fig. 2 *Major blood supply to the cervical somites, spinal cord, and brain at about 29 days of development. Note that the vertebral artery has not yet formed. Solid arrows indicate direction of blood flow. (Reproduced with permission from Bavinck JN, Weaver DD: Subclavian artery supply disruption sequence: Hypothesis of a vascular etiology for Poland, Klippel-Feil, and Mobius anomalies. Am J Med Genet 1986;23:903–918. Reprinted by permission of Wiley-Liss, Inc., a subsidiary of John Wiley & Sons, Inc.)*

intersegmental arteries (Fig. 2). These vessels arise from the dorsal aorta and supply blood to the somites and corresponding regions of the neural tube. During days 32 through 42, the first nine of these dorsal intersegmental arteries, the seven cervical and first two thoracic arteries, develop anastomoses between themselves at right angles (Figs. 1 and 3). The completion of these perpendicular anastomoses marks the establishment of the vertebral arteries cranial to and the superior intercostal arteries (Fig. 1) caudal to the seventh dorsal intersegmental arteries. During this time, the seventh dorsal intersegmental arteries enlarge and become the subclavian arteries. At their cranial ends, the vertebral arteries fuse to form the basilar artery, which in turn connects with the cerebral posterior arteries. The latter two arteries form parts of the circle of Willis.

The proximal portions of the first six cervical and the first two thoracic dorsal intersegmental arteries regress (Fig. 3), leaving the somites and neural tube in these regions supplied by the vertebral and superior intercostal arteries. Slightly distal to the origin of these latter two vessels, the internal thoracic (mammary) arteries originate from the subclavian arteries (Fig. 1). These internal thoracic arteries supply blood to the sternocostal heads of the pectoralis major, the breasts, the anterior chest wall, and the scapulae. By the end of day 48 or thereabout, the subclavian arteries are supplying blood to the anterior chest wall, the posterior shoulder girdles, the arms, the neck, and the hindbrain (Fig. 1). Vascular changes similar to those described above

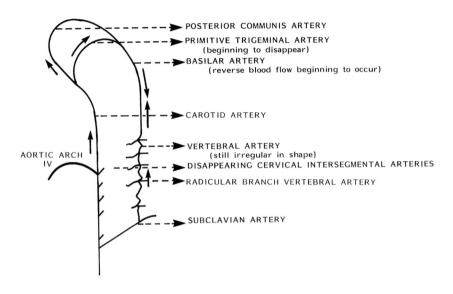

Fig. 3 *Major blood supply to the cervical somites, spinal cord, and brain at about 42 days of development. Note that the proximal portions of the first six cervical intersegmental arteries have regressed and disappeared. The hind brain is now supplied with blood from the vertebral artery, and the subclavian artery has developed from the seven intrasegmental arteries. (Reproduced with permission from Bavinck JN, Weaver DD: Subclavian artery supply disruption sequence: Hypothesis of a vascular etiology for Poland, Klippel-Feil, and Mobius anomalies.* Am J Med Genet *1986;23:903–918. Reprinted by permission of Wiley-Liss, Inc., a subsidiary of John Wiley & Sons, Inc.)*

occur in all other parts of the developing embryo. Moore[12] and Sadler[13] provide specific detail for these regions.

The Subclavian Artery Supply Disruption Sequence

Poland's syndrome consists of unilateral absence of the sternocostal head of the pectoralis major, ipsilateral absence or hypoplasia of the breast, and ipsilateral terminal transverse limb defects that are characterized by absence or hypoplasia of distal limb structures that involve fingers, the hand, and occasionally the forearm.[11] In some cases, the hand essentially is missing, with minute, incompletely formed digits present at the distal end of the arm. In terminal transverse limb defects, the proximal arm structures usually are normal. Klippel-Feil syndrome involves segmentation defects of the cervical and upper thoracic vertebrae with malformation and/or fusion of two or more vertebrae.[11] As a result of these vertebral defects, the affected individual may have a short neck, a low posterior hairline, neck pterygia, and decreased neck motion. Möbius' syndrome refers to unilateral or bilateral palsies of the sixth and usually the seventh cranial nerves, but other cranial nerves also may be

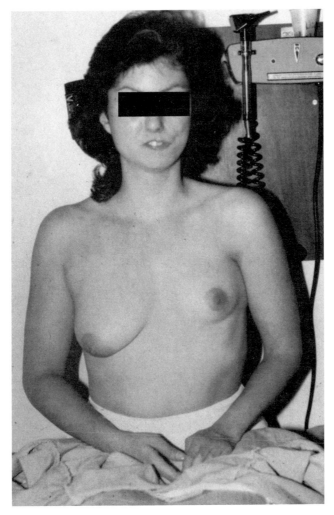

Fig. 4 An adult female with left-sided Möbius' and Poland's syndromes. Note deficiency of the sternocostal heads of the pectoralis major and the breast and the hypoplasia of the left hand.

involved.[11] The affected individual has abducens paresis, facial weakness, and other craniofacial problems. Sprengel anomaly is winging and abnormal positioning of the scapula.[11] One or both scapulae may be hypoplastic and in a congenitally high position with the lower angle turned toward the spine.

The above described conditions are interrelated in that patients with one of them may also have features of the other conditions. For instance, a person with Klippel-Feil syndrome may have terminal transverse limb defects in addition to the vertebral defects, or an individual with Poland's syndrome

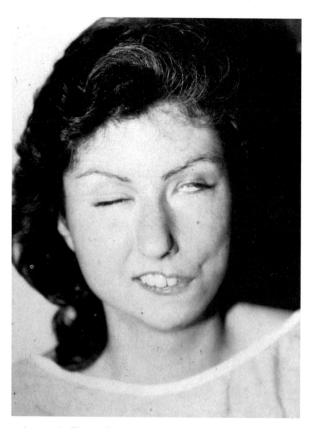

Fig. 5 Same patient as in Figure 4. Note the left-side facial weakness.

may have cervical vertebral defects and Sprengel anomaly.[11] Patients have had both Möbius' and Poland's syndromes (Figs. 4 and 5) and others have had both Klippel-Feil and Möbius' syndromes as well as terminal transverse limb defects. The overlapping of conditions in these patients suggests that there may be a common etiology or pathogenesis for Möbius', Klippel-Feil and Poland's syndromes, terminal transverse limb defects,[11] and Sprengel anomaly.

The Subclavian Artery Supply Disruption Sequence Hypothesis

Based on the development of the vascular system in the head, neck, chest, and arms, and the observations that features often overlap in patients with these disorders, Bavinck and Weaver[11] proposed the subclavian artery supply disruption sequence hypothesis.[11] This hypothesis states that the pathogenesis of

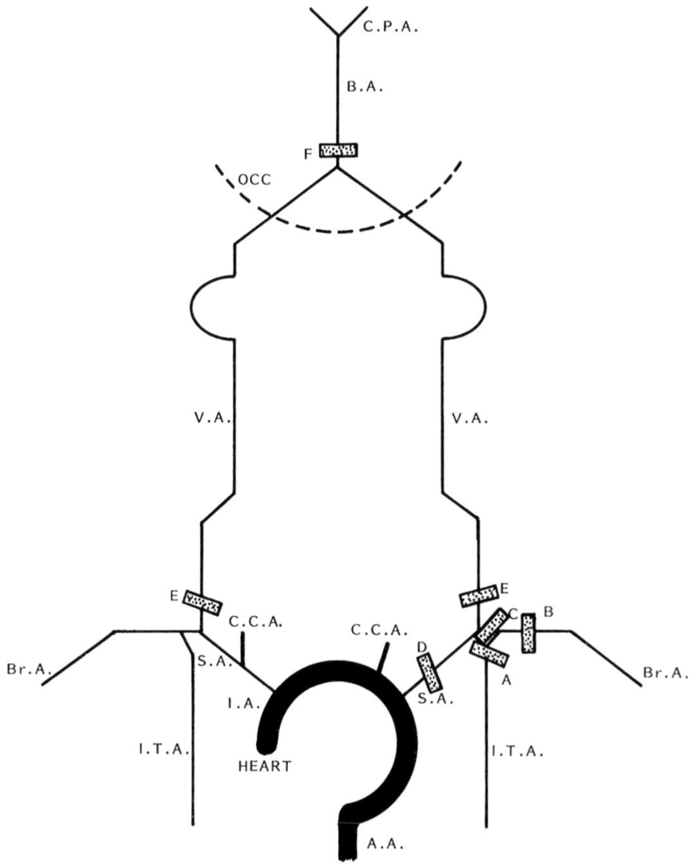

Fig. 6 *The subclavian artery supply disruption sequence: locations of vascular inter-ruption with resulting conditions. A, isolated pectoralis major absence with breast hypoplasia; B, isolated terminal transverse limb defects; C, Poland's syndrome; D, subclavian steal "syndrome"; between E and F, Klippel-Feil syndrome; F, Möbius' syndrome. A.A. = arch of the aorta; B.A. = basilar artery; Br.A. = branchial arteries; C.C.A. = common carotid arteries; C.P.A. = cerebral posterior arteries; I.A. = innomi-nate artery; I.T.A. = internal thoracic arteries; OCC = occipital bone; S.A. = subcla-vian arteries; V.A. = vertebral arteries. (Reproduced with permission from Bavinck JN, Weaver DD: Subclavian artery supply disruption sequence: Hypothesis of a vascular etiology for Poland, Klippel-Feil, and Mobius anomalies. Am J Med Genet 1986;23:903–918. Reprinted by permission of Wiley-Liss, Inc., a subsidiary of John Wiley & Sons, Inc.)*

the above conditions is the result of an interruption of the early embryonic blood supply in the subclavian, vertebral, and/or their branch arteries. Furthermore, this interruption occurs during the fifth through the eighth week of development, and the resulting specific pattern of abnormalities depends

33

on the location(s) of the blockage(s), the extent and the timing of occurrence(s), and the duration of the obstruction(s).

Interruption of the internal thoracic artery (Fig. 6, point A) will lead to ipsilateral absence of the costosternal heads of the pectoralis major and hypoplasia or aplasia of the breast. Interruption of the subclavian artery distal to the origin of the internal thoracic artery will result in isolated terminal transverse limb defects (Fig. 6, point B). Obstruction of the subclavian artery proximal to the internal thoracic artery, but distal to the vertebral artery will cause Poland's syndrome (Fig. 6, point C). Klippel-Feil syndrome is produced by interruption of blood flow at the origin or at any segment along the developing vertebral artery and/or the radicular branches (Fig. 6, point E). Möbius' syndrome develops from premature regression of one or more of the early arteries of the brain, probably the primitive trigeminal arteries, and/or obstruction in the basilar (Fig. 6, point F) and/or the vertebral arteries (Fig. 6, point E). Sprengel anomaly results from a partial or complete obstruction of the subclavian, the internal thoracic, and/or the suprascapular artery. Obstruction of one or more of these vessels will lead to hypoplasia of the scapula and to lack of development of the upper portion of the serratus anterior. This problem, in turn, will lead to failure of descent of the scapula, an elevated position and winging of the scapula, and to scapular hypoplasia.

Obstruction of the subclavian arteries proximal to the branching of the vertebral arteries (Fig 6, point D) probably does not result in abnormalities. If this situation does arise, there may be "subclavian steal" in which blood is supplied to the distal subclavian artery by reverse blood flow in the vertebral artery on the affected side. In this situation, the blood supply would be either from the basilar artery and/or the vertebral artery from the opposite side.

Clinical Correlation

The above hypothesis can explain much of the clinical overlap observed in Möbius', Klippel-Feil, and Poland's syndromes, terminal transverse limb defects, and Sprengel anomaly. Any combination of physical findings could be achieved by various combinations of obstructions of the subclavian and/or branch arteries. For instance, obstruction of the vertebral artery and a concomitant blockage of the subclavian artery distal to the origin of the internal thoracic artery would produce Klippel-Feil syndrome and terminal transverse limb defects.

The variation in the pattern of vertebral anomalies seen in Klippel-Feil syndrome could be explained by premature regression or obstruction of one or more of the cervical and thoracic intersegmental arteries, delay in development of one or more of the anastomotic vessels that form between these intersegmental arteries, obstruction of the newly formed vertebral artery at any location along its course, or any combination of these possibilities. The severity and extent of the vertebral defects would relate to the type and location of the blockage. For instance, massive fusion of most or all of the cervical vertebrae would result from interruption of blood supply near the origin of the vertebral artery, while the fusion of two vertebrae would likely result from premature regression or obstruction of a single dorsal intersegmental artery.

Partial or complete destruction of the cranial nerve nuclei has been found consistently in Möbius' syndrome. These pathologic changes could result from ischemia during crucial development times, such as the ischemia that might be produced by premature regression of primitive brain vessels or temporary obstruction in the basilar and/or vertebral arteries.[14,15] Depending on the timing and location(s) of the obstructive event(s), various cranial nuclei, including those of the sixth and seventh cranial nerves, could be destroyed. The combination of affected nuclei would account for the clinical variation seen in patients with Möbius' syndrome.

The sternocostal portions of the pectoralis major, the upper portion of the serratus anterior, the breast, and portions of the anterior chest wall are supplied with blood from the internal thoracic arteries. Interruption of blood supply at a critical period in the embryonic development of these areas would lead to absence or hypoplasia of the supplied structures. Absence of the sternocostal portions of the pectoralis and breast aplasia/hypoplasia are found not only in Poland's syndrome but also as an isolated finding without limb involvement. Presumably, this latter situation is explained by isolated obstruction of the internal thoracic artery. The severity of breast involvement would be related to the time in development at which the obstructive event occurred. Support for some of the above contentions comes from the fact that the pectoralis major differentiates as a muscle at approximately days 40 to 42.

There is considerable variation in the severity of the limb defect seen in terminal transverse limb defects either as an isolated defect or in association with Poland's, Klippel-Feil, or Möbius' syndromes. The variation ranges from mild reduction of the hand size with no disability to severe reduction in size of the hand, fingers, and forearms, with no useful hand function. Upper limb development begins at about 27 days after fertilization, and cutaneous separation of the fingers is completed by about day 52.[11] If a vascular disruption were to produce a limb defect, then the severity could be explained by the timing of the ischemic event. For instance, if the obstruction occurred between days 36 and 40, then development of the hand and fingers would be arrested at a relatively early stage, and the individual would be left with a severe terminal transverse limb defect. If the obstruction occurred later, say at day 50, when the fingers are well differentiated, then only relatively mild hypoplasia to the fingers would ensue. Chorionic villus sampling (CVS) was most commonly done between 8 and 12 weeks from the last menstrual period. The beginning of the 8-week period is equal to approximately 42 days after conception, and obviously is during the time of limb/hand development. Limb defects associated with CVS may be related to obstruction of the subclavian or other arteries, or to some other vascular phenomenon, say those reported by Webster and associates.[7]

Poland's syndrome may occur on either the right or the left side, but normally not both. When the condition is present on the left side, there is an increased chance of finding dextrocardia (10%).[1] The presence of dextro-cardia supports the contention that abnormal vascular development is the cause of Poland's syndrome. Bilateral Poland's syndrome may not exist because if it were to occur, it might lead to death in utero.

Mechanisms Producing the Subclavian Artery Supply Disruption Sequence

There is at this time no direct evidence for the mechanism(s) leading to the vascular disruption in the subclavian artery supply disruption sequence.[11] A number of possibilities have been put forth, including blood vessel edema, thrombi, or emboli that obstruct the vessel's lumen, or obstruction through external pressure on the vessel by edema of the surrounding tissue, local hemorrhage, a cervical rib, an aberrant muscle, amniotic band, a tumor, or embryonic intrauterine compression.[11] Premature regression of vessels or delay in vessel formation could result from several different environmental factors, such as drugs, chemicals, generalized hypoxia, and hyperthermia.[11] Genetic factors do not seem to play a significant role as a mechanism because there is a low recurrence of the subclavian artery supply disruption sequence in siblings.

Conclusion

Probably many of the birth defects that orthopaedic surgeons encounter represent vascular disruptions of one kind or another. Because the events leading to these defects occur prenatally and, perhaps, in the early part of the pregnancy, it may be impossible to distinguish vascular disruptions from malformations, let alone identify the initiating pathologic event. More refined methods of identifying birth defects caused by vascular pathogenesis in human will need to await advancement in technology or further experimental data from animal studies. However, the physician needs to keep in mind the possibility of a vascular mechanism when seeing birth defects because most birth defects of vascular origin are not inherited and as such have low risks of recurrence. This latter information may be important to the parents of affected children.

References

1. Cohen MM Jr (ed): *The Child With Multiple Birth Defects,* ed 2. New York, NY, Oxford University Press, 1997, pp 15–54.

2. Hoyme HE, Jones KL, Van Allen MI, Saunders BS, Benirschke K: Vascular pathogenesis of transverse limb reduction defects. *J Pediatr* 1982;101:839–843.

3. Van Allen MI: Fetal vascular disruptions: Mechanisms and some resulting birth defects. *Pediatr Ann* 1981;10:219–233.

4. Van Allen MI, Hoyme HE, Jones KL: Vascular pathogenesis of limb defects: I. Radial artery anatomy in radial aplasia. *J Pediatr* 1982;101:832–838.

5. Van Allen MI: Structural anomalies resulting from vascular disruption. *Pediatr Clin North Am* 1992;39:255–277.

6. Van Allen MI, Smith DW, Shepard TH: Twin reversed arterial perfusion (TRAP) sequence: A study of 14 twin pregnancies with acardius. *Semin Perinatol* 1983;7:285–293.

7. Webster WS, Lipson AH, Brown-Woodman PD: Uterine trauma and limb defects. *Teratology* 1987;35:253–260.

8. Mastroiacovo P, Tozzi AE, Agosti S, et al: Transverse limb reduction defects after chorion villus sampling: A retrospective cohort study. GIDEF: Gruppo Italiano Diagnosi Embrio-Fetali. *Prenat Diagn* 1993;13:1051–1056.

9. Holmes LB: Report of National Institute of Child Health and Human Development Workshop on Chorionic Villus Sampling and Limb and Other Defects, October 20, 1992. *Teratology* 1993;48:7–13.

10. Moore CA, Weaver DD, Bull MJ: Fetal brain disruption sequence. *J Pediatr* 1990;116:383–386.

11. Bavinck JN, Weaver DD: Subclavian artery supply disruption sequence: Hypothesis of a vascular etiology for Poland, Klippel-Feil, and Mobius anomalies. *Am J Med Genet* 1986;23:903–918.

12. Moore KL (ed): *The Developing Human: Clinically Oriented Embryology*, ed 4. Philadelphia, PA, WB Saunders, 1988, pp 286–333.

13. Sadler TW: Cardiovascular system, in Sadler TW (ed): *Langman's Medical Embryology*, ed 7. Baltimore, MD, Williams & Wilkins, 1995, pp 183–231.

14. Lipson AH, Webster WS, Brown-Woodman PD, Osborn RA: Moebius syndrome: Animal model-human correlations and evidence for a brainstem vascular etiology. *Teratology* 1989;40:339–350.

15. St. Charles S, DiMario FJ Jr, Grunnet ML: Mobius sequence: Further in vivo support or the subclavian artery supply disruption sequence. *Am J Med Genet* 1993;47:289–293.

Chapter 4
Heritable Limb Deficiencies

Golder N. Wilson MD, PhD

A striking discovery of modern dysmorphology is that most congenital anomalies have a genetic basis. Even when birth defects occur without a family history, informed chromosomal or DNA analysis may provide evidence for a spontaneous genetic change. The substantial genetic contribution to limb anomalies can be appreciated by analysis of the on-line catalogue of mendelian disorders established by Victor McKusick.[1] Of almost 4,000 genetic diseases listed in the catalogue, 1,836 have birth defects and 652 of these (36%) include limb anomalies.[2] I will analyze the 205 mendelian forms of limb deficiencies contained in the McKusick catalogue, contrast them with sporadic deficiencies, and consider how attention to associated anomalies may yield insights into the classification and causes of limb deficiencies.

Incidence and Classification of Limb Deficiencies

Although many authors have used the term "limb reduction defects," limb deficiency is a more accurate term that incorporates both absence and size reduction of the 120 human limb bones. Froster[3] has reviewed the myriad schemes for classification of limb deficiency. Frantz and O'Rahilly[4] used descriptive terms such as amelia (absence of limbs), hemimelia (medial or lateral limb rays), acheiria or apodia (absences of hands or feet), adactyly (absence of fingers), or phocomelia (absence of middle limb segments with retention of distal segments). Some authors prefer the use of amelia for complete and meromelia for partial absence of the limb.[5] Meromelias can be further subdivided into terminal, intercalary (eg, phocomelia), transverse, longitudinal (ie, hemimelia), pre- or postaxial, or central (eg, split hand/foot, ectrodactyly) deficiencies.[5] Mixtures of the older and revised nomenclature are often used for clinical description, but difficulty can arise when precise categorization of limb deficiencies is needed for the purpose of epidemiologic or mechanistic studies.

Table 1 lists the incidence over an 18-year period of various limb deficiencies among 1,213,913 live births in British Columbia.[6] Known genetic or teratogenic syndromes (eg, Fanconi anemia or thalidomide embryopathy) were excluded. The classification listed in the left column of Table 1 is hierarchical and follows the ontogeny of limb segments (upper extremity before lower, proximal segment before distal). A patient with absent humeri, radioulnar synostosis, and hypoplastic femur would thus be classified under

Table 1 Limb deficiencies: population incidence and occurrence in heritable disorders

Limb Deficiencies	British Columbia Survey[6]			Heritable Disorders[1]		
	Cases*	Fraction (%)	Syndromic† (%)	Total (No.)	Fraction (%)	Syndromic†
All limb deficiencies	6.0	100	53	205	100	80
Amelia	0.15	2.5	61	11	5.4	91
Upper limb	3.4	57	38	66	32	73
Lower limb	1.1	18	20	15	7.3	80
Upper/lower limb	0.95	16	—	124	61	87
Transverse	1.3	22	30	35	17	80
Amniotic bands	0.19	3.2	25	0	0	0
Humerus	0.090	1.5	64	6	2.9	83
Radius	0.92	15.3	54	26	13	96
Ulna	0.074	1.2	33	13	6.3	77
Hand	0.91	15	28	5	2.4	80
Phalanges, preaxial	0.50	8.3	46	8	3.9	88
Phalanges, postaxial	0.33	5.5	30	2	1.0	100
Phalanges, middle	0.61	10.2	26	2	1.0	100
Phalanges, unspecified	0	0	0	51	25	76
Femur	0.26	4.3	16	9	4.4	89
Tibia	0.07	1.2	25	7	3.4	71
Tibia/fibula	0.11	1.0	28	0	0	0
Fibula	0.06	1.1	14	11	5.4	82
Foot	0.26	0.83	26	0	0	0
Phalanges, preaxial	0.05	1.3	0	5	2.4	80
Phalanges, postaxial	0.08	1.7	30	3	1.5	67
Phalanges, middle	0.10	1.7	25	1	0.5	100
Phalanges, unspecified	0.09	1.5	—	14	6.8	64

* Cases per 10,000 live births
† Anomalies outside of the musculoskeletal system; many cases had deficiency at several limb sites

humeral defects, with the other limb changes recognized as additional musculoskeletal anomalies.[6] When a hierarchical classification is not used, the frequent coexistence of multiple limb deficiencies causes between 8% and 33% of cases to be labeled as mixed or unclassified. Among the 659 cases of limb deficiencies ascertained in British Columbia, 190 (29%) had involvement of more than one limb, and only 93 (14%) were bilaterally symmetric.[6]

The overall incidence of limb deficiencies was 6.0 per 10,000 live births, with 3.4 per 10,000 affecting the upper limbs and 1.1 per 10,000 affecting only the lower limbs (Table 1). Other epidemiologic surveys have yielded similar incidence figures for limb deficiencies, ranging from 5 to 9.7 per 10,000 live births and an approximate 3:1 ratio of upper to lower limb deficiencies.[7,8] The incidence of deficiencies affecting particular sites within the limb are also listed in Table 1. There is a higher incidence for middle ray versus pre- or postaxial phalangeal deficiencies in both the hands and feet. These trends are also reported in other epidemiologic surveys, but the numbers of cases lacking particular limb components depends on the classification system.[3,6–8]

Comparison of Heritable Limb Deficiencies With Those in a Birth Registry

The right panels of Table 1 summarize the characteristics of inherited limb deficiency disorders as gathered from the McKusick catalogue of mendelian disorders.[1,2] Some 205 limb deficiency disorders were identified, their component anomalies were encoded in a database, and their principal deficiencies were categorized hierarchically by the method of Froster-Iskenius and Baird.[6] There were 80 autosomal dominant, 85 autosomal recessive, and seven X-linked limb deficiency disorders; 32 were of uncertain inheritance. The McKusick catalogue includes 165 skeletal dysplasias, but only two had concurrent limb deficiencies (one transverse, one longitudinal). Limb duplications were present in 57 (28%) of the genetic limb deficiencies, and only three of the genetic group had transverse deficiencies. Syndactyly (30%) was also common in heritable limb deficiencies, as was synostosis, carpal/tarsal coalition, or symphalangism (18%).

Inspection of Table 1 reveals some interesting contrasts between limb deficiencies ascertained through a birth registry[6-8] and those ascertained as part of recognized heritable disorders. Upper limb deficiencies are more predominant in the birth registry (57%) compared to the genetic database (32%). Sixty-one percent of the genetic disorders involve both upper and lower limbs compared to 16% of the birth registry cases. Unilateral involvement is rare in genetic disorders (2%) but frequent in the birth registry cases (86%); the expected action of mutant genes on all four limb buds is supported by this comparison. Using symmetry as a guide, more than 15% of the sporadic limb deficiencies noted in the British Columbia survey are likely to be genetically determined.

The proportionate involvement of limb segments is very similar between the birth registry and genetic cases (eg, humerus 1.5%, radius-ulna 16.5%, hand 39% of birth registry cases; humerus 2.9%, radius-ulna 19.3%, hand 33% of genetic disorders). Genetic disorders are less likely to have the hand than the digits involved (2.4% versus 15% of birth registry cases). However, the frequency of transverse deficiencies in the genetic disorders (17%) is almost as high as that of birth registry cases (22%). Acheiria or diffuse metacarpal/carpal deficiencies are thus unlikely to be genetic, but other transverse deficiencies may be unless amniotic band remnants or constrictions are observed. Amelias occur in a higher proportion of genetic disorders (5.4%) than of birth registry cases (2.5%).

Insights Into Limb Deficiencies From Associated Anomalies

More than 80% of heritable limb deficiencies are associated with anomalies outside the musculoskeletal system (Table 1). Limb deficiencies ascertained by birth registry have a lesser but still considerable 53% likelihood of being part of a multiple anomaly syndrome.

Upper limb deficiencies are most likely to have associated anomalies, particularly in genetic disorders. Radial deficiencies are likely to be syndromic in birth registry cases or in genetic disorders. Humeral deficiencies were the most predictive of additional anomalies in the registry cases. Humeral deficiencies conferred a grim prognosis for affected infants, because five of the 11 cases (45%) died in the neonatal period.[6]

Table 2 shows the distribution of associated anomalies by organ system. The birth registry cases are more likely to be associated with respiratory, genitourinary, and additional musculoskeletal anomalies (syndactyly in particular) whereas the genetic disorders are more likely to be associated with craniofacial and cardiovascular disorders or polydactyly. The child with limb deficiency should have careful assessment of the craniofacial, cardiac, gastrointestinal, genitourinary, integumentary, and nervous systems. Peripheral blood counts, skeletal radiographic survey, urinalyses, hearing, vision, and growth should be monitored during infancy and early childhood until it is clear that the limb deficiency is isolated.

In a further breakdown of anomaly associations (Table 3), categories of mendelian limb deficiencies are examined for patterns of associated anomalies. Amelias are associated with craniofacial and genital anomalies, whereas transverse meromelias are highly associated with cardiovascular anomalies and are more likely than longitudinal deficiencies to have coexistent gastrointestinal anomalies. The latter associations would fit with the suspected vascular nature of many transverse limb deficiencies. Mendelian disorders with longitudinal limb deficiencies are particularly associated with craniofacial and genitourinary anomalies. Deficiencies of the upper extremity are more likely than lower limb deficiencies to be associated with cardiovascular defects. The percentage of associated craniofacial, integumentary, and particularly genitourinary anomalies increased with progression from deficient proximal to distal limb segments, but anomalies associated with deficiency of the middle segments of upper or lower limbs were quite similar. There were also similarities between anomalies associated with preaxial or postaxial longitudinal deficiencies, but central deficiencies of the hands were associated with integumentary defects.

In general, the data in Table 3 do not reveal striking associations between sites of limb deficiencies and defects of particular organ systems. The data of Froster and Baird[6-8] reveal the general associations of limb deficiencies with craniofacial, cardiac, gastrointestinal, and genitourinary anomalies shown in Table 2, but there are few correlations of anomaly pattern with the sites of limb deficiency. Exceptions to this rule in the birth registry data[6-8] include associations of amelia with omphalocele and diaphragmatic hernia, and of radial ray deficiencies with cardiac anomalies and imperforate anus. The latter correlation undoubtedly reflects the presence of many patients with VATER (vertebral, anal, tracheoesophageal, renal, and radial limb anomalies) association in the birth registry data.[6-8]

Table 2 Spectrum of associated anomalies in limb deficiency cases and disorders

Associated Anomalies by System	British Columbia Survey[6]		Hereditable Disorders[1]	
	Cases (No.)	Fraction (%)	Disorders (No.)	Fraction (%)
Limb deficiencies*	348	100	164	100
Craniofacial	97	28	130	79
Cardiovascular	62	18	65	40
Respiratory	21	6	8	4.9
Gastrointestinal	72	21	18	11
Genitourinary	70	20	33	20
Integumentary	42	12	43	26
Hematologic	13	3.7	14	8.5
Endocrinologic	9	2.6	5	3.0
Nervous	47	14	58	36
Musculoskeletal	130	37	57	35
Polydactyly	7	2	51	31
Syndactyly	88	25	54	33
Synostosis	—	—	30	19

*Only syndromic limb deficiencies are included

Fibular and Tibial Deficiencies

Fibular deficiencies are listed in Table 3 and in the miniatlas (Outline 1). Fibula and tibia deficiencies are more common in the genetic data (3% to 5% of limb deficiency disorders) than in the birth survey data (1.1% to 1.2% of cases with limb deficiency). The low incidence in the population study of Froster and Baird[8] contrasts with the data from several orthopaedic reviews of older patients that describe fibular deficiency as the most common anomaly of long bones.[9] In the orthopaedic reviews, about one third of fibular deficiencies are bilateral and very few are inherited or associated with other anomalies.[10] Lewin and Opitz[9] interpret the common, isolated deficiencies of the fibula to mean that the bone is undergoing regressive evolution and, therefore, is developmentally unstable. Most genetic disorders with fibular deficiency are syndromic (Table 2), and they are more often associated with cardiac anomalies and genitourinary defects than disorders with tibial deficiencies (Table 3).

Insights Into the Mechanisms of Limb Deficiency By Genetic Analysis

Rapid advances in molecular and developmental biology have identified genes relevant to limb development (Chapters 1 and 2). One productive route of investigation has been to characterize developmental genes in

Table 3 Anomalies associated with specific types of limb deficiency

Type of Deficiency*	Site	Total† (No.)	Cf (%)	Card (%)	GI (%)	Integ. (%)	GU (%)	Ns (%)
Amelia	UL or LL	10	50	20	10	30	50	10
Transverse	UL or LL	25	44	88	32	36	32	28
Longitudinal	UL or LL	160	34	22	7.5	24	38	16
	UL	84	31	30	4.8	13	39	17
	LL	37	43	19	5.4	16	14	19
	Proximal	12	50	33	36	36	17	17
	Middle UL	34	59	44	8.9	2.7	8.9	26
	Middle LL	17	47	35	0	17	17	23
	Distal	111	83	36	5.4	28	41	35
	R,T, preaxial	78	77	40	2.6	1.3	13	9.0
	Mesaxial	9	33	11	11	33	22	22
	U, Fib., postax.	30	70	43	6.7	6.7	0	6.7
	Tibial deficiency	5	60	20	0	0	0	40
	Fibular deficiency	9	66	33	0	11	22	11

* UL, upper limb; LL, lower limb; Cf, craniofacial; Card, cardiovascular; GI, gastrointestinal;
Integ, integumentary; GU, genitourinary, Ns, nervous system
† Only syndromic limb deficiencies are included

Drosophila and then to evaluate their role in vertebrate limb development. A dramatic success was the discovery that a particular inherited syndactyly was caused by a mutation in a human homeotic gene. Homeotic mutations replace one normal structure with another.[10] Other genes important for limb development have been revealed by transgenic mouse experiments, exemplified by identification of the formin gene responsible for the mouse phenotype *limb deformity*.[11]

Another approach for understanding limb development is to characterize heritable limb deficiencies in humans. When families are sufficiently large or numerous, the putative gene causing a limb deficiency can be mapped to a specific chromosome region through linkage analysis. Then, the arduous but increasingly successful approach of positional cloning is used to sort through the genes in that chromosomal region until a DNA mutation is identified. Examples of this approach are the craniosynostosis/limb defect syndromes that have been related to fibroblast growth factor receptor genes.[12] The 205 mendelian limb deficiency disorders described here are thus vehicles for gene isolation using the appropriate molecular techniques, and a battery of DNA diagnostic tests should soon be available to aid in the classification of patients with limb deficiency.

Although the identification of limb patterning genes is important, it is also necessary to understand how these genes interact to form embryonic pathways that are impacted in genetic limb deficiencies. The registry of heritable limb anomalies (Tables 1 and 2) can reveal developmental relationships based on simultaneous disruption of limbs and other organs. Survey of the associated anomalies can provide a map of the early human blastocyst and delineate the progression from early genes that control embryonic domains to later genes that act specifically on the limb. In this way, limb patterning genes that are revealed by human genetic and transgenic mouse experiments can be placed in their embryonic context.

For example, the frequent concurrence of cardiac anomalies with longitudinal limb deficiencies suggests a shared embryonic heritage.[13] Factors regulating early orientation of the embryo (anteroposterior, dorsoventral, and lateral axis formation) may impact a heart-limb domain before these primordia arise separately from the lateral mesoderm. From this perspective, higher frequencies of cardiac anomalies in upper limb deficiencies might relate to the anterior position of both heart and upper limbs. Similarly, the striking patient with mirror limb anomalies, situs inversus, and complex heart disease (Sandrow syndrome;[14] Outline 1) may reflect common factors in the genesis of heart-limb symmetry (laterality).

If a heart-limb field exists, as suggested by clinical review, then future research should focus on molecules expressed in both heart and limb primordia as a rich source of limb patterning genes. Candidates include the *activin*, *sonic hedgehog*, and *retinoic acid receptor* genes that are expressed in heart and limb, as well as the *Holt-Oram* gene that maps to chromosome region 12q24.[13,15] This combined medical and molecular approach emphasizes the role of clinical delineation in scientific understanding as well as for preventive management of limb deficiency associations.

Outline 1 A miniatlas of heritable limb deficiencies*

Amelias (transverse deficiency, all limb segments)

Roberts syndrome (AR, 268300)—limb deficiency varying from amelia or phocomelia, most severe in the upper extremities, to less pronounced hypoplasia or absence of radii, ulnae, carpals, and tibiae. Associated anomalies include microcephaly, cleft lip/palate, and cryptorchidism. An unusual separation of centromeric chromatin can be seen by chromosome analysis.

Transverse deficiencies (intercalary, phocomelic; proximal limb segment)

Antley-Bixler syndrome (AR, 207410)—limb deficiencies include hypoplastic humerus with radiohumeral synostosis and bowing of the femurs. Associated anomalies include craniosynostosis, choanal atresia, and cardiac and renal defects.

Femur-fibula-ulna complex (?AR, 228200)—absence or hypoplasia of the femur with variable deficiencies of the upper and lower limbs, particularly of the postaxial rays. Most cases are not familial, and the intercalary femoral deficiency is similar to that in the femoral hypoplasia-unusual facies syndrome that is associated with maternal diabetes.

Transverse deficiencies (intercalary, distal segment)

Aarskog syndrome (XL, 305400)—brachydactyly of all digital rays with "swan-neck" deformities of the fingers. Associated problems include short stature, hypertelorism, and shawl scrotum with cryptorchidism.

Acrodysostosis (AD, 101800; AR, 201150)—brachydactyly with short metacarpals and metatarsals. Associated anomalies include nasal hypoplasia and short stature. Families suggestive of AD and AR inheritance have been described.

Camptobrachydactyly (AD, 114150)—broad, short hands with short metacarpals, short metatarsals, supernumerary metatarsals, and digital contractures.

Heart-hand syndrome, Spanish type (AD, 140450)—short metatarsals and brachydactyly with associated cardiac conduction defects.

Juberg-Hayward syndrome (AR, 216100)—brachydactyly with short metacarpals and thumb hypoplasia. Associated anomalies include microcephaly and cleft lip/palate.

Martsolf syndrome (AR, 212720)—brachydactyly and short metacarpals with associated short stature, microcephaly, hypogonadism, and cataracts.

Saethre-Chotzen syndrome (AD, 101400)—brachydactyly with hypoplasia of the distal phalanges and syndactyly. Associated anomalies include craniosynostosis with facial asymmetry.

Trichorhinophalangeal syndrome I (AD, 190350)—short metacarpals and metatarsals with syndactyly and digital asymmetry. Associated anomalies include sparse hair and a bulbous nose.

Trichorhinophalangeal syndrome II, Langer-Giedion syndrome (AD, 150230)—short metacarpals and metatarsals with associated sparse hair, bulbous nose, multiple exostoses, and mental retardation.

Transverse deficiencies (terminal, middle or distal limb segment)

Acheiropodia, Brazilian type (AR, 200500)—absence of the hands and feet, with a characteristic bone remnant in the upper limb that is parallel to the humerus (Bohomoletz bone). There are no associated anomalies.

Adams-Oliver syndrome (AD, 100300)—limb deficiencies of the lower legs, feet, hands, or digits combined with cutis aplasia of the scalp. Additional anomalies may include strabismus, microphthalmia, and duplicated urinary collecting system.

Aglossia-hypodactyly, Hanhart syndrome complex (?AD, 103300)—a group of disorders with extremely variable limb deficiency ranging from the characteristic transverse deficiency of digits to terminal deficiencies of the middle or upper limb segments. Associated anomalies include small or absent tongue, small jaw, and a spectrum of cranial nerve palsies, pectoral muscle hypoplasia, and syndactylies that merge with the Mobius or Poland sequences. Inheritance is not well defined, and the asymmetry of limb deficiency in many individuals provides evidence for multifactorial determination.

CHILD syndrome (XL, 308050)—the acronym denotes congenital hemidysplasia, ichthyosiform erythroderma, and limb defects, which include asymmetric transverse deficiencies of upper and lower limbs. The limb deficiencies occur ipsilateral to the skin changes, and other associated anomalies can include unilateral hypoplasia of the brain, cleft lip, and hearing loss.

Splenogonadal fusion-limb deficiency (?AD, 183300)—variable transverse limb deficiencies or amelia associated with splenogonadal fusion, micrognathia, and abnormal dentition. Most cases are sporadic.

Transverse deficiencies (terminal, distal segment; brachydactyly)

Anophthalmia, type Waardenburg (AR, 206920)—short terminal phalanges with syndactly associated with anophthalmia.

Borjeson-Forssman-Lehman syndrome (XL, 301900)—brachydactyly with short middle and terminal phalanges. Associated anomalies include coarse facies with hypogenitalism, obesity, and mental retardation.

Coffin-Siris syndrome (AR, 135900)—brachydactyly with short terminal phalanges (particularly the fifth digit) associated with growth and mental retardation, coarse facies, and hypoplastic nails.

Kallman syndrome with brachydactyly (AR, 211750)—brachydactyly with hypoplastic terminal phalangies. Associated anomalies include hypogonadotrophic hypogonadism and anosmia.

Martsolf syndrome (AR, 212720)—brachydactyly and short metacarpals with associated short stature, microcephaly, hypogonadism, and cataracts.

Saethre-Chotzen syndrome (AD, 101400)—brachydactyly with hypoplasia of the distal phalanges and syndactyly. Associated anomalies include craniosynostosis with facial asymmetry.

Schinzel-Giedion syndrome (AR, 269150)—brachydactyly with short terminal phalanges and short metacarpals. Associated anomalies include midface hypoplasia,
cardiac defects, renal defects, and mental retardation.

Longitudinal deficiencies (preaxial, radial and tibial)

Aase syndrome (AR, 205600)—radial aplasia associated with anemia.

Baller-Gerold syndrome (AR, 218600)—radial aplasia with hypoplasia of the phalanges and metacarpals, associated with craniosynostosis.

Fanconi syndrome (AR, 227650)—upper limb deficiencies of the thumb and radius
with occasional developmental dysplasia of the hip. Other problems include pancytopenia, cardiac anomalies, urogenital anomalies, eye anomalies, and predisposition
to leukemia.

Nager syndrome (?AD, 154400)—radial ray deficiency with thumb hypoplasia associated with mandibulofacial dysostosis.

Radial deficiency-choanal stenosis (AD, 179270)—absent or hypoplastic radial ray
with esotropia and choanal stenosis.

Sandrow preaxial deficiency with mirror duplication (AD, 13575)—absent first digit
with mirror duplication of digits two to five, and eight to ten total digits on the
hands and feet. Associated anomalies may include deficiencies of the radii and tibiae, duplications of the ulnae and fibulae and, in one patient,13 situs ambiguus with
complex heart defects, pulmonary isometry, mesoliver, and asplenia.

Thrombocytopenia-absent radius (TAR) syndrome (AR, 274000)—radial aplasia with
preservation of the thumbs and associated ulnar hypoplasia are the rule. Associated
anomalies include short stature, strabismus, micrognathia, dislocated hip, club foot,
and occasional lower limb deficiency.

WT-limb-blood syndrome (AD, 194350)—radial deficiency with bifid or hypoplastic
thumbs and occasional ulnar hypoplasia. There is associated pancytopenia.

Longitudinal deficiencies (postaxial, ulnar and fibular)

Brachydactyly E-atrial septal defect (AD, 113301)—short fourth and fifth metacarpals
associated with a round facies and atrial septal defect.

Ulnar-mammary syndrome (AD, 181450)—ulnar ray deficiencies associated with
hypoplasia of the apocrine and mammary glands, hypogonadism, and short stature.

Longitudinal deficiencies (mesaxial or central, ectrodactylies)

Ectrodactyly, isolated (AD, 183600)—deficiency of the central rays of both hands and
feet. The disorder is notorious for incomplete penetrance, which can complicate its
distinction from autosomal recessive ectrodactyly.

Ectrodactyly, isolated (AR, 225300)—upper and lower limb ectrodactyly.

Ectrodactyly-ectodermal dysplasia-clefting (EEC) syndrome (AD, 129900)—upper and
lower limb deficiencies of the central ray varying from syndactyly to absence of the
metacarpals and digits (ectrodactyly). There is associated cleft palate, sparse hair,
light pigmentation with photosensitivity, and lacrimal duct hypogenesis.

Ectrodactyly-ectodermal dysplasia-macular dystrophy (EEM) syndrome (AR,
225280)—ectrodactyly associated with ectodermal dysplasia and progressive macu-
lar dystrophy.

Ectrodactyly-ectodermal dysplasia-clefting (Rosselli-Gulienetti) syndrome (AR,
225000)—ectrodactyly of the upper and lower limbs with anhidrosis, hypotrichosis,
microdontia, nail dysplasia, genitourinary anomalies, and popliteal or perineal pterygia.

Longitudinal deficiencies (intercalary, sometimes phocomelic; middle segment)

Holt-Oram syndrome (AD, 142900)—upper limb deficiencies varying from hypoplastic
thumb or radial aplasia to severe hypoplasia of the entire forearm and defects of the
humerus, clavicle, scapula or sternum. Associated anomalies include cardiac and
vertebral defects.

Pillay ophthalmomandibulomelic dysplasia (AD, 164900)—ulnar deficiency and short
forearms are associated with temporomandibular fusion and corneal opacities.

Cortada scoliosis-ulnar hypoplasia syndrome (AR, no McKusick number)[16]—ulnar hypoplasia and small hands are associated with scoliosis, microcephaly, and mental retardation.

Tibial aplasias

Gollop-Wolfgang complex (AR, 228250)—tibial deficiency with bifid femurs and upper limb ectrodactyly.

Mohr-Majewski orofaciodigital syndrome type IV (AR, 258860)—hypoplasia of the tibiae with deviation and bowing of the tibiae; associated with duplications of the radial or ulnar rays and sensorineural deafness.

Richieri-Costa cleft hand, absent tibiae syndrome (AD, 119100)—tibial deficiency associated with upper limb ectrodactyly.

Tibial absence with polydactyly (AD, 188740)—tibial deficiency with duplications of the radial ray and cardiac defects.

Tibial aplasia (AR, 275220)—absence or hypoplasia of the tibias produces short and bowed lower limbs with club feet, angulation, and skin dimpling at the apex of the bowed limb.

Tibial aplasia with deafness (AR, 275230)—tibial deficiency associated with sensorineural deafness.

Werner tibial hypoplasia with polydactyly (AD, 188770)—tibial deficiency with duplications of the ulnar ray and accessory phalanges of the radial ray.

Fibular aplasias

Brahimi syndrome (AR, no McKusick number)16—fibular aplasia and short forearms.

Camptodactyly syndrome, Guadalajara type (AR, 211910)—fibular hypoplasia and hallux valgus with associated broad nasal bridge, intrauterine growth retardation, and camptodactyly.

Craniosynostosis with fibular aplasia (AR, 218550)—absence of the fibula with craniosynostosis.

Dupan syndrome (AR, 228900)—fibular deficiency with brachydactyly of the terminal phalanges and short metacarpals.

Fibuloulnar aplasia with renal anomalies (AR, 228940)—fibular agenesis with oligosyndactyly and hypoplastic ulnae. Associated anomalies include renal cystic disease, pulmonary hypoplasia, cardiac anomalies, and early death.

Fuhrmann syndrome (AR, 228930)—hypoplasia or absence of the fibulas, bowing of the femurs, and tarsal coalition associated with other bony anomalies including polydactyly, syndactyly, and oligodactyly.

Kozlowski syndrome (unknown inheritance)16—hypoplasia of the fibulas with duplication of the thumb and cardiac defects.

McKusick-Weilbacher limb deficiency (AR, 246000)—unilateral deficiency or hypoplasia of the femur and fibula. Scoliosis and cataracts are associated.

Oto-onychoperoneal syndrome (AR, 259780)—aplasia or hypoplasia of the fibulae associated with abnormal ears, limb contractures, and absent nails.

* Limb deficiencies are grouped according to their distribution of bony defects, with inheritance indicated as AD (autosomal recessive), AR (autosomal recessive), or XL (X-linked). Tibial and fibular deficiencies are listed separately at the end. The six-digit McKusick number (in parentheses) serves as a reference that can be accessed through the print or on-line version of the McKusick catalogue.[1] The McKusick numbers for AD, AR, and XL diseases begin with 1, 2, and 3, respectively. Listing in the McKusick catalogue does not imply that all or even most cases of a disorder are genetic; it merely indicates that familial aggregation of the disorder has been reported.

References

1. McKusick VA (ed): *Mendelian Inheritance in Man: A Catalog of Human Genes and Genetic Disorders*, ed 11. Baltimore, MD, Johns Hopkins University Press, 1994.

2. Wilson GN: Genomics of dysmorphogenesis. *Am J Med Genet* 1992;42:187–196.

3. Froster UG: Letter: Academicians are more likely to share each other's toothbrush than each other's nomenclature. *Am J Med Genet* 1996;66:471–474.

4. Frantz CH, O'Rahilly R: Congenital skeletal limb deficiencies. *J Bone Joint Surg* 1961;43A:1202–1224.

5. Swanson AB: A classification for congenital limb malformations. *J Hand Surg* 1976;1A:8–22.

6. Froster-Iskenius UG, Baird PA: Limb reduction defects in over one million consecutive livebirths. *Teratology* 1989;39:127–135.

7. Froster UG, Baird PA: Upper limb deficiencies and associated malformations: A population-based study. *Am J Med Genet* 1992;44:767–781.

8. Froster UG, Baird PA: Congenital defects of lower limbs and associated malformations: A population based study. *Am J Med Genet* 1993;45:60–64.

9. Lewin SO, Opitz JM: Fibular a/hypoplasia: Review and documentation of the fibular developmental field. *Am J Med Genet* 1986;2(suppl):215–238.

10. Manak JR, Scott MP: A class act: Conservation of homeodomain protein functions. *Development* 1994;(suppl):61–71.

11. Vogt TF, Jackson-Grusby L, Rush J, Leder P: Formins: Phosphoprotein isoforms encoded by the mouse limb deformity locus. *Proc Natl Acad Sci USA* 1993;90:5554–5558.

12. Muenke M, Schell U, Hehr A, et al: A common mutation in the fibroblast growth factor receptor 1 gene in Pfeiffer syndrome. *Nat Genet* 1994;8:269–274.

13. Wilson GN: Why developmental fields are important: An appreciation by way of Holt-Oram and a putative heart-limb develomental field. *Proc Greenwood Genet Center* 1996;15:163.

14. Nowaczyk MJM, Clarke H, Smith C, Siegel-Bartelt J: Genetic heterogeneity in forelimb duplication. *Am J Hum Genet* 1996;59:544.

15. Bonnet D, Pelet A, Legeai-Mallet L, et al: A gene for Holt-Oram syndrome maps to the distal long arm of chromosome 12. *Nat Genet* 1994;6:405–408.

16. Stevenson RE, Meyer LC: The limbs, in Stevenson RE, Hall JG, Goodman RM (eds): *Human Malformations and Related Anomalies*. New York, NY, Oxford University Press, 1993, pp 699–804.

Chapter 5
Medical Conditions Associated With Congenital Limb Deficiencies

Yoshio Setoguchi, MD

Introduction

Fortunately for the rehabilitation team treating children with limb reduction deformities, most of the patients with congenital deficiencies do not present with other associated medical problems. Their growth and development are normal, and all the efforts of the rehabilitation team are directed towards normalizing the child's functional abilities.

In most clinics for children with congenital limb deficiencies, the routine pediatric care is referred to a local pediatrician. However, the knowledge that certain conditions may have associated medical problems can often be picked up by the rehabilitation team when they are aware of these particular congenital anomalies. The identifications of these associated problems and their treatment requires the coordinated efforts of the rehabilitation team and the community-based pediatrician. Therefore, the initial team evaluation must include a complete medical history as well as a physical examination. Knowledge of syndromes, associations in which the limb deficiencies are part of a scope of medical problems, helps to identify them. Then, a rehabilitation program should consider all aspects of the patient's medical needs, and the team needs to ensure that the total treatment program is coordinated and prioritized.

Several approaches to classifications of associated medical anomalies are available. However, none of these approaches are based specifically on the involved limb deficiency. This chapter will not attempt to cover all associations, but will cover those that frequently are seen in clinics for children with limb deficiencies. These associations will be reviewed from the perspective of the limb or limb structures involved.

Upper Extremities

Hands

Early Amnion Rupture Sequence[1]
This condition, which also is called congenital constriction band syndrome or Streeter band syndrome, is believed to be secondary to early rupture of the amniotic membrane with subsequent malformation caused by early

compression of the embryo. The resultant aberrant amnion bands (strands) can cause disruption of structures in the craniofacial areas, abdominal wall, and/or the limbs. The type and extent of the resultant deformities relate to the timing of the amnion rupture.[2] Clinically, each case seen is unique in terms of its manifestations, but also is distinguishable by the constriction bands and terminal amputations of the extremities. Typically, the digits of the hands and feet are affected; however, a greater portion of the limbs may be involved. When the constriction band is severe, with restriction of the vascular supply to the distal extremity, there is distal hypoplasia or aplasia.

Most cases of early amnion have been reported to result in spontaneous abortions. In these early cases, involvement of craniofacial structures is more common. The patients most commonly seen in the clinic at the Shriners Hospital for Children, Los Angeles Unit, have amniotic constriction bands with or without amputations and tufting of the terminal digits. This condition is believed to be sporadic in nature, and therefore, recurrence risk is believed to be negligible.

It is rare that a patient with this condition has only one limb involved. Usually, more than one limb is involved, although the degree of involvement varies from almost complete amputation to only distal digital amputation. If digits are involved, syndactylism and terminal tufting usually are present. Treatment requires the coordinated efforts of a hand surgeon and/or plastic surgeon, orthopaedic surgeon, and the prosthetic/rehabilitation team.

Poland's Anomaly[3]

This condition consists of unilateral absence of the pectoralis minor and the sternal portion of the pectoralis major muscles associated with some type of abnormality of the ipsilateral hand. The hand deformities could vary from hypoplasia of the hand and digits with syndactyly, brachydactyly, and reduction deformities. Involvement of the nipple and rib defects are rarely seen. A complete workup in these cases should include spine radiographs and ultrasound studies to rule out renal anomalies.

Oromandibular-Limb Hypogenesis Spectrum[4]

Previously, this group of associated malformations were grouped under seven different conditions or syndromes. These include aglossia-aglossia syndrome (probably more correctly called hypoglossia-hypodactyly syndrome); Hanhart syndrome; Moebius syndrome; Charlie M. syndrome; facial-limb disruptive spectrum; glossopalatine ankylosis syndrome; and limb deficiency-splenogonadal fusion syndrome. Although some dysmorphologists discuss these conditions as distinct entities, there is considerable overlapping of the features such that they are now all listed under the above title. For purposes of this report, I will describe the distinct features of each of the seven conditions. Etiology for each of the conditions is unknown. Limb reduction deformities in these conditions vary considerably. However, in my experience, it is most common for the limb deformities to occur distally in the hands and feet.

***Moebius Syndrome*[5]** Classically, this condition presents with multiple congenital cranial nerve palsies, but it most often involves the sixth and seventh nerves. The patients who are referred to clinics for amputees have limb deficiencies as well as varying degrees of mental retardation.

Often, these patients are not considered for prosthetic rehabilitation because of the mask-like facies resulting from the bilateral facial paralysis. However, I find that most of these patients are excellent prosthetic users.

The characteristic facial features include the bilateral facial nerve involvements; however, the degree of involvement on each side varies with frequent asymmetry. Because of the involvement of the sixth cranial nerve, the patients cannot abduct either eye beyond the midline. Ptosis, nystagmus, and strabismus may also be present. Typically, the opening of the mouth is small. Poor feeding may be a problem, which can be exacerbated by the involvement of the fifth, ninth, and twelfth nerves. Unilateral tongue hypoplasia is frequent and may be associated with muscle fasciculations. Thus, there may be speech problems in addition to the feeding problems.

The limb defects occur in approximately 50% of cases. The most common deficiencies include hypoplasia of digits, syndactyly, and clinodactyly, but more severe deficiencies do occur.

Hypoglossia-Hypodactylia Syndrome[6,7] The classic clinical features include small tongue, usually with an absent anterior portion, which gives the appearance of ankylosis of the tongue; small mandible with absence of the mandibular incisors and associated underdevelopment or atrophy of the mandibular alveolar ridge; and limb anomalies.

The limb anomalies can be quite variable and often more than one limb is affected. Most often, the limb defects are distal and involve primarily the hands and feet. However, more severe deficiencies have been reported. These patients, as do most in this category, require not only the multidisciplinary team to manage the prosthetic needs but also a craniofacial team.

Hanhart Syndrome[8] Classically this syndrome described patients with micrognathia and limb deficiencies involving primarily the hands and feet—foreshortened digits and oligodactyly. The difference from the above syndrome is that the tongue is relatively normal.

Glossopalatine Ankylosis Syndrome[2] Limb anomalies in this condition are quite variable. It may affect both hands and feet. Greater degree of limb deficiencies is rare. The major defect is one of intraoral attachments between tongue and palate, tongue and other intraoral structures, or maxilla and mandible.

Limb Deficiency-Splenogonadal Fusion Syndrome[9] This condition presents with a cord-like structure connecting the spleen with the gonadal structures on the same side. As with other syndromes in this group, associated anomalies include craniofacial anomalies, such as micrognathia, malformed low set ears, microglossia, and abnormal tooth eruptions. The limb deficiencies are again variable but involve the upper extremities more than the lower extremities.

Charlie M. Syndrome Patients with this condition present with hypertelorism, facial paralysis on occasion, absent or conically shaped incisors, cleft palate, and involvement of hands and feet.

Facial-Limb Disruptive Sequence[1] This is another description for congenital constrictive band syndrome, and I believe it does not fit in this group of conditions. It is distinct and is related to a disruption of facial and limb structures.

Adams-Oliver Syndrome[2]

This rare condition, aplasia cutia congenita with terminal transverse defects of limbs, involves aplastic scalp with absence of hair (alopecia), usually in the posterior parietal area with or without involvement of the cranium. The limb deficiencies are usually terminal types involving the digits of both hands and feet and may include complete absences. Other anomalies include small lower jaw, undescended testicles, eye muscle anomalies, and cleft lip.

During the initial phase of lower extremity prosthetic fitting, if skull defects are present, helmet therapy might avoid serious head injuries. This condition is autosomal dominant with variability in expression.

Ectrodactyly-Ectodermal Dysplasia-Clefting Syndrome (EEC syndrome)[11]

The clinical features are quite evident with the exception of the skin manifestations, which are quite variable. Involvement includes the skin, hair, lacrimal system, and nails. Sweating and heat regulation may be problems. Limb anomalies usually do not require prosthetic intervention. Patients, however, will need the services of hand/plastic surgery and a craniofacial team.

Ulna

Grebe Syndrome[11]

This is a rare syndrome with short stature due to foreshortened limbs. Both upper and lower extremities are involved but more often the ulna in the upper and tibia in the lower extremities. Usually, the shortening is greater in the lower extremities.

DeLange Syndrome (Brachmann-deLange syndrome)[11]

These patients present with classic craniofacial features including microcephaly, bushy eyebrows with synophrys, long eyelashes, long philtrum (upper lip), high arched palate, and micrognathia. Skin manifestations include hirsutism, perioral cyanosis, and cutis marmorata. The limb deficiencies can range from phocomelia to micromelia, but a very common finding is that of ulnar absence with a single digit.

These patients are usually severely mentally retarded and there is considerable growth retardation. Therefore, they usually are not candidates for prosthetic rehabilitation.

Miller Syndrome (post-axial acrofacial dysostosis syndrome)

The limb deficiencies are postaxial, ie, the ulnar aspect ivolves the ulna and corresponding lateral rays, and may include syndactyly. The craniofacial features include malar hypoplasia, sometimes showing radiologic evidence of a bony cleft; down-slanting of the palpebral fissures; coloboma of the eyelids; micrognathia; and abnormal external ears. Cleft lip and palate and conductive hearing loss may also occur.

Radius

TAR (thrombocytopenia-absent radii)[12]

This syndrome requires immediate diagnosis and treatment in the newborn period. Any signs of bleeding require a platelet count. There may be absence or hypoplasia of the megakaryocytes. Treatment with platelet transfusion is required to try to prevent or minimize any central nervous system damage resulting from intraventricular bleeding.

The limb deficiencies are usually absence or hypoplasia of the radius with radially clubbed hand with deformities of or absence of the thumb. The limb defects can be unilateral or bilateral.

Other features can include congenital heart disease, small stature, foreshortened humeri and hypoplastic shoulder girdles, and lower extremity deformities. If the child survives the neonatal period, usually after a period of platelet transfusion, the hematologic problem usually improves. This condition is believed to be autosomal recessive although most of the cases seen are first cases.

Fanconi's Pancytopenia Syndrome[13]

Dysmorphic and limb reduction defects are quite variable and some patients have only the hematologic disorders. The skeletal anomalies include hypoplastic to absent thumbs, radial hypoplasia, and congenital hip dislocations. Infants with this condition are relatively small at birth and are born with the limb defects and patchy brown discoloration of the skin.

The onset of the hematologic disorder of bleeding, pallor, and/or recurrent infections occurs at anywhere from 5 to 10 years of age. Many of these patients, if diagnosed correctly, respond to testosterone and hydrocortisone analogue therapy.

This condition is autosomal recessive. Early prenatal and postnatal diagnosis can be made even with little or no hematologic manifestations by demonstrating a high frequency diepoxy-butane induced chromosomal breakage in peripheral blood lymphocytes as well as in cultured amniotic fluid cells.

Holt-Oram (Hand-Heart) Syndrome[14]

The limb anomalies can range from radial deficiencies, partial or complete with absence of the thumb, radially clubbed hand with or without elbow function to complete humeral, radioulnar phocomelia. Although the syndrome usually is asymmetric, both sides are involved.

The cardiac lesion is classically an atrial septal defect but other anomalies have been reported, such as ventricular septal defects and tetrology of Fallot (Lewis-Franceschiti syndrome). Other less frequent anomalies include hypertelorism, Poland's anomaly, pectus excavatum, and scoliosis. This condition is autosomal dominant with variable penitrance.

VATER Association (VACTERL)[15]

The classic features of this group of associated anomalies include vertebral defects, imperforate anus, tracheoesophageal fistula with esophageal atresia, and radial and renal dysplasia. The new nomenclature includes the addition of cardiac defects and separation of the "R" defect to renal and limb anomalies. In addition, the physician often finds prenatal growth deficiency, single umbilical artery, and defects of the external genitalia. The majority of these patients do not have any central nervous system involvement, and intellectual development is good.

Etiology is unknown, and the patterns of malformation have been generally sporadic in occurrence. However, this condition has been noted with greater frequency in offspring of diabetic mothers.

Baller-Gerold Syndrome[2]

This is a relatively rare condition in which radial deficiencies from absent radial digits to partial or complete absence of the radius are associated with craniosynostosis. The cranial sutures that usually are affected are the coronal sutures.

These patients require early referral to a neurosurgeon and plastic surgeon for treatment of the craniosynostosis. Later in the first year, the patient may require hand surgery, but these patients rarely require prosthetic treatment.

Trisomy 18

This condition rarely is seen in a children's amputation or pediatric rehabilitation clinic because these patients have multiple congenital anomalies, including severe growth defects and mental retardation. The limb anomalies usually include middle and distal ray deficiency, usually unilateral, with or without radial and tibial involvement.

Other quite unusual conditions with radial deficiencies include Blackfin-Diamond syndrome, which has an associated hematologic disorder, and Aase syndrome, which includes anemia with variable leukopenia.

Humerus

Roberts Syndrome (SC phocomelia syndrome)[16]

This condition, also called pseudothalidomide, includes marked skeletal and mental retardation with microcephaly, cleft lip and/or palate, hypotelorism, facial hemangioma, malformed ears, cryptorchidism, and cardiac defects.

This condition is felt to be autosomal dominant. Many of these children, if not stillborn, die in early infancy. Prosthetic fitting depends on the residual function in the extremities and the developmental age of the child.

Lower Extremities

Feet

See the section on deficiencies of the hands. Often, patients with hand deformities of a transverse type also have foot deformities.

Tibia and Fibula

Tibial Absence–Congenital Deafness

Absence of the tibia, with or without absences of the toes, along with congenital deafness has been noted in some families. The features are variable in penitrance. Some cases involve only deafness and others involve only the tibial defects.

Recently, at the Shriners Hospital for Children, Los Angeles, we have seen two patients with bilateral tibial absences that have not been previously reported. These two children have very distinct craniofacial features, hand anomalies, and the typical absent tibiae with severe varus deformities of the feet and ankles. The craniofacial features include brachycephaly, frontal bossing, hypertelorbitism, protuberant ears, and mild micrognathia. The hand anomalies are quite unusual in that there is little or no flexion-extension of the digits, and both the palmar and volar aspects of the hands look alike except for the nails, which are on the correct side. These children are both developmentally delayed with very late speech and language development.

In addition to these two distinct group of cases with tibial deficiencies, we have seen a number of patients with tibial absenses, usually bilateral, with hand anomalies. Some patients have no defects other than the tibial defects. However, a number of patients have ectrodactyly with absence of the central rays, and others have polydactyly with reduplication of the ulnar rays.

There is a familiar tibial absence pattern in which the fibula and fibular digits are reduplicated. This results in very unstable knee and ankle joints with either six or seven toes. No other anomalies are noted, and the child's development is normal.

Fibular Deficiency

This is the most common lower extremity limb deficiency. This defect often is seen with deformities or deficiencies in part or all of the femur. However, the majority of these cases do not present with other organ system involvement.

Femur

Roberts Syndrome

See section on humeral deficiencies.

Femoral Hypoplasia–Unusual Facies Syndrome[2]

The limb defects can range from hypoplastic to absent femora and fibulae. They also may involve the humeri with restricted elbow motion. Deformities may also be noted in the pelvis and lower spine. The distinctive facial features include short nose with hypoplastic aloe nasi, long philtrum and thin upper lip, micrognathia, cleft palate, and up-slanting of the palpebral fissures. In spite of the hip deformities and short lower limbs, these patients are able to ambulate. They may want to try prostheses to obtain normal height.

Summary

Most children with congenital limb deficiencies do not fall into any of the above conditions, which present with other anomalies. However, they all deserve a complete evaluation to rule out these syndromes. A comprehensive rehabilitation program requires a coordinated treatment program for all of the medical problems presented by the child with a limb deficiency.

References

1. Jones KL, Smith DW, Hall BD, et al: A pattern of craniofacial and limb defects secondary to aberrant tissue bands. *J Pediatr* 1974;84:90–95.

2. Smith D: *Recognizable Patterns of Human Malformation.* Philadelphia, PA, WB Saunders, 1994.

3. Mace JW, Kaplan JM, Schanberger JE, Gotlin RW: Poland's syndrome: Report of seven cases and review of the literature. *Clin Pediatr* 1972;11:98–102.

4. Chicarilli ZN, Polayes IM: Oromandibular limb hypogenesis syndromes. *Plast Reconstr Surg* 1985;76:13–24.

5. Steigner M, Stewart RE, Setoguchi Y: Combined limb deficiencies and cranial nerve dysfunction: Report of six cases. *Birth Defects* 1975;11:133–141.

6. Cohen MM Jr, Pantke H, Siris E: Nosologic and genetic considerations in the aglossy-adactyly syndrome. *Birth Defects* 1971;7:237–240.

7. Hall BD: Aglossia-adactylia. *Birth Defects* 1971;7:233–236.

8. Wexler MR, Novark BW: Hanhart's syndrome: Case report. *Plast Reconstr Surg* 1974;54:99–101.

9. Given HF, Guiney EJ: Splenic-gonadal fusion. *J Pediatr Surg* 1978;13:341.

10. Rudiger RA, Haase W, Passarge E: Association of ecrtodactyly, ectodermal dysplasia, and cleft lip-palate. *Am J Dis Child* 1970;120:160–163.

11. Romeo G, Zonana J, Rimoin DL, et al: Heterogeneity of nonlethal severe short-limbed dwarfism. *J Pediatr* 1977;91:918–923.

12. Hall JG, Levin J, Kuhn JP, Ottenheimer EJ, van Berkum KA, McKusick VA: Thrombocytopenia with absent radius (TAR). *Medicine* 1969;48:411–439.

13. Glanz A, Fraser FC: Spectrum of anomalies in Fanconi anaemia. *J Med Genet* 1982;19:412–416.

14. Holt M, Oram S: Familial heart disease with skeletal malformations. *Br Heart J* 1960;22:236–242.

15. Quan L, Smith DW: The VATER Association: Vertebral defects, Anal-atresia, T-E fistula with esophageal atresia, Radial and Renal dysplasia: A spectrum of associated defects. *J Pediatr* 1973;82:104–107.

16. Herrmann MJ, Feingold M, Tuffli GA, Opitz JM: A familial dysmorphogenetic syndrome of limb deformities, characteristic facial appearance and associated anomalies: The "pseudothalidomide" or "SC-Syndrome." *Birth Defects* 1969;5:81–89.

Section 2
Congenital Femoral Deficiency

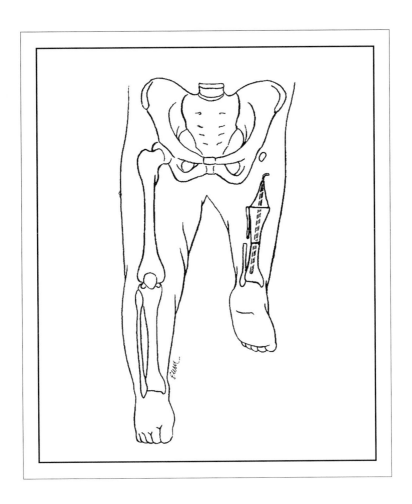

Consensus

Classification of Congenital Deficiency of the Femur (Including PFFD and Congenital Short Femur)

The disorder commonly termed proximal focal femoral deficiency is misnamed. We suggest the condition be called congenital deficiency of the femur. This disorder includes intact femora as well as those with defects. Current radiologic classifications are inadequate for treatment planning. The classification of Gillespie and Torode is useful for planning treatment. However, it should be modified as follows: A, femur long enough (> 50% present) and foot level at mid tibia or below (taking into consideration the flexion contractures) with good knee function or bad knee function and mobility; B, femur not long enough (< 50% present) and foot between knee and mid tibia level or above with a good or bad knee and a good or bad foot; and C, virtual absence of femur with the foot at knee joint level or above.

Chapter 6

Classification of Congenital Abnormalities of the Femur

Robert Gillespie, MB,ChB, FRCSC, FRCS(Ed)

Introduction

There are a number of problems with the existing classifications of congenital abnormalities of the femur. They tend to be based on detailed analyses of a large number of radiographs without the associated clinical information, such as degree of flexion contracture of the hip and knee, knee stability, absolute leg-length discrepancy, and other clinical facts that bear strongly on decisions regarding surgical and prosthetic management.

Nomenclature is a problem as it generally is in limb deficiency literature. The acronym PFFD (proximal femoral focal deficiency) has been embedded solidly in the literature since the 1968 symposium on the subject.[1] This descriptive term often is used to describe a femur that is very short but has no defect, a femur with a defect that is distal rather than proximal, and a femur with a subtotal rather than focal defect.

Radiographs are likely to be misleading, especially in an infant with a congenital short femur in which the proximal unossified head, neck, and greater trochanter are in moderate varus. Radiographs of such an infant are often taken with the hip somewhat flexed, and the resulting foreshortened appearance gives the impression of a very short Aitken type A or even type B PFFD, when in reality the femur is intact and 60% of the length of the normal side. I have known this kind of misclassification to lead to early ablation of the foot in a child whose limb may have been capable of reconstruction and leg equalization. Early classification of an infant's radiographs introduces a tendency to exaggerate the severity of the anomaly in the less severe cases and creates a meaningless multiplicity of types and subtypes in more complex cases.

There is need for a classification based on clinical information, sophisticated imaging, and radiographs put together in such a way that aggressive surgical decisions can be delayed to at least age 2 1/2 years. Ideally, such a classification should provide a guide to prosthetic and surgical care.

Further difficulty in classification results from the subgroup of cases with multiple limb deficiencies and often bilateral femoral anomalies, which include recognizable syndromes, such as femoral hypoplasia-unusual facies syndrome,[2,3] and other multimembral cases that are genetic, thalidomide-induced, or otherwise induced by fetal injury. In my experience, the femurs in these cases may have bizarre additional qualities, such as true hip dislocation and unusual angular deformities of the femoral shaft. It is tempting, therefore, to place these in a separate group.

A review of the literature plus my own experience reinforces the notion that the number of reasonably distinct forms of femoral reduction deformities that can be described is proportionate to the number of radiographs reviewed and, in a sense, is limitless. This leads me to think that any useful classification needs to be based on "lumping" rather than "splitting" if it is to be helpful to the clinician and capable of gaining wide acceptance.

Preexisting Classifications

Probably the best known classification is that described by Aitken. Aitken intended his classification to apply to true PFFD, but only too often others have referred to the congenital short femur as type A PFFD. Aitken did not intend this and regarded the short femur with coxa vara as a different condition.

The Amstutz[4] (Fig. 1) classification and that of Pappas[5] (Fig. 2) provide very extensive "splitting" type portrayal of the many radiologic forms they encountered. The Fixsen and Lloyd-Roberts[6] classification of very early radiologic appearances has proved very helpful in early recognition of the congenital short femur.

Torode and I,[7] working with a prosthetist in a large limb-deficiency clinic, recognized essentially only two broad groups that presented clearly different management problems; namely, the congenital short femur and the true PFFD sydrome. It seemed to us important to separate the congenital short femur once and for all from true PFFD to avoid the risk of ablation of the foot in infancy in cases in which much more idealistic reconstruction is possible at a later date.

The classification of Hamanishi[8] (Fig. 3) is very appealing in portraying a progressive reduction of the femur all the way from simple shortening to subtotal absence. I have come to recognize that the flaw in Haminishi's classification is the implication that the shorter the femur, the more varus there is, which simply is not true. I have encountered a well-formed hip and proximal femur with almost nothing else.

Can the proposed international terminology for the classification of congenital limb deficiency be used? The late Hector Kay chaired an international committee in an attempt to unify terminology in this area in 1973.[9] The committees included members from the United States, West Germany, and Great Britain. The major problem faced by the committee was the reconciliation of the Frantz-O'Rahilly nomenclature,[10] then commonly accepted in the United States, with the German nomenclature, which used such terms as meromelia and ectromelia.

The recommendation of this working group of the International Society for Prosthetics and Orthotics was to eliminate confusing terms of Latin and Greek derivation (hemimelia, meromelia, etc) and use simple, easily-translated English terms. Thus, the basic descriptive term for femoral reduction deformities would simply become longitudinal deficiency of the femur; the

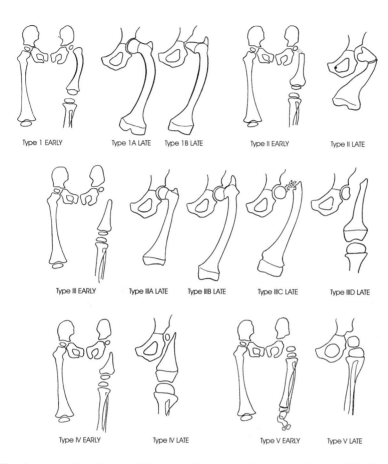

Type 1 EARLY   Type 1A LATE   Type 1B LATE   Type II EARLY   Type II LATE

Type III EARLY   Type IIIA LATE   Type IIIB LATE   Type IIIC LATE   Type IIID LATE

Type IV EARLY   Type IV LATE   Type V EARLY   Type V LATE

Fig. 1 Amstutz classification. (Reproduced with permission from Amstutz HC: The morphology, natural history, and treatment of proximal femoral focal deficiencies, in Aitken GT (ed): Proximal Femoral Focal Deficiency: A Congenital Anomaly. Washington, DC, National Academy of Sciences, 1968, pp 50–76.)

terms intercalary, phocomelia, and ectromelia were dispensed with. The term could be rendered more specific by the addition of the words partial, proximal, central, and distal. The condition referred to as a PFFD Aitken D would be called a longitudinal deficiency femur, partial, proximal.

There would not seem to be much benefit in this classification other than the elimination of the PFFD acronym. The term proximal femoral focal deficiency brings to mind a classic clinical picture: a child with a profoundly short femur, a bulbous thigh segment lying in external rotation and flexion with a flexed knee, and the foot lying at the level of the contralateral normal knee or just below it. The radiograph reveals some sort of failure of bone formation proximally, at the very least a subtrochanteric pseudarthrosis and at

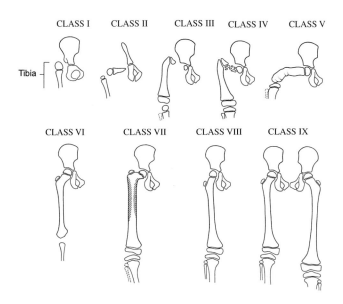

Fig. 2 *Pappas classification. (Reproduced with permission from Pappas AM: Congenital abnormalities of the femur and related lower extremity malformations: Classification and treatment.* J Pediatr Orthop *1983;3:45–60.)*

the worst, complete absence of the proximal femur and acetabulum. The child will require a prosthesis and any surgical maneuvers can only improve hip stability or prosthetic function. There exists, therefore, a PFFD "syndrome" and this familiar term serves well to communicate its existence between pediatric orthopaedists and prosthetists.

The problem is that the term PFFD is used in published classifications and everyday orthopaedic usage to describe the congenital short femur, a condition that has a profoundly different functional potential. The simple fact is that it is a misnomer. In all cases, the entire femur is abnormal rather than purely proximally and the abnormality is never focal.

If yet another classification of reduction deformities of the femur, or of longitudinal deficiencies of the femur were to be attempted, it should separate clinical patterns in a fashion helpful to planning case management and should include indicators of total leg length; nature of deformity of hip and knee, such as hip and knee fixed flexion and external rotation; and the weightbearing line of the tibial shaft in relation to the center of gravity.

The extremely helpful observations of Fixsen and Lloyd-Roberts[6] enable inference of the stability of the proximal femur and the development of the hip in very early radiographs. Furthermore, none of these descriptions takes into account soft-tissue anatomy, as recently studied by Pirani and associates,[11] who used magnetic resonance imaging (MRI).

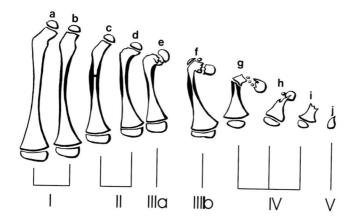

Fig. 3 Hamanishi classification. (Reproduced with permission from Hamanishi C: Congenital short femur: Clinical, genetic and epidemiological comparison of the naturally occurring condition with that caused by Thalidomide. J Bone Joint Surg *1980;62B:307–320.)*

The lesser degrees of femoral deficiency, the so-called congenital short femur, presents at birth with a clinical picture fairly typical of classical PFFD. The thigh is obviously short and a little thicker in appearance. The hip and knee are slightly flexed and tend to lie in external rotation. In overall length, however, there is a significant difference. The foot on the affected side, when pulled down gently, lies at or below the midpoint of the contralateral normal tibia, implying immediately that the femur is 50% or more of the normal length.

Radiographs at birth typically show a bowed femur with a smooth, rounded proximal end lying a little higher and further lateral to the pelvis than the normal side. The early radiographs frequently exaggerate the shortness of the bone because of foreshortening caused by the hip lying in flexion at the moment of x-ray exposure.

By the time the child is walking, it is clear that the hip and knee flexion contractures are rapidly resolving and the true features of this type of congenital short femur are clear. The femur is slightly bowed, there is moderate coxa vara in most but not all cases. The length of the femur is typically about 60% that of the normal side. There is some valgus at the knee, and the knee joint is unstable in the anteroposterior (AP) plane. The limb tends to lie in some external rotation and can be rotated to neutral but typically there is no internal rotation at the hip because of some degree of femoral retroversion.

The final leg-length discrepancy in a tall male with a normal 50-cm femur will be around 20 cm, and in a short female it will be about 15 or 16 cm, which curiously enough closely approximates the length of the foot. This type of case then is, by modern standards, at least theoretically capable of leg equalization. Some cases with the same features in regards to length and hip and knee architecture have a subtrochanteric pseudarthrosis, which if dealt with promptly and efficiently by surgery can have the same prognosis.

The more severe group, those in which the femur is less than 50% of the normal femur, make up that infinitely variable series of cases that typically is thought of as "true" PFFD. Early radiographs may show any of the signs described by Fixsen and Lloyd-Roberts.[6] The final appearance at maturity varies from a very intact mini femur through those with a "Shepherd's crook" deformity in extreme varus, those with an intact femoral head, neck, and trochanter with a pseudarthrotic gap separating the proximal elements from a distal segment consisting only of the femoral condyles to the typical Aitken C and D varieties in which no acetabulum exists and all that is seen of the femur is a variably shaped distal end sometimes fused to the tibial epiphysis.

All of these radiologic varieties in this group share one of the most important features from the prosthetist's point of view; namely, the short thigh segment in most cases lies in a significant degree of flexion. The knee, which is always dysplastic, also exhibits a fixed flexion contracture. The net effect of these deformities is that, in the standing position, the knee center is displaced anterior to the pelvis and the weightbearing line of the tibia must fall well anterior to the patient's center of gravity. The prosthetist, therefore, must struggle to achieve ischial weightbearing in the prosthesis and, inevitably, when the child bears weight on the prosthetic side, the hip and knee are pushed into further flexion, greatly exaggerating the inevitable lurching Trendelenburg gait.

This combined flexion deformity of hip and knee could be caused by the absence of true hip extensors and the structural block to knee extension, with the hamstrings working only to flex the knee without the mechanical advantage of hip stability that would allow the hamstrings to help in hip extension. In those cases with an intact "mini femur," the displacement of the knee is much less. At the other extreme, those cases in which the femur is almost completely absent, paradoxically the problem is minimized because the thigh segment is so short that no significant anterior displacement of the weightbearing line of the tibia occurs and the prosthetist's task is easier.

Another aspect of this group of severe deficiencies is the "reconstructability" of the hip. In my experience, achieving union across defects, cartilaginous or pseudarthrotic, in the proximal femur achieves nothing functionally unless a greater trochanter exists or significant medialization of the limb can be achieved to bring the weightbearing line of the tibia closer to the midline.

Suggested Approach to a New Clinical Classification

If it is accepted that from the surgical and prosthetic viewpoint three categories of a child with longitudinal deficiency of the femur are seen, then a true clinical rather than radiologic classification may be possible (Fig. 4).

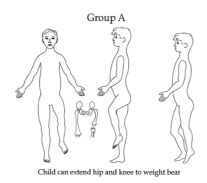

Group A

Child can extend hip and knee to weight bear

Group B   Group C

Horizontal line indicates length relationship to contralateral limb
Vertical line indicates anterior displacement of weight bearing axis of tibia

Fig. 4 Proposed classification.

Group A

This group consists of those cases thought of as congenital short femur, which have the following features.

Clinical Features

In infancy, the hip and knee lie in some flexion. The femur is obviously short, the thigh segment appears wider. There is limited internal rotation at the hip so that the thigh tends to lie in some external rotation. Abduction of the hip is limited compared to the normal side. All of these features are very similar to the more severe PFFD.

However, the distinguishing features are a sense of proximal stability in that there is no "pistoning" of the femur. The knee joint can be almost fully extended and, most importantly, when the baby's feet are gently pulled down, the foot lies opposite the midpoint of the contralateral tibia or lower, indicating an overall leg-length discrepancy of 20% or less.

Radiologic Features

In infancy, the radiograph shows typically the stable appearance described by Fixsen and Lloyd-Roberts;[6] namely, a smooth, rounded, bulbous proximal end often lying more proximally and laterally than normal. By age 2 years, the radiographic appearance is revealed as a typical short femur that has a well-formed proximal end with a good hip joint and some variable coxa vara with lateral bowing of the shaft. In some cases, there may be a cartilaginous defect in the subtrochanteric area or proximal shaft that may heal spontaneously or readily with surgical attention.

Rarely the short femur is very normal in appearance or may demonstrate coxa valga. There is commonly some valgus at the knee, with the deformity in the distal femur.

Prognosis

If the femur is 60% the length of the contralateral femur, then leg-length equalization is a possibility. Surgical correction of coxa vara and retroversion of the proximal femur are readily achieved, as is correction of the knee valgus by distal femoral osteotomy. The knee is always somewhat dysplastic and always shows some AP laxity, which puts it at risk during lengthening procedures, and care has to be taken to avoid posterior subluxation of the knee.

If the femur is 50% or less of the length of the contralateral femur then, in my view at least, van Nes rotationplasty done through an arthrodesis of the knee joint and prosthetic fitting can provide a very functional result.

Group B

This group consists of those cases Aitken classified as PFFD types A, B, and C.

Clinical Features

In infancy, the clinical features represent an exaggeration of those seen in group A. The thigh is very short, bulbous, and lies in some external rotation with some flexion at the hip, and more importantly, some fixed flexion at the knee. There is usually a sense of proximal instability with pistoning of the thigh segment.

When the feet are gently pulled down, the foot lies at a point between the knee and the midpoint of the contralateral femur, and the knee flexion contracture persists. The overall leg-length discrepancy is in the order of 40%. As the child begins to stand, the outstanding clinical feature of this group becomes apparent; namely, the characteristic anterior projection of the thigh and flexed knee.

Radiographic Features

In infancy, the radiograph shows the unstable signs of Fixsen and Lloyd-Roberts,[6] a "tufted" appearance of the proximal femur or a pointed end. As the hip matures, a great variety of appearances may develop from an intact "mini femur" through various forms of tenuous cartilaginous, partially ossified femoral necks to pointed proximal ends terminating above an apparently empty acetabulum.

Prognosis

This group of cases must be treated prosthetically. The surgeon's task is to modify the limb where indicated to facilitate and maximize prosthetic function.

Some of these cases may offer the opportunity to improve the alignment and stability of the proximal femur and hip by osteotomy or procedures to obtain bony continuity between the shafts and head of the femur. The truth is that in the absence of a greater trochanter, the result of these procedures is often disappointing in terms of the elimination of Trendelenburg lurch, but can be helpful in diminishing it by simple medialization of the femur and creating better pelvifemoral stability.

The most striking feature of these children is anterior projection of the thigh segment, which places the weightbearing line of the tibia well anterior to the body's center of gravity. Paradoxically, this problem becomes greater as the flexed thigh segment is longer, forcing the prosthetist to use the "ship's funnel" type of socket to gain some control of the unstable hip and knee complex and gain ischial weightbearing.

Fusion of the knee to create a single tibiofemoral lever arm as recommended by King[12] is a most useful form of surgical intervention for these cases, allowing much improved prosthetic fit and alignment. If the overall length of the limb brings the foot well below the contralateral knee, then Van Nes rotationplasty is an option; otherwise, Syme or Boyd amputation of the foot with length adjustment can allow a good end-bearing stump.

Group C

This group of cases represents the Aitken D form of PFFD, which really is a subtotal absence of the femur.[1]

Clinical Features

The thigh segment of the infant is very short and bulbous. The leg lies in external rotation with the foot at or proximal to the level of the contralateral knee. There is a sense of marked proximal instability and pistoning.

Radiographic Features

In infancy, the femur is represented by a rounded or triangular ossified area, which is the distal end of the femur, sometimes fused to the tibial epiphyses. There is often dysplasia of the hemipelvis and no acetabular development. As time passes, no further ossified tissue appears.

Prognosis

This group of cases must be fitted prosthetically, and because of shortness of the limb and the fact that, unlike group B cases, there is no significant anterior displacement of the tibia, it is relatively easy for the prosthetist to fit. There is no indication for arthrodesis of the knee and, in some of the shortest cases, the prosthetist may prefer to retain the foot within the socket for better suspension and control. There may be a place for fusing the femoral condyles to the pelvis as described by Steel and associates,[13] but I have no experience with that procedure.

Conclusion

In summary, I suggest that there is some benefit in classifying longitudinal deficiencies of the femur according to all of the clinical manifestations observed between 1 and 2 years of age as the child is beginning to walk, rather than on radiographic findings alone.

The suggested classification applies only to children with monomelic involvement. Bilateral femoral deficiencies and other multilimb deficiencies are frequently part of heritable syndromes or patterns of intrauterine injury with a multiplicity of problems beyond those of prosthetic and orthopaedic management and should be viewed as unique case-management challenges. In many cases, management is complicated by deficiency of the leg below the knee, typically a fibular hemimelia, which, of course, will alter surgical planning appropriately.

References

1. Aitken GT: Proximal femoral focal deficiency: Definition, classification and management, in Aitken GT (ed): *Proximal Femoral Focal Deficiency: A Congenital Anomaly.* Washington, DC, National Academy of Sciences, 1969, pp 1–22.

2. Johnson JP, Carey JC, Gooch WM III, Petersen J, Beattie JF: Femoral hypoplasia: Unusual facies syndrome in infants of diabetic mothers. *J Pediatr* 1983;102: 866–872.

3. Burn J, Winter RM, Baraitser M, Hall CM, Fixsen J: The femoral hypoplasia: Unusual facies syndrome. *J Med Genet* 1984;21:331–340.

4. Amstutz HC: The morphology, natural history and treatment of proximal femoral focal deficiencies, in Aitken GT (ed): *Proximal Femoral Focal Deficiency: A Congenital Anomaly.* Washington, DC, National Academy of Sciences, 1969, pp 50–76.

5. Pappas AM: Congenital abnormalities of the femur and related lower extremity malformations: Classification and treatment. *J Pediatr Orthop* 1983;3:45–60.

6. Fixsen JA, Lloyd-Roberts GC: The natural history and early treatment of proximal femoral dysplasia. *J Bone Joint Surg* 1974;56B:86–95.

7. Gillespie R, Torode IP: Classification and management of congenital abnormalities of the femur. *J Bone Joint Surg* 1983;65B:557–568.

8. Hamanishi C: Congenital short femur: Clinical, genetic and epidemiological comparison of the naturally occurring condition with that caused by Thalidomide. *J Bone Joint Surg* 1980;62B:307–320.

9. Kay HW, Day HJ, Henkel HL, et al: The proposed international terminology for the classification of congenital limb deficiencies. *Dev Med Child Neurol* 1975;34(suppl):1–12.

10. Frantz CH, O'Rahilly R: Congenital skeletal limb deficiencies. *J Bone Joint Surg* 1961;43A:1202–1224.

11. Pirani S, Beauchamp RD, Li D, Sawatzky B: Soft tissue anatomy of proximal femoral focal deficiency. *J Pediatr Orthop* 1991;11:563–570.

12. King RE: Some concepts of proximal femoral focal deficiency, in Aitken GT (ed): *Proximal Femoral Focal Deficiency: A Congenital Anomaly.* Washington, DC, National Academy of Sciences, 1969.

13. Steel HH, Lin PS, Betz RR, Kalamchi A, Clancy M: Iliofemoral fusion for proximal femoral focal deficiency. *J Bone Joint Surg* 1987;69A:837–843.

Chapter 7

Overview and Comparison of Syme's Amputation and Knee Fusion With the van Nes Rotationplasty Procedure in Proximal Femoral Focal Deficiency

William L. Oppenheim, MD
Yoshio Setoguchi, MD
Eileen Fowler, PhD, PT

Introduction

Proximal femoral focal deficiency (PFFD) is a congenital orthopaedic condition involving the upper femur, adjacent soft tissues, and frequently, the acetabulum as well as distal portions of the limb. The incidence ranges from one in 50,000 to one in 200,000. The condition does not appear to be genetically transmitted, and other than those cases associated with thalidomide administration, the etiology remains unknown. Boden and associates[1] postulated a defect in proliferation and maturation of chondrocytes in the proximal growth plate, whereas Epps[2] felt that the condition could be the result of a neural crest injury at the L4-5 level. Whatever the etiology, a clinical hallmark is subtrochanteric bowing as contrasted with the varus deformity of the femoral neck seen in congenital coxa vara. Current classification schemes attempt to subcategorize various morphologic aspects of the bony anlage in order to predict future development, but the simple four-part Aitken classification[3] seems to have stood the test of time. Clearly, there is a continuum of severity from simple congenital shortening of the femur, through coxa vara and PFFD, to near total agenesis. Treatment will vary according to the degree of involvement, remaining growth, and the presence of associated anomalies. It is essential that the clinician understand the breadth of the deformity and the complexity of potential treatment decisions.

Largely due to the abnormal appearance, the birth of a child with PFFD is often viewed as tragic, engendering feelings of guilt, disappointment, fear, and anxiety in parents and physicians alike. Facility with dealing with these psychosocial aspects comes with experience. Fortunately, most children are treated in prosthetic centers where they and their parents can meet other similarly affected families, view the condition at a later age, and thus have many of their fears allayed.

Clinical Presentation

At birth there is a short bulky thigh (ship's ventilator appearance) held in flexion, abduction, and external rotation. The level of the foot with respect to the opposite limb varies from midtibia to above the knee. The condition is bilateral in 15%. Up to 70% have associated congenital defects, the most common of which is associated paraxial fibula deficiency.[4,5] Valgus positioning of the foot at the ankle implies total absence of the fibula. The lateral foot rays may also be absent or hypoplastic. Hip instability is usually present in cases of acetabular incompetence, but the fact that the knee may be only a few centimeters below the hip complicates the examination. Soft-tissue deficiencies range from the total absence of some muscles to partial reduction in muscle mass or length.[6] Nevertheless, the severe shortening of the proximal femur gives a bulky appearance to the soft-tissue envelope so that the severity of the loss may not be immediately apparent.

Radiology and Classification

Radiographs will reveal shortening, subtrochanteric bowing, and retardation of capital femoral epiphyseal ossification. Imaging studies, such as ultrasound, arthrography, or magnetic resonance, may also be helpful in determining the true situation prior to bony ossification, but do not change the prognosis. Although an ossification center may develop over time, bony continuity with the femoral shaft still is not assured. Spontaneous 'healing' takes place in the majority as late as 7 to 8 years of age, by which time the subtrochanteric bowing can be readily appreciated.

Management

Aitken[3,7] has referred to four major biomechanical losses that need to be addressed in the treatment of PFFD: (1) inequality of leg lengths, (2) malrotation, (3) inadequate proximal musculature, and (4) instability of the proximal joints. The vast majority of unilaterally affected children will need a prosthesis regardless of the treatment adopted. Surgical treatment will be influenced by the projected limb-length inequality at the end of growth. An estimate is possible because the percent difference remains constant throughout growth. Thus, if the femur is 45% short at birth, it will be 45% short at the completion of growth. If the sound contralateral femur is deemed by standard growth charts to be 40 cm, the involved femur would be just 22 cm at skeletal maturity, leaving an 18 cm discrepancy without considering the possibility of an associated fibula deficiency. Most authors rarely suggest lengthening for projected discrepancies beyond 12 to 15 cm. However, in mild cases where leg-length discrepancy is the main consideration, standard leg lengthening techniques may be used for projected differences up to approximately 6 cm at full growth. Lengthening of the short side combined with epiphysiodesis of the long side can be very effective.

Perhaps an additional 5 cm may be made up by contralateral epiphysiodesis at the cost of some loss of stature. In view of the difficulties of lengthening congenital as contrasted to acquired conditions, this approach thus becomes a viable alternative for up to 12 cm of projected discrepancy.

All children will start with nonsurgical treatment consisting of an extension prosthesis at walking age (between 9 to 12 months). Fitting of a prosthesis is complicated by the proximal bulkiness and shortness of the thigh, instability of the hip, and the presence of a foot at the level where a prosthetic knee joint frequently needs to be incorporated, usually by ages 3 to 4 years. To aid with prosthetic fitting, when the knee is situated close to the hip and surgical treatment beyond simple leg lengthening is entertained, a knee fusion with or without ablation of the foot by Boyd or Syme's amputation has become the most widely used procedure. The knee fusion converts the proximal femur into a single skeletal lever, a term coined by King.[8] Use of a prosthesis after knee fusion slowly eliminates the abduction and rotational contractures spontaneously. Foot amputation is performed to facilitate prosthetic fitting, but many families prefer to have the foot maintained, and many European prosthetists pride themselves in being able to effectively fit around the foot. In North America, foot ablation is more widely accepted and generally carried out before 2 years of age to avoid the child having grief reactions to the loss. With or without the foot, the child functions as an above-knee amputee. This situation can theoretically be improved by preserving, but rotating the foot 180° to serve as a surrogate knee and, thus, allow the child to function as a below-knee amputee (Fig. 1).

The procedure of fusing the knee and simultaneously, or later rotating the foot was described by Borggreve[9] in 1930, and then by van Nes[10] in 1950. It has remained a controversial approach, in part because of the cosmetic consideration of having the foot on "backward." Westin and Gunderson[11] in 1969 reported only two successful outcomes in eight patients. Four of the eight did not achieve satisfactory rotation, and two others derotated after full rotation. In 1975, Kostuik and associates[12] stated that while it might improve function, it should be postponed until age 12 years because of frequent problems associated with derotation. Koman and associates[4] believed that it should not be performed, but offered no data.

A review by Torode and Gillespie[13] was more encouraging. They used a technique that combined arthrodesis of the knee and tibial osteotomy. By achieving most of the rotation at the knee, the muscles crossing the leg were stretched to a lesser degree, reducing the tendency toward derotation over time. Friscia and associates[14] reported a series of 13 patients treated similarly to the technique of Torode and Gillespie (Fig. 1). The results were excellent or satisfactory in ten of 12 unilateral cases (Fig. 2). Five required repeat surgery as a result of spontaneous derotation. The prerequisites for the procedure were a reasonably normal foot and ankle, presence of a fibula, and an active arc of motion of the ankle of at least 45°. Although the procedure was performed in both limbs of one patient, function did not appear improved, and it was not again considered for such patients. In unilateral cases, although a stable hip improved the final result, an unstable hip was not viewed as a contraindication. None of the patients, including six

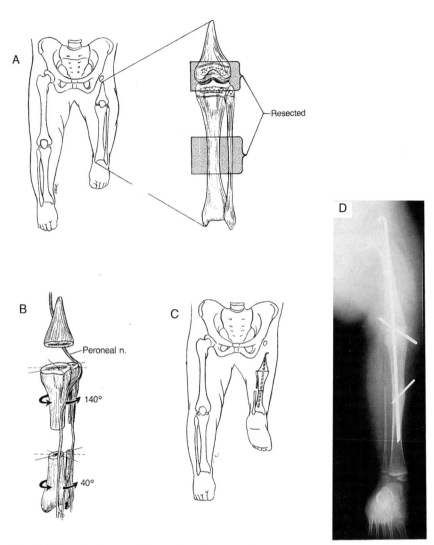

Fig. *1 Schematic diagrams illustrating the surgical conversion to a van Nes rotation-plasty.* **A,** *Plan for level of resections. We include the distal femoral physis as part of our initial procedure.* **B,** *Showing the resected areas and the direction and magnitude of the initial resections.* **C,** *Final schematic appearance.* **D,** *Typical x-ray appearance. (Reproduced with permission from Oppenheim WL, Setoguchi Y: Congenital lower limb deficiencies, in Chapman HW, Madison M (eds):* Operative Orthopaedics, *ed 2. Philadelphia, PA, JB Lippincott, 1993, vol 4, p 3246.)*

females, felt that the leg was cosmetically unacceptable. If a patient should object to the cosmetic appearance or suffer psychologically, ablation could always be performed with conversion to a Syme's or Boyd amputation and above-knee function.

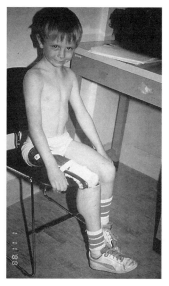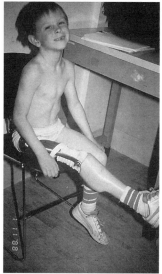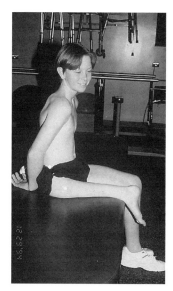

*Fig. 2 Below knee function can be simulated by the rotated ankle after the van Nes rotationplasty procedure. Clinical appearance in the prosthesis. **Left,** Flexion with patient seated. **Center,** Active prosthetic knee extension performed by the ankle plantarflexors. **Right,** Cosmetic appearance with the foot facing rearward.*

Most limbs treated with the van Nes procedure end up too long, requiring procedures to limit their length so that the surrogate foot is at a level opposite the contralateral knee. For this reason, we always sacrifice the distal femoral growth plate at the time of knee fusion. Because we fuse the distal femoral shaft into the proximal tibial ossification center, this procedure is done from 18 months to 2 years of age, once the proximal tibial epiphysis, often delayed in its appearance in this condition, has ossified.

Syme's Amputation Versus van Nes Rotationplasty

Intuitively, one would expect that foot preservation with below-knee function in PFFD should be better than the more widely used knee fusion and foot ablation that results in above-knee function (Fig. 3). However, because patients with PFFD, as contrasted to the usual amputee, exhibit associated defects in hip musculature, external rotation contractures, and associated leg and foot anomalies, the situation often is not so simple. In an effort to address these issues, we studied patients with PFFD in our functional assessment laboratory. Gait analysis and oxygen consumption data were compared for seven patients who had undergone the van Nes procedure and nine patients who had undergone Syme's amputation.

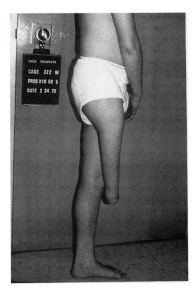

Fig. 3 *An alternative to rotationplasty. Typical appearance of a Syme's conversion and knee fusion case with the knee level (thigh segment) slightly long.*

Gait Mechanics

Our subjects were recruited from the Child Amputee Prosthetic Programs at Shriners Hospital, Los Angeles and the University of California at Los Angeles (UCLA). All subjects who had a van Nes procedure wore an exoskeletal prosthesis with a corset style attachment at the thigh, a hinged knee, and a socket for the foot. All subjects who had a Syme's procedure had a constant friction, single axis prosthetic knee joint. van Nes subjects exhibited adequate rotation at the time of data collection. The patients did not have energy-storing prosthetic feet. Patients were videotaped as they walked at their preferred speed across a walkway that concealed a force platform. Standard procedures for the collection and calculation of biomechanical data were used.[15] The patients who had undergone the van Nes procedure demonstrated improved prosthetic limb function and fewer contralateral sound limb compensations compared to those with Syme's amputations.

Differences in Prosthetic Limb Function

An analysis of the ground reaction forces revealed that both groups exhibited a decrease in the amount of prosthetic limb weightbearing as compared to their contralateral sound limbs (Fig. 4). Data from the van Nes group were closer to normative data. Their vertical component exhibited a more customary bimodal shape and the mean duration of weightbearing was longer. The two mean peak vertical components were greater and the unloading phase, or valley, was less. In contrast, the Syme's group tended

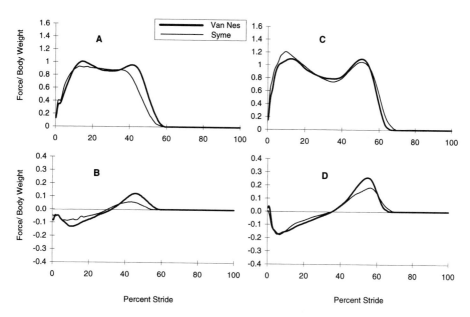

Fig. 4 *Mean ground reaction forces normalized to body weight for patients who have had van Nes rotationplasty or Syme's amputations. The vertical components of the ground reaction force vector are shown in **A** for the prosthetic limbs and **C** for the contralateral sound limbs. Contralateral sound limb mean vertical components for both groups were similar to those of unaffected subjects. The prosthetic limb vertical components were lower for both groups as compared to the contalateral sound limbs. The Syme's group has a flatter, more abnormal loading response. The mean horizontal components are shown in **B** for the prosthetic limbs and **D** for the contralateral sound limbs. Negative values indicate the braking phase and positive values, the propulsive phase. Contralateral sound limb mean curves for both groups were similar to those of unaffected subjects. Mean prosthetic horizontal components were diminished for each group compared to the natural limbs and normative data, but to a greater degree for the Syme's amputation group.*

to avoid forces due to acceleration. The Syme's group also exhibited lower peak braking and propulsive forces.

Evidence for prosthetic knee function influenced by the anatomic ankle in the van Nes group could be seen by examining the joint angular and moment data during walking. Patients who had a van Nes rotationplasty were able to maintain a flexed knee posture during single-limb support in midstance, whereas the Syme's group demonstrated knee hyperextension during stance (Fig. 5, *top*). This was expected since prosthetic knee joint hyperextension kept the ground reaction force vector anterior to the mechanical knee, ensuring its stability. van Nes patients produced knee extensor moments during single limb support. All patients in the Syme's amputation group produced knee flexor moments during this phase of gait (Fig. 5, *bottom*) because the passive properties of the mechanical knee joint resisted the external extensor moment.

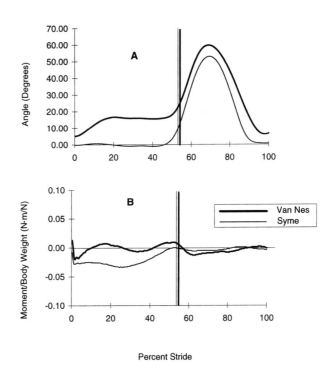

Fig. 5 *Mean prosthetic knee joint angles (**top**) and moments (**bottom**) for patients who have had Van Nes rotationplasties or Syme's amputations. The vertical lines represent toe off. Extensor moments are positive and flexor moments are negative. The mean data for van Nes patients indicates prosthetic knee function during midstance as demonstrated by knee flexion angles and knee extensor moments. All Syme's patients kept their knees in hyperextension to stabilize their mechanical knee joints and exhibited knee flexor moments during stance.*

Contralateral Sound Limb Compensations

The functional deficit due to the missing limb musculature must be compensated by the remaining uninvolved or contralateral sound limb; ie, the extra work done to compensate for the missing limb is performed by the sound limb. Differences between the two surgical approaches can be inferred by examining the extent of the sound limb compensations necessary for the patient to optimize his or her gait. Compensatory mechanisms, such as vaulting and excessive joint moment and power generation, were observed in both groups, but were seen to a greater extent in the Syme's amputation group.

Vaulting, or stance phase plantarflexion of the contralateral sound limb, was a compensation used to ensure prosthetic limb clearance during swing in many subjects. However, the prevalence and magnitude of plantarflexion was highest for the Syme's amputation group (Fig. 6, *top*). The mean ankle

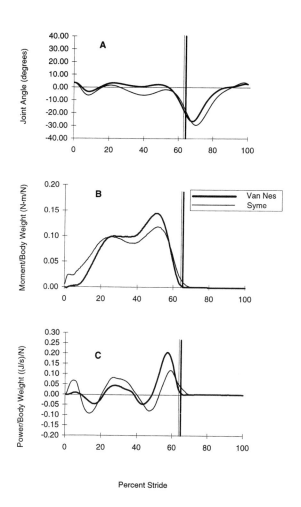

Fig. 6 *Mean contralateral sound limb ankle joint angles* **(top)**, *moments* **(center)**, *and powers* **(bottom)**, *for patients who have had van Nes rotationplasties or Syme's amputations. Dorsiflexion is positive and plantarflexion is negative. Extensor moments are positive and flexor moments are negative. Power generation is shown as positive and absorption as negative. The vertical lines represent toe off. Evidence of compensatory natural limb vaulting was observed for both groups but to a greater degree for the Syme's amputation group. Instead of continued dorsiflexion during midstance, the joint angle reversed in order to clear the prosthetic limb, which was in swing at this time, and prevent tripping. This ankle action resulted in a plateau in continued ankle extensor moments and inappropriate power production during this phase of gait.*

joint angle for these patients exhibited a reversal into plantarflexion during stance between 20% to 50% of the stride cycle. Patients who had a van Nes rotationplasty exhibited a plateau rather than continued dorsiflexion, as would be seen in unaffected subjects.

81

Contralateral sound limb ankle joint moments and powers also reflected evidence of vaulting. The mean ankle joint moment for the van Nes rotationplasty group exhibited a delay in what normally should have been a continuous increase in the ankle joint moment during stance (Fig. 6, *center*). The Syme's amputation group moment minimum was coincident with peak ankle joint plantarflexion during this phase, moving the ground reaction force vector closer to the ankle joint and decreasing the moment arm. Excessive ankle joint power generation as a result of vaulting was observed in both groups during this phase of gait, but was greatest in the patients who had a Syme's amputation (Fig. 6, *bottom*). Ankle joint power absorption rather than generation should have occurred at this time.

Mean peak knee flexor and hip extensor moments in the beginning of stance phase were excessive for the contralateral limb in the Syme's amputation group (Fig. 7, *left*). Because the prosthetic limb for this group did not exhibit adequate propulsive ground reaction forces, the contralateral limb had to "pull" the individual's center of mass forward onto itself. This action resulted in greater knee and hip power generation during initial stance (Fig. 7, *right*). Thus, the Syme's patients as a group required greater compensation by the contralateral sound limb than did the van Nes patients.

The gait analysis data suggest that a functioning van Nes patient more closely mimics the contralateral sound limb or an unaffected patient's limb in terms of ground reaction forces, forward propulsion, and active knee control. The contralateral limb of the van Nes patient does not need to generate as much of a power profile to compensate for the loss of the missing limb. van Nes patients exhibited less vaulting, a smoother gait overall, and less inappropriate power generation.

Oxygen Consumption Studies

The gait analysis data suggested greater energy requirements for the Syme's group. To determine whether this analysis could be supported by examining oxygen consumption directly, we recruited 16 patients with PFFD and used the UCLA Pulmonary Function Laboratory. Nine van Nes patients were compared to seven patients who had undergone the Syme's procedure with knee fusion. The groups were comparable in terms of the numbers of Aitken class A, B, and C patients. Oxygen cost was significantly lower in the van Nes group (Fig. 8), while patient selected walking speeds tended to be higher.[16] The difference in oxygen cost between the groups, 0.12 ml/kg/ml, is comparable to data in the literature measuring the differences between below knee and above knee amputees (0.09 ml/kg/ml).[17] In one recent study,[18] oxygen cost was approximately 10% lower in the van Nes group, but the difference was not statistically significant. The study did not take into account the fact that younger children have a greater metabolism and a greater oxygen consumption. Such studies must consider the effects of age in order to make a proper comparison. We were able to do this as demonstrated in Figure 8.

Based on our clinical experience, and supported by these laboratory data, we continue to offer the van Nes procedure as the preferable choice, all other factors being equal. As pointed out by Hall (JE Hall, MD, personal commu-

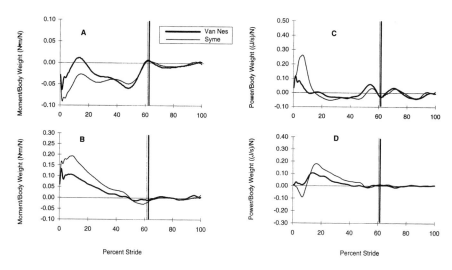

Fig. 7 *Mean contralateral sound limb knee joint moment (**top left**), hip joint moment (**bottom left**), knee joint power (**top right**), and hip joint power (**bottom right**) for patients who have had van Nes rotationplasty or Syme's amputations. Excessive hip extensor and knee flexor moments were observed for the Syme's group after initial contact. Minimal propulsive ground reaction forces for the prosthetic limb were also observed at this time (see Fig. 1), requiring more effort on the part of the contralateral sound limb to bring the body's center of mass forward on itself.*

nication, New Orleans, LA, 1990), the concept of discarding a potentially useful body part, such as an ankle joint, is the position that perhaps should require defense.

The Hip Joint

Although much attention has been focused on the conversion to either a van Nes or above-knee functional Syme's procedure, the crux of the matter in terms of function frequently remains focused at the hip joint. Surgery has been directed to healing the pseudarthrosis and to restoring the neck shaft angle by valgus osteotomy.[19] Those cases with severe involvement are usually left alone save for the fusion of very short segments into the ilium.[20] Each of these issues is addressed elsewhere in this symposium. As usual, the best results have been in Aitken classes A and B. Most series report a high rate of recurrence with a high reoperation rate as well. If valgus osteotomies are performed, Krajbich[21] recommends obtaining 155° to 170° of valgus. The timing of hip surgery remains controversial. Usually, surgeons wait until there is sufficient bone for fixation, frequently after the age of 5 years. A recent report once again raises the issue of earlier surgery in an effort to promote more normal growth.[22] Improvement in gait depends on the abductor strength more than on adductor tightness. In approaching pseudarthrosis, the

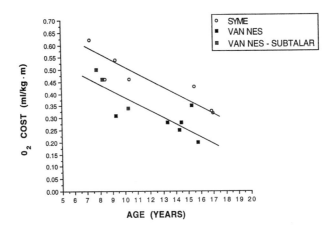

Fig. 8 *Graph showing the relationship between the oxygen cost, the subject's age, and the type of operative procedure. van Nes-Subtalar refers to those subjects that had at least 90° of rotation back toward the original position at the time of data collection. According to the multivariate linear aregression analysis, younger children and subjects who had had a Syme's amputation had a significantly greater mean oxygen cost (p = 0.0001 and p = 0001; respectively). The r² value was 0.79, and the difference between the two operative groups was 0.12 milliliters per kilogram of body mass per meter at each age. (Reproduced with permission from Fowler E, Zernicke R, Setoguchi Y, Oppenheim W: Energy expenditure during walking by children who have proximal femoral focal deficiency. J Bone Joint Surg 1996;78A:1857–1862.)*

potential loss of motion must be weighed against the presumed burden of instability. Surgery should be delayed until it is certain that bone-to-bone healing will be feasible once the pseudarthrosis is resected.

Conclusion

PFFD encompasses a complicated spectrum of pathology. No one approach is applicable for all cases. Treatment must be individualized. The goal of treatment is to maximize function. For mild cases the femur can be lengthened, or the opposite site shortened by epiphysiodesis. In the more involved child, Aitken classes A and B are the most salvageable and will receive the most attention from both a surgical and nonsurgical standpoint. Prosthetic fitting can be facilitated by knee fusion accompanied by either a van Nes rotationplasty or a Syme's or Boyd amputation. The absence of a fully stable hip is not in itself a contraindication for these procedures. For those children with a good hip and adequate foot and ankle function, the van Nes procedure allows more normal function as documented by clinical observation, gait analysis, and oxygen consumption studies. However, because the cosmetic appearance can be disturbing to some, a good psychological assessment is integral to preoperative planning. Regardless of which treatment is chosen, most children will require a prosthesis. The prosthetic limb will generally be too long for the prosthetic knee to lie at a level comparable to the opposite member, so shortening procedures must be considered for the involved side. Once the proximal femur has ossified, we consider valgus osteotomy of the hip. In those cases of severe shortening without hip stability, usually Aitken classes C and D, iliofemoral fusion with use of the knee as a surrogate hip can be weighed. Although the costs, both monetary and psychological, can be trying, as a group these children do well and function to the full potential that they are given, both from a mechanical standpoint and from the standpoint of socialization and productivity.

References

1. Boden SD, Fallon MD, Davidson R, Mennuti MT, Kaplan FS: Proximal femoral focal deficiency: Evidence for a defect in proliferation and maturation of chondrocytes. *J Bone Joint Surg* 1989;71A:1119–1129.

2. Epps CH Jr: Proximal femoral focal deficiency. *J Bone Joint Surg*1983;65A:867–870.

3. Aitken GT: Amputation as a treatment for certain lower-extremity congenital abnormalities. *J Bone Joint Surg* 1959;41A:1267–1285.

4. Koman LA, Meyer LC, Warren FH: Proximal femoral focal deficiency: Natural history and treatment. *Clin Orthop* 1982;162:135–143.

5. Hillmann JS, Mesgarzadeh M, Revesz G, Bonakdarpour A, Clancy M, Betz RR: Proximal femoral focal deficiency: Radiologic analysis of 49 cases. *Radiology* 1987;165:769–773.

6. Pirani S, Beauchamp RD, Li D, Sawatzky B: Soft tissue anatomy of proximal femoral focal deficiency. *J Pediatr Orthop* 1991;11:563–570.

7. Aitken GT: Proximal femoral focal deficiency: Definition, classification and management, in Aitken GT (ed): *Proximal Femoral Focal Deficiency: A Congenital Anomaly.* Washington, DC, National Academy of Sciences, 1969, pp 1–22.

8. King RE: Some concepts of proximal femoral focal deficiency, in Aitken GT (ed): *Proximal Femoral Focal Deficiency: A Congenital Anomaly.* Washington, DC, National Academy of Sciences, 1969, pp 23–49.

9. Borggreve J: Kniegelenksersatz durch das in der Beinlängsachse um 180° gedrehte Fussgelenk. *Arch F Orthop* 1930;28:175–178.

10. van Nes CP: Rotation-plasty for congenital defects of the femur: Making use of the ankle of the shortened limb to control the knee joint of a prosthesis. *J Bone Joint Surg* 1950;32B:12–16.

11. Westin GW, Gunderson FO: Proximal femoral focal deficiency: Review of treatment experience, in Aitken GT (ed): *Proximal Femoral Focal Deficiency: A Congenital Anomaly.* Washington, DC, National Academy of Sciences, 1969, pp 100–110.

12. Kostuik JP, Gillespie R, Hall JE, Hubbard S: Van Nes rotational osteotomy for treatment of proximal femoral focal deficiency and congenital short femur. *J Bone Joint Surg* 1975;57A:1039–1046.

13. Torode IP, Gillespie R: Rotationplasty of the lower limb for congenital defects of the femur. *J Bone Joint Surg* 1983;65B:569–573.

14. Friscia DA, Moseley CF, Oppenheim WL: Rotational osteotomy for proximal femoral focal deficiency. *J Bone Joint Surg* 1989;71A:1386–1392.

15. Schneider K, Hart T, Zernicke RF, Setoguchi Y, Oppenheim W: Dynamics of below-knee child amputee gait: SACH foot versus Flex foot. *J Biomech* 1993;26:1191–1204.

16. Fowler E, Zernicke R, Setoguchi Y, Oppenheim W: Energy expenditure during walking by children who have proximal femoral focal deficiency. *J Bone Joint Surg* 1996;78A:1857–1862.

17. Waters RL, Perry J, Antonelli D, Hislop H: Energy cost of walking of amputees: The influence of level of amputation. *J Bone Joint Surg* 1976;58A:42–46.

18. Alman BA, Krajbich JI, Hubbard S: Proximal femoral focal deficiency: Results of rotationplasty and Syme amputation. *J Bone Joint Surg* 1995;77:1876–1882.

19. Lange DR, Schoenecker PL, Baker CL: Proximal femoral focal deficiency: Treatment and classification in forty-two cases. *Clin Orthop* 1978;135:15–25.

20. Steel HH, Lin PS, Betz RR, Kalamchi A, Clancy M: Iliofemoral fusion for proximal femoral focal deficiency. *J Bone Joint Surg* 1987;69A:837–843.

21. Krajbich I: Proximal femoral focal deficiency, in Kalamchi A (ed): *Congenital Lower Limb Deficiencies.* New York, NY, Springer-Verlag, 1989, pp 108–127.

22. Tonnis D, Stanitski DF: Early conservative and operative treatment to gain early normal growth in proximal femoral focal deficiency. *J Pediatr Orthop* 1997;6:59–67.

Chapter 8

Rotationplasty in the Management of Proximal Femoral Focal Deficiency

J. Ivan Krajbich, MD, FRCSC

Introduction

The management of proximal femoral focal deficiency (PFFD) remains a major challenge to the treatment team. A multidisciplinary team approach is the cornerstone of modern management of this condition and its impact on the patients and their families. The pediatric orthopedic surgeon frequently has a role not only as a provider of surgical expertise, but also as a leader of the treatment team and a major source of information to the family and the health care providers.[1] It is important that the child's caregivers receive realistic information regarding the child's condition, type of treatment available, and expected outcome. Unfortunately, complete restoration of the affected extremity is rarely possible.[2–5] Currently, in the majority of children afflicted by PFFD, the goal of surgical treatment necessarily remains to obtain a functionally optimal residual limb to power a lower leg prosthesis.[6–11] It is to the definition and achievement of this goal that this chapter is dedicated.

Barring a complete limb restoration, the "ideal" residual lower extremity in a child with PFFD would have: (1) a stable, painless, functional hip joint; (2) a stable, painless, functional, biologic knee joint; and, (3) an end weight-bearing stump with no potential for bony overgrowth. This ideal, however, may not be accomplishable in some more severely involved extremities.

Success of hip reconstruction depends largely on the severity of the PFFD. The Aitken classification[1] is a very useful guide as far as hip reconstruction is concerned, and its implications vis-à-vis hip reconstruction are discussed elsewhere.[12,13] On the other hand, reconstruction and/or creation of a biologic, functional knee is not necessarily dependent on the severity of the proximal deficiency. With rare exceptions, when the involved femur is Aitken type A, the deficiency can be restored and at least partially lengthened to a sufficient degree for the patient's anatomic knee to function as a true knee. The creation of a biologic knee depends on the integrity of the distal part of the extremity because a relatively normal lower leg, with functioning foot and ankle, can be used to reconstruct a functional knee joint.[13] This reconstructive procedure is variously called van Nes rotationplasty, Borggreve procedure, tibial rotationplasty or simply rotationplasty.[14,15] Its principle is to use the patient's relatively normal foot and ankle as a functional knee joint by rotating the distal part of the extremity 180° and bringing the ankle up to the level of the contralateral normal knee. The ankle joint thus substitutes for the knee joint and the foot pointing posteriorly substitutes for the proximal tibia. Limbs so reconstructed can be fitted with an external prosthesis that allows extremity function similar to that of the below knee amputee. The "ankle/knee" joint is thus powered by the patient's own leg muscles. Ankle dorsiflexors provide knee flexion and the gastrocnemius-soleus group provides knee extension, substituting for the absent or dysplasic quadriceps. Additional advantages of this procedure are that the new ankle/knee retains its proprioceptive qualities and the foot provides for a good weightbearing stump. Because of the presence of the foot on the end of the extremity, many patients do not view this procedure as an amputation.[16] If, for any reason, the outcome of the procedure is not acceptable to the patient or the family, the rotationplasty can easily be converted to more traditional Syme's amputation. Thus, no bridges are burned.

Historic Review

The procedure was first reported by Borggreve in 1930.[17] He used it to substitute for a knee destroyed by tuberculosis. van Nes was the first to describe this procedure in the English literature in 1950.[18] He used the procedure for patients with congenital femoral deficiencies. The procedure subsequently has been used in several centers of pediatric orthopaedics in North America, and in 1966, Hall[19] reported on his experience with his modification of this procedure. The procedure was performed by osteotomizing the tibia and fibula in mid-diaphysis. A segment of the bone was resected to allow 180° rotation without undue tension on the neurovascular bundle.[20] In many centers the rotationplasty is still performed in this fashion.[21] However, Gillespie and Torode[22] pointed out the advantages of combining the rotationplasty with a knee fusion, accomplishing most of the rotation at the knee level and leaving only a small amount of rotation to be performed through the tibial osteomy.[23] Their procedure provides the patient with a solid "one bone" thigh in more anatomic position for weightbearing instead of the "double hip joint" of patients with an unfused knee and a short residual femur. In the latter circumstance, the residual limb is aligned anteriorly and laterally to normal anatomic positions as a result of the flexion, abduction, and external rotation contracture of the PFFD hip. This poor position is often aggravated by a knee flexion contracture. The Gillespie-Torode procedure further allows for easier adjustment of the thigh length without weakening leg musculature through excessive shortening, and finally, it allows most of the leg muscles to exercise their function in more or less a straight line, decreasing the tendency for subsequent derotation.[16]

Based on my experiences with the Gillespie-Torode modification of rotationplasty and with rotationplasty in resection of malignant bone tumors around the knee,[24,25] I have further modified the procedure to obtain all of the rotation through the knee, with simultaneous knee arthrodesis. All the muscles crossing the knee joint are detached and transferred into a new position so they all pull in a straight line across the rotated, arthrodesed knee to prevent late derotation.[13,16] The experience with this modification has been very positive and it is this version of the procedure that is described in detail in this chapter.

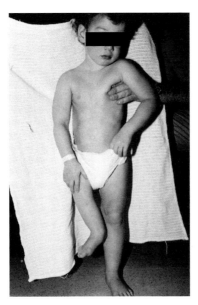

Fig. 1 *Typical degree of a limb shortening in a child with PFFD (Gillespie-Torode, Class B).*

Indications and Prerequisites

Any child born with a unilateral PFFD can be viewed as a potential candidate for rotationplasty provided that certain criteria are met. The child and the family should be carefully assessed by the entire pediatric limb-deficiency team to arrive at an accurate diagnosis regarding the limb deficiency and all other possible associated abnormalities. Psychological factors in the family unit need to be assessed as well.

It is important to distinguish between the more severe form of a congenital short femur and a true PFFD,[22] because many children with congenital short femur may be candidates for limb equalization procedures using modern techniques of limb lengthening.[26] Children with a true PFFD (Gillespie-Torode, Class B) are only rarely candidates for limb lengthening, and optimizing their limb as a functional stump for prosthetic fitting is the primary goal of the surgical treatment (Fig. 1). van Nes rotationplasty can be used in all types of PFFD (Fig. 2), including the more severe ones (Aitken types C and D).[13] The factor that determines the feasibility of rotationplasty is not so much the severity of the femoral deficiency as the status of the extremity distal to the knee. For the rotationplasty to be functionally successful the child must have a relatively normal ankle and foot. Hence, children with no or only very mild fibular deficiency are ideal candidates. More severe ipsilateral fibular deficiencies, present in many children with PFFD, can be a contraindication to rotationplasty. A stiff ankle and subtalar joint, markedly

89

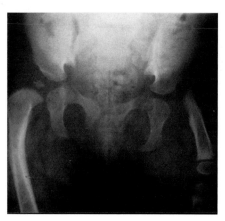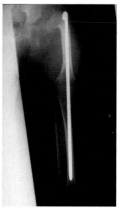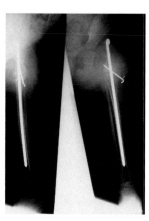

*Fig. 2 Left, Aitken Type A PFFD with a reconstructable hip joint. **Center,** Same patient following van Nes rotationplasty. Note improved ossification of the trochanteric and cervical area. **Right,** van Nes rotationplasty in Aitken Type B PFFD.*

dysplastic foot, and/or marked tibial shortening and bow with dysfunctional muscles all preclude successful rotationplasty. However, some degree of ankle joint valgus and moderate plantarflexion contracture and even absence of the lateral ray of the foot can be accommodated, provided that combined ankle and subtalar joint motion is in the vicinity of 50° to 60°. Occasionally, this requirement can be met by lengthening lateral and posterior soft-tissue structures prior to rotationplasty.

Acceptance of rotationplasty by the treating surgeon is, in my opinion, still the most important reason why this operation is not used more widely. It is a technically significantly more demanding procedure than Syme's amputation. Relative rarity of the condition leaves most orthopaedic surgeons with scant experience with van Nes rotationplasty, and therefore, they are somewhat reluctant to recommend it as a treatment choice. Parents of the child afflicted with PFFD are also faced with an unfamiliar, stressful situation. Unless rotationplasty is described to them with full confidence and the advantages and disadvantages clearly pointed out, parents will tend to view rotationplasty as an experimental procedure with unpredictable results. The need for an unconventional prosthesis is yet another factor in reluctance to pursue rotationplasty as a mode of treatment.[20] Most of these points are, of course, quite valid. Poorly performed operations, compromised by complications, or a badly functioning prosthesis are a poor alternative to Syme's amputation and knee fusions with traditional prosthetic fitting. Therefore, lack of surgical and/or prosthetic expertise is a relative contraindication to rotationplasty. However, referral to a center where such expertise is available should be strongly encouraged because the functional advantage of a well-functioning rotationplasty over the lifetime of the PFFD patient can be quite significant. Therefore, the child should be given every opportunity to explore this option or, at least, be objectively informed regarding rotationplasty.[16,27]

Timing of the Surgical Treatment

There are no definitive guidelines as to the timing of the rotationplasty. Early literature suggested that the best time for surgery was late childhood or adolescence. The reason for this was an attempt to minimize derotation and correctly estimate final thigh length. More recent literature suggests that the procedure should be carried out before the child reaches preschool or kindergarten age; I share this view. Early surgery lessens the impact of the altered anatomy both psychologically and functionally. With use of the more recently modified surgical techniques, both late derotation and thigh length have become much less of an issue. My preferred time for surgery is between ages 2 and 3 years. However, the procedure can be carried out at any time afterward, and sometimes is done so for various reasons, such as referral or parental preference.

Surgical Technique

The surgical technique described is my preferred technique, with appreciation that other modifications and versions exist and are successfully practiced by pediatric orthopaedic surgeons around the world.

The child is given general anesthesia. With the child in a supine position, the involved extremity is free draped from the foot to the umbilicus. A radiotransparent table is used so fluoroscopy can be used if and when needed. An S-shaped incision is made, starting longitudinally on the lateral aspect of the thigh. At the level of the knee it is curved somewhat anteriorly and medially, then it is continued longitudinally and distally into the leg for about 2 to 3 in. This part of the incision is quite anterior (Fig. 3). A lateral flap usually is developed first, with the goal of identifying, dissecting free, and protecting the peroneal nerve. This step may sometimes be less than completely routine because an associated fibular deficiency can alter the normal anatomic relations. Once the peroneal nerve is protected, the iliotibial band and tendon of the biceps femoris can be detached from their insertions on the tibia and the lateral head of the gastrocnemius from its origin on the femoral condyle. All the detached tendons and muscles are carefully marked. The popliteal neurovascular bundle can now be identified, dissected free at the back of the knee, and gently retracted posteriorly. Next, the medial flap is developed, including the retinaculum layer.

The patellar tendon is detached from the tibia and elevated anteriorly and proximally. The capsule of the knee joint is then incised circumferentially, carefully protecting the posterior neurovascular bundle and the peroneal nerve. The knee joint is then inspected and remaining connecting intra-articular structures are divided. Most knee joints in patients with PFFD are grossly abnormal with absent cruciate ligaments (Fig. 4). Next, the medial hamstrings, gracilis, and sartorius are detached from their insertion on the tibia, and the medial head of the gastrocnemius from its origin on the distal femur. The popliteus is divided at the level of the joint. Tendons and muscle ends are labeled with sutures.

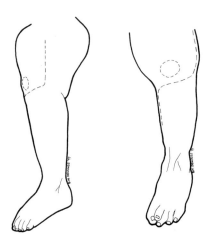

Fig. 3 *Skin incision.*

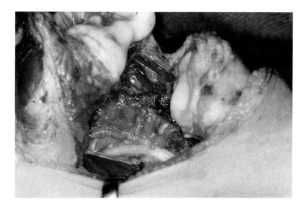

Fig. 4 *Knee in a child with proximal femoral focal deficiency. Note a complete absence of any cruciate ligament structures. The peroneal nerve is seen at the lower edge of the wound.*

The distal femur is exposed by retracting the soft tissues proximally, and it is transected using a surgical saw. Osteotomy is carried out about 0.5 to 1.0 cm proximal to the distal femoral growth plate (Fig. 5). Longer or shorter segments may need to be taken depending on overall length of the extremity, as the goal is to make the van Nes rotationplasty extremity equal in length to or slightly longer than the contralateral thigh (Fig. 6). In virtually every case the distal femoral growth plate needs to be removed to prevent the

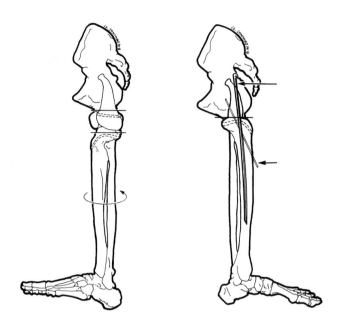

Fig. 5 Left, *Schematic drawing of osteotomy cuts as related to the epiphyseal plates and the knee joint.* **Right,** *The distal segment is rotated 180° and fixed with intramedulary rod (long arrow) and optional cross-pin (short arrow).*

van Nes thigh from growing too long and to obtain enough shortening so that the rotation can be carried out without undue tension on the neurovascular bundle. Next the articular surface of the tibia is removed by cutting through the subchondral bone 4 to 5 mm proximal to the tibial growth plate. Popliteal vessels are again carefully identified and further dissected proximally into the adductor hiatus. Adductor tendon insertion is best divided to allow the vessels to swing freely medially and anteriorly. Then, 180° of external rotation is attempted through the resected knee carefully identifying the neurovascular structures and checking them for evidence of excessive tension or pressure. Any vascular compromise warrants further dissection of the bundle, freeing it further proximally (usually around the adductor hiatus) until it is free of tension and distal pulses are present. Occasionally, further shortening of the femur is necessary to accomplish this.

The rotation arthrodesis is completed by using an intramedullary rod for internal fixation. Either a Rush rod or a Kirschner wire (K-wire) is usually introduced into the femur through a retrograde channel, thus assuring a central placement at the arthrodesis site. The final position is checked by fluoroscopy. The exact desired rotation is carefully checked and any final adjustments to it are made at this time. The final rotational position is then secured by one cross K-wire. The previously detached muscles are reattached across the arthodesis, paying particular attention to the heads of the

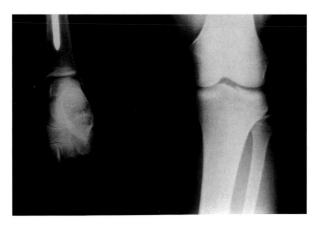

Fig. 6 *van Nes rotationplasty ankle-knee at the level of the contralateral knee.*

gastrocnemius. Final check of the vascular status is made and the wound is closed in a routine fashion. Skin flaps sometimes look somewhat unyielding as a result of the rotation but invariably close satisfactorily.

The extremity is immobilized in a one and one-half well-padded hip spica cast for 4 to 6 weeks. Following the removal of the cast, the child is started on a physical therapy rehabilitation program to regain range of motion and strength in his or her hip and new "ankle/knee." Two to 3 weeks following cast removal, a mold is taken of the child's leg and foot for manufacture of a rotationplasty prosthesis. Once the prosthesis is manufactured and fitted, the child is started on therapy sessions for gait training to obtain the maximum functional advantage of his or her new functional knee. It is not unusual to have to adjust the prosthetic alignment and socket orientation several times over the first year or so as the child's range of motion in the ankle/knee increases.

Conclusion

Rotationplasty is a valuable addition to the treatment armamentarium of orthopaedic surgeons treating children with PFFD. Recent long term follow-up studies, together with biomechanical and energy consumption studies consistently show the advantage of rotationplasty over Syme's amputation with no psychological or self-image problems.[28–30] In experienced hands, the procedure carries very low complication rate and its long term advantages well outweigh the initial disadvantage of a more complex and longer operation as compared to a Syme's amputation.[14,16,23]

References

1. Aitken GT (ed): Proximal femoral deficiency: Definition, classification and management, in *Proximal Femoral Focal Deficiency: A Congenital Anomaly.* Washington, DC, National Academy of Sciences, 1969.

2. Amstutz HC: Abstract: Prognosis for growth and development of congenital anomalies of the lower extremities. *J Bone Joint Surg* 1967;49A:1011.

3. Koman LA, Meyer LC, Warren FH: Proximal femoral focal deficiency: A 50-year experience. *Dev Med Child Neurol* 1982;24:344–355.

4. Lange DR, Schoenecker PL, Baker CL: Proximal femoral focal deficiency: Treatment and classification in forty-two cases. *Clin Orthop* 1978;135:15–25.

5. Lloyd-Roberts GC, Stone KH: Congenital hypoplasia of the upper femur. *J Bone Joint Surg* 1963;45B:557–560.

6. Aitken GT: Amputation as a treatment for certain lower-extremity congenital abnormalities. *J Bone Joint Surg* 1959;41A:1267–1285.

7. Damsin JP, Pous JG, Ghanem I: Therapeutic approach to severe congenital lower limb length discrepancies: Surgical treatment versus prosthetic management. *J Pediatr Orthop B* 1995;4:164–170.

8. Fixsen JA, Lloyd-Roberts GC: The natural history and early treatment of proximal femoral dysplasia. *J Bone Joint Surg* 1974;56B:86–95.

9. Kalamchi A, Cowell HR, Kim KI: Congenital deficiency of the femur. *J Pediatr Orthop* 1985;5:129–134.

10. King RE: Some concepts of proximal femoral focal deficiency, in Aitken GT (ed): *Proximal Femoral Focal Deficiency: A Congenital Anomaly.* Washington, DC, National Academy of Sciences, 1969.

11. King RE: Providing a single skeletal lever in proximal femoral focal deficiency. *Inter Clin Info Bull* 1966;6:23.

12. Steel HH, Lin PS, Betz RR, Kalamchi A, Clancy M: Iliofemoral fusion for proximal femoral focal deficiency. *J Bone Joint Surg* 1987;69A:837–843.

13. Krajbich I: Proximal femoral focal deficiency, in Kalamchi A (ed): *Congenital Lower Limb Deficiencies.* New York, NY, Springer-Verlag, 1989, pp 108–127.

14. Friscia DA, Moseley CF, Oppenheim WL: Rotational osteotomy for proximal femoral focal deficiency. *J Bone Joint Surg* 1989;71A:1386–1392.

15. Kostuik JP, Gillespie R, Hall JE, Hubbard S: Van Nes rotational osteotomy for the treatment of proximal femoral focal deficiency and congenital short femur. *J Bone Joint Surg* 1975;57A:1039–1046.

16. Alman BA, Krajbich JI, Hubbard S: Proximal femoral focal deficiency: Results of rotationplasty and Syme amputation. *J Bone Joint Surg* 1995;77A:1876–1882.

17. Borggreve J: Kniegelenksersatz durch das in der Beinlängsachse um 180 degree gedrehte Fussgelenk. *Arch Orthop* 1930;28:175–178.

18. Van Nes CP: Rotation-plasty for congenital defects of the femur: Making use of the ankle of the shortened limb to control the knee joint of a prosthesis. *J Bone Joint Surg* 1950;32B:12–16.

19. Hall JE: Rotation of congenitally hypoplastic lower limbsto use the ankle joint as a knee. *Inter Clin Info Bull* 1966;6:3.

20. Hall JE, Bochmann D: The surgical and prosthetic management of proximal femoral focal deficiency, in Aitken GT (ed): *Proximal Femoral Focal Deficiency: A Congenital Anomaly.* Washington, DC, National Academy of Sciences, 1969.

21. Kritter AE: Tibial rotation-plasty for proximal femoral focal deficiency, in Kalamchi A (ed): *Congenital Lower Limb Deficiencies*. New York, NY, Springer-Verlag, 1989, pp 152–162.

22. Gillespie R, Torode IP: Classification and management of congenital abnormalities of the femur. *J Bone Joint Surg* 1983;65B:557–568.

23. Torode IP, Gillespie R: Rotationplasty of the lower limb for congenital defects of the femur. *J Bone Joint Surg* 1983;65B:569–573.

24. de Bari A, Krajbich JI, Langer F, Hamilton EL, Hubbard S: Modified van Nes rotationplasty for osteosarcoma of the proximal tibia in children. *J Bone Joint Surg* 1990;72B:1065–1069.

25. Kotz R, Salzer M: Rotation-plasty for childhood osteosarcoma of the distal part of the femur. *J Bone Joint Surg* 1982;64A:959–969.

26. Saleh M, Goonatillake HD: Management of congenital leg length inequality: Value of early axis correction. *J Pediatr Orthop* 1995;4B:150–158.

27. Harter S (ed): *Manual for the Self-Perception Profile for Adolescents*. Denver, CO, University of Denver, 1988.

28. McClenaghan BA, Krajbich JI, Pirone AM, Koheil R, Longmuir P: Comparative assessment of gait after limb-salvage procedures. *J Bone Joint Surg* 1989;71A:1178–1182.

29. Varni JW, Setoguchi Y: Correlates of perceived physical appearance in children with congenital/acquired limb deficiencies. *J Dev Behav Pediatr* 1991;12:171–176.

30. Waters RL, Perry J, Antonelli D, Hislop H: Energy cost of walking of amputees: The influence of level of amputation. *J Bone Joint Surg* 1976;58A:42–46.

Consensus

The Role of Rotationplasty in Congenital Deficiency of the Femur

Properly performed rotationplasty with appropriate fitting and training has functional advantages over amputation. This procedure may be combined with other procedures, such as knee fusion and hip stabilization.

Potential disadvantages of rotationplasty include derotation over time and cosmetic problems. Derotation can be minimized by performing the rotation through the knee arthrodesis. Patient education, especially by discussions with other patients, is essential for informed decision-making.

Major foot and ankle deformities such as fibular deficiency are relative contraindications, and bilateral deficiency is a definite contraindication.

Chapter 9

Iliofemoral Fusion for Proximal Femoral Focal Deficiency

Howard H. Steel, MD, PhD

Introduction

There are indications for iliofemoral fusion for femoral deficiency.[1] The procedure is indicated in an Aitken class B deficiency (Fig. 1), which is characterized by a short femur that has no continuity with the hip joint and is associated with a significantly dysplastic acetabulum, and in class D, in which the acetabulum and femoral head are absent and the femoral shaft is shortened. Briefly put, it will work in a femoral deficiency in which there is an unstable acetabulum with a very short femoral shaft and a deficient acetabulum.

The fusion is done to establish a stable relationship between the femur and the pelvis, which eliminates disabling pistoning, making prosthetic fitting much less difficult and the gait more steady. The additional reason for fusing the femur parallel to the floor and perpendicular to the coronal plane, in line with the triradiate epiphysis, is that in this position (Fig. 2), when the patient's anatomic knee extends the effect is that of a flexing hip and when the knee flexes the effect is that of an extending hip. The patient's highly placed knee then maintains motion, although it is converted into the flexion and extension range expected from the hip.

The fusion also provides the option of doing a rotationplasty on the tibia so the ankle can act as a knee, thereby allowing the patient effectively to have a below-knee-amputation prosthesis. This would be the ideal situation, but orthopaedic surgeons are aware of the lack of acceptance of the van Nes procedure, particularly in females. They dislike the bizarre appearance of the rotationplasty and, more scientifically, there is currently some uncertainty as to whether the flexion and extension mechanisms of the ex-ankle are actively functioning as a new knee. Nevertheless, the gait does seem to be better than that achieved with a Syme's amputation and an above-knee prosthesis.

The Surgical Technique

It should be accepted from the start that the surgical approach to this procedure is a great adventure in the abnormalities of surgical anatomy; ie, nothing was put together in a normal fashion. The Smith-Peterson approach is used along the iliac crest to the anteroinferior spine and extended distally and laterally. The iliac apophysis is split, and the origins of the gluteus medius and tensor fascia lata muscles are reflected subperiostally from the

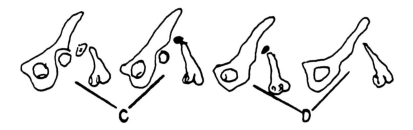

Fig. 1 *Aitken class C short femur and significant dysplasia of the acetabulum with no shaft/hip joint continuity. Aitken class D with a shortened femur and absent femoral head and acetabulum.*

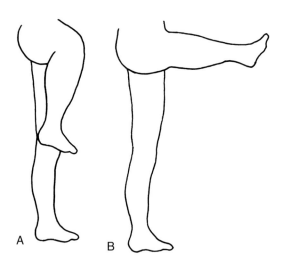

Fig. 2 *Range of motion of new knee/hip after fusion of femur to acetabulum parallel to the floor and perpendicular to the coronal plane.* **A,** *The knee in flexion functions as a hip extending.* **B,** *The knee in extension functions as a hip flexing. (Reproduced with permission from Steel HH, Lin PS, Betz RR, Kalamchi A, Clancy M: Iliofemoral fusion for proximal femoral focal deficiency. J Bone Joint Surg 1987;65A:837–842.)*

lateral wall of the ilium. A dissection is further carried through the available identifiable planes to the level of the acetabulum and to the proximal femur. Retract the muscles necessary to get complete exposure of both the acetabulum and the proximal femur, and protect neurovascular structures. The area of the dysplastic hip can sometimes be identified, but intraoperative radiography certainly is recommended. The atrophic proximal part of the femur and acetabulum are cleaned of soft tissue and decorticated to bleeding bone. The proximal end of the femur is then plugged into the pelvis at the acetabular level, parallel to the floor and perpendicular to the coronal plane, and affixed there with screws or pins. The fascia and muscles are approximated to as normal a position as possible. The skin is closed, and the patient is placed in a hip spica until there is evidence of osseous union.

It became evident, as the procedure was developed, that the new femur/knee joint should be no further in front of the symphysis pubis than 2 cm. This problem was solved by shortening the femur so that it protruded no further than 2 cm and, if considerable growth was left in the distal femoral epiphysis, closing it at the time of hip fusion. Initially, these steps were taken with some temerity because of apprehension that if the distal femoral epiphysis was closed the distal femoral condyle would not grow and, therefore, its relation with the tibia would be distorted. This was not the case because of the appositional bone growth that remained in the cartilaginous cover of the femoral condyle. Therefore, the best case scenario was realized when femoral growth was stopped at the time of fusion. If this is not done, the femur grows into abduction and extension, and osteotomy is required to restore it to its more functional position perpendicular to the coronal plane.

Materials

Eight patients in the Shriners Hospital system had femoral fusion for Aitken class C and D deficiencies. The records on two of these are irretrievable. Sixteen other patients were found who have had the procedure in various children's centers throughout the United States. Records have been made available on all patients with at least a 10-year follow-up, and the oldest patient in the series is now 25 years of age and 23 years post iliofemoral fusion, distal femoral epiphysiodesis, and a Syme's amputation. The pool is not very large, but several conclusions are warranted from clinical evaluation and radiographs where possible, and chart review where patients could not be evaluated personally.

All patients had a solid bony fusion of their femur to the acetabulum on the first operation and none of the 22 patients, at skeletal maturity, had the fusion taken down or revised to an arthroplasty. Ten of the patients, in whom the femur was fused to the acetabulum parallel to the floor and perpendicular to the coronal plane and the distal femoral epiphysis was closed during the same operation, had no further procedures done at the hip/knee level. Eight patients had either femoral shortening or osteotomy to correct unacceptable angulation, and four children underwent distal femoral epiphysiodesis as a secondary procedure.

Ten children underwent hip fusion between the ages of 1 1/2 and 3 years. Twelve patients had hip fusion between the ages of 5 and 7 years. Five of the children fused between 1 1/2 and 3 years had a van Nes rotationplasty done between age 7 and 8 years, and three of these patients, who were rotated at age 7 years, required a revision because of external rotatory drift of the foot. The other five patients had a Syme's amputation. Four of these patients required no revisions for either the Syme's or the hip procedure. Two patients who had a Syme's amputation in the 1 1/2 to 3 year period, required tibiofibular shortening because at the end of growth, the prosthetic knee was 10 to 12 cm below the contralateral knee.

At the end of growth, two patients were dissatisfied with the appearance of the backward placed foot from their van Nes rotationplasty and were converted to a Syme's amputation. One patient in the van Nes series had removal of all the toenails for persistent and recurrent onychocryptosis.

Overall, the 22 patients were all happy with their hip and were interested in no further revision or change. Two patients felt that their knees were not at the correct level and would have been more pleased had this not resulted, but they were not interested in surgical intervention to alleviate the situation. Only two of the 22 were felt to have a Trendelenburg gait. The etiology of this was obscure because the hip was stable and the knee was not unstable. Both of these patients had a Syme's amputation and it was believed that, perhaps, the pseudo-Trendelenburg gait was the result of pistoning in the socket.

Conclusion

I have reviewed the results of an iliofemoral fusion with the femur parallel to the floor and have found good functional results that last into adulthood. The Trendelenburg gait is eliminated in almost all patients and joint motion is maintained. Certain technical details are important in obtaining a good result. The femoral condyles should not protrude more than 2 cm anterior to the symphesis pubis. The distal femoral physis should be fused at the initial procedure to prevent growth that displaces the extremity anterior to the weightbearing axis.

The procedure works well with either a Syme's amputation or a van Nes rotationplasty. There are significant functional advantages to the rotationplasty, which allows some degree of active control of the prosthetic knee with proprioceptive feedback. Gradual derotation may occur and repeated rotationplasty may be necessary. The appearance of the rotated foot is a significant problem for some patients, and two patients requested and had later amputations of the backward foot. These two patients noted no functional loss after amputation. The decision for rotation or amputation is complex and should be discussed at length with patients and parents.

Reference

1. Steel HH, Lin PS, Betz RR, Kalamchi A, Clancy M: Iliofemoral fusion for proximal femoral focal deficiency. *J Bone Joint Surg* 1987;69A:837–843.

Chapter 10

Rotationplasty With Hip Stabilization in Congenital Femoral Deficiency

Kenneth L.B. Brown, MD, MSc, FRCSC

Introduction

Conventional treatment for severe types of congenital femoral deficiency is Syme's amputation of the foot when the patient begins to stand. When older, the patient usually has a knee fusion to allow elimination of the knee flexion contracture and produce a longer lever arm to facilitate prosthetic fitting. The patient then functions as an above-knee amputee and often has an unsightly gait because of pistoning of the unstable proximal femur.

van Nes[1] described a rotationplasty whereby the leg is rotated so that the foot lies 180° posterior to its normal axis. The ankle then becomes a knee joint and the patient functions as a below knee amputee. When rotation is done through the tibia in a young child, derotation often occurs.[2-5] Absence of hip stability is not addressed by this procedure.

This is a report of a patient who underwent a new form of rotationplasty 12 months ago. The proximal, abnormal part of the femur was resected along with some thigh muscles. The limb was completely amputated except for the femoral vessels and sciatic nerve. The limb was then rotated externally 180° and the remaining distal femur was fused to the ilium so that the knee functions as a uniplanar hip joint while the rotated ankle functions as a knee joint. The normal lower leg anatomy was not disturbed.

Case Report

A 16-year-old boy recently moved from India, where he was born with a short and externally rotated right lower extremity. He was in good health and had no prior operations, injuries, or infections in his extremity. The patient began to walk independently at 16 months of age. In India, an attempt was made to fit a prosthesis but he could not tolerate its weight. The patient developed a gait whereby he walked with the externally rotated leg in extreme equinus and he shifted his body laterally to be able to touch the floor. The gait was very unsightly, and he was able to walk only two to three blocks before tiring. The lower limbs measured 87.5 cm on the left and 63 cm on the right, resulting in a 24.5-cm discrepancy. Two centimeters of the discrepancy were in the tibia. The foot was at the level of the proximal calf of the normal leg.

The affected limb was externally rotated with a shortened funnel shaped thigh and a relatively normal lower leg, foot, and ankle (Fig. 1, *A* and *B*). Examination of the hips revealed a painless and noncrepitant range of motion. The right hip had a 25° flexion deformity with further flexion to 95°. There was no gross telescoping of the right hip. There was no flexion contracture of the knee, but it was moderately unstable in the mediolateral and anteroposterior planes. The ankle had a somewhat decreased range of motion, not quite reaching the neutral position in maximum extension. There was a slight decrease in strength in the right quadriceps. Ankle dorsiflexors and plantarflexors were strong (grade 5/5). Multiple radiographic views of the pelvis, foot, and ankle revealed a congenital femoral deficiency (Fig. 1, *C*). There was a mild hypoplasia of the knee, fibular deficiency, and a ball-and-socket ankle.

After discussion of the surgical options including Boyd amputation or limb lengthening, the patient opted for an amputation-reimplantation rotationplasty and iliofemoral fusion. Both lower extremities were draped free to aid in determining the position of the rotated limb. A circumferential incision was made in the thigh just above the knee crease. An anterolateral longitudinal proximal extension was made perpendicular to the circumferential incision between the anterior superior iliac spine and the greater trochanter to aid exposure of the pelvis. It is important to include the superficial fascia of the thigh with the skin flaps to preserve their blood supply. The quadriceps, adductors, and hamstring muscles were transected proximally and distally, just past their musculotendinous junctions. The gastrocnemius muscle was dissected from the femur, protecting its nerve and blood supply. The femoral artery and vein were identified at the pelvic brim and followed distally to Hunter's canal. Side branches were ligated and cut to prevent kinking and tethering of the vessels after rotation. The sciatic nerve was identified and dissected distally. The proximal femur was freed and the ilium was exposed subperiosteally. The final shortening of the femur was done following fixation to the pelvis. Some of the resected bone from the femoral shaft was used as bone graft to form a bridge from the femur to the pelvis. The leg was rotated externally 180° and the leg pushed as far proximal as possible for reattachment. A longitudinal incision was made perpendicular and distal to the incision on the medial aspect of the leg (former lateral anatomic aspect of the leg) to facilitate attachment of the femoral condyle to the pelvis. A sterile Doppler pulsimeter was useful to monitor the circulation in the foot of the rotated leg. As much of the thigh musculature as necessary was removed so that there was no obstruction to the blood flow to the rotated leg. If there is poor circulation, the leg can be derotated for a few minutes to reestablish flow and ensure that no kinking of the vessels occurs. Fixation was made with screws. An oval-shaped window was cut into the ilium, to pass the femoral shaft through to aid stabilization. The femoral shaft was notched to allow the femur to lie in a more direct vertical position.

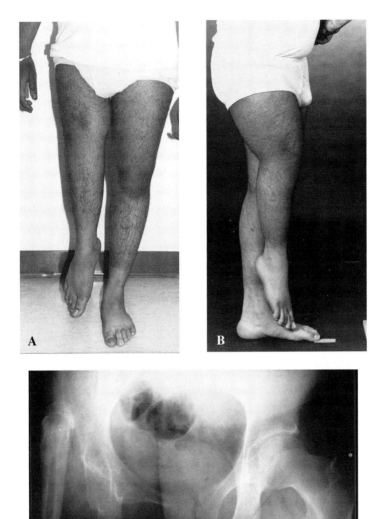

Fig. 1 A, *Frontal photograph of a 16-year-old boy with congenital femoral deficiency.* **B,** *Lateral view showing the marked shortening of the limb and a relatively normal foot.* **C,** *Radiographic appearance of the affected right hip. There is poor acetabular development.*

The rotated leg was attached in neutral to slight abduction and neutral to slight external rotation. An intraoperative radiograph was done to confirm

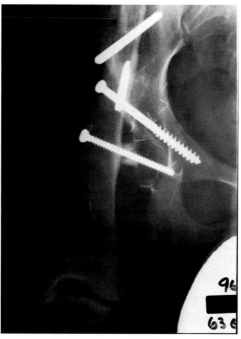

Fig. 2 *The radiographic appearance after surgery shows the position of the rotated limb. An oval has been made in the ilium to allow the residual femoral shaft to fit through for added stability. The oval shape allows the femoral segment to be moved in any direction prior to fixation. The internal fixation was supplemented by an external fixator from the pelvis to the tibia. The femur could not be attached more proximally because of the very thick layer of subcutanous fat that impeded migration.*

the position of the limb. The medial hamstrings were attached to the anterior lateral muscles of the rotated leg. The gastrocnemius muscle bellies were attached to the iliopsoas, rectus femoris, and sartorius stumps on the pelvic side of the incision. The quadriceps tendon was attached to the remaining stumps of hamstring muscles. The redundant vessels and sciatic nerve were gently coiled beneath the muscles with a special note taken of their position should further surgery become necessary. Excess skin and subcutaneous soft tissues were trimmed to allow closure of the wound. An external fixator from the pelvis to the tibia was used to supplement the internal fixation.

The patient was discharged from the hospital 9 days after surgery. He developed a deep wound infection that grew Enterobacter species. Three surgical debridements were required at 12, 18, and 20 days after the original surgery to control the infection. After the third debridement, the wound was closed, the external fixator removed, and a hip spica applied. The cast was removed at 8 weeks and range-of-motion exercises were instituted after radiographs showed adequate healing (Fig. 2). The patient received his pros-

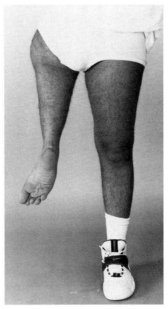
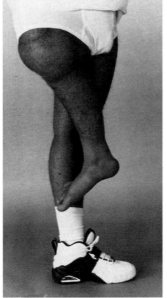
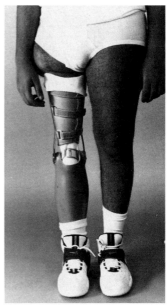
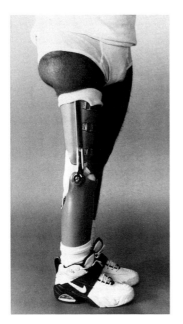
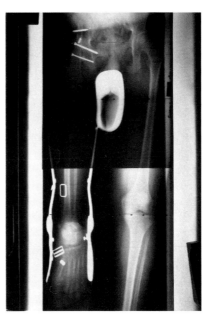

Fig. 3 Top left, A frontal photograph following rotationplasty showing the position of the limb. ***Top center,*** The lateral view of the rotated leg. The anatomic knee has become the hip and the anatomic ankle is the knee. ***Top right,*** A frontal view of the patient wearing his prosthesis. ***Bottom left,*** A lateral photograph of the patient standing in his prosthesis. ***Bottom right,*** A standing radiograph from hip to ankle showing the alignment of the rotated limb in the prosthesis.

thesis and began partial to full weightbearing as tolerated 10 weeks follow-ing surgery. Examination of the patient 7 months following surgery showed a good alignment of the rotated limb (Fig. 3). The range of hip motion was 90° passive and 60° active flexion. The active hip flexion appeared 6 months after surgery and was still improving at review. The ankle range of motion before surgery was maintained because free active motion was started imme-diately following rotationplasty.

Discussion

Borggreve[6] was the first to describe rotationplasty in 1929 when he operat-ed on a 12-year-old girl with tuberculosis. Recently, this type of rotation-plasty has been used for limb reconstruction in patients following resection of malignant tumors of the distal femur,[7-10] proximal tibia,[11] and proximal femur.[12] van Nes[1] was the first to describe rotationplasty for patients with congenital femoral deficiency. In this procedure, the tibia is cut and the muscles are rotated with the bone. More recently, other authors have described the results of this procedure,[2,4,13,14] including the problem of grad-ual derotation of the tibia. As the leg derotates, the foot is pointed to the side; therefore, the plane of axis is wrong for good function as a below-knee amputee. The exteme rotation can weaken ankle and foot flexion and exten-sion. Some of these problems can be eliminated when rotation takes place during knee fusion, although tibial rotation is still necessary to complete rotation in many cases. Despite these drawbacks, patients with a van Nes rotationplasty have several functional benefits compared to those with a Syme's amputation.[2,9,15] However, even when successful, this procedure does not address the problem of the unstable hip. In 1987, Steel and asso-ciates[5] described a procedure in four patients with Aitken class C and D congenital femoral deficiency in which the distal femur was fused to the pelvis in 90° of flexion without rotation.

Follow-up of the four patients with the amputation-reimplantation rota-tionplasty is still relatively short.[16] This rotationplasty with hip stabilization does improve the gait of patients because of their stable hip and a strong ankle and foot flexion and extension that allow them to function as below-knee amputees. Further follow-up is needed to determine the long-term effects of the arthrodesis and rotation on the anatomic knee.

References

1. van Nes CP: Rotation-plasty for congenital defects of the femur: Making use of the ankle of the shortened limb to control the knee joint of a prosthesis. *J Bone Joint Surg* 1950;32B:12–16.
2. Fowler E, Zernicke R, Setoguchi Y, Oppenheim W: Energy expenditure during walking by children who have proximal femoral focal deficiency. *J Bone Joint Surg* 1996;78A:1857–1862.
3. Friscia DA, Moseley CF, Oppenheim WL: Rotational osteotomy for proximal femoral focal deficiency. *J Bone Joint Surg* 1989;71A:1386–1392.

4. Kostuik JP, Gillespie R, Hall JE, Hubbard S: Van Nes rotational osteotomy for treatment of proximal femoral focal deficiency and congenital short femur. *J Bone Joint Surg* 1975;57A:1039–1046.

5. Steel HH, Lin PS, Betz RR, Kalamchi A, Clancy M: Iliofemoral fusion for proximal femoral focal deficiency. *J Bone Joint Surg* 1987;69A:837–843.

6. Borggreve J: Kniegelenksersatz durch das in der Beinlängsachse um 180° gedrehte Fussgelenk. *Arch f Orthop* 1930;28:175–178.

7. Kotz R, Salzer M: Rotation-plasty for childhood osteosarcoma of the distal part of the femur. *J Bone Joint Surg* 1982;64A:959–969.

8. Jacobs PA: Limb salvage and rotationplasty for osteosarcoma in children. *Clin Orthop* 1984;188:217–222.

9. Cammisa FP Jr, Glasser DB, Otis JC, Kroll MA, Lane JM, Healey JH: The Van Nes tibial rotationplasty: A functionally viable reconstructive procedure in children who have a tumor of the distal end of the femur. *J Bone Joint Surg* 1990;72A:1541–1547.

10. Gottsauner-Wolf F, Kotz R, Knahr K, Kristen H, Ritschl P, Salzer M: Rotationplasty for limb salvage in the treatment of malignant tumors at the knee: A follow-up study of seventy patients. *J Bone Joint Surg* 1991;73A:1365–1375.

11. de Bari A, Krajbich JI, Langer F, Hamilton EL, Hubbard S: Modified Van Nes rotationplasty for osteosarcoma of the proximal tibia in children. *J Bone Joint Surg* 1990;72B:1065–1069.

12. Winkelmann WW: Hip rotationplasty for malignant tumors of the proximal part of the femur. *J Bone Joint Surg* 1986;68A:362–369.

13. Kritter AE: Tibial rotation-plasty for proximal femoral focal deficiency. *J Bone Joint Surg* 1977;59A:927–934.

14. Torode IP, Gillespie R: Rotationplasty of the lower limb for congenital defects of the femur. *J Bone Joint Surg* 1983;65B:569–573.

15. Alman BA, Krajbich JI, Hubbard S: Proximal femoral focal deficiency: Results of rotationplasty and Syme amputation. *J Bone Joint Surg* 1995;77A:1876–1882.

16. Brown KLB: Amputation-reimplantation rotationplasty and iliofemoral arthrodesis for patients with severe congenital femoral deficiency. *J Bone Joint Surg,* in press.

Consensus

Iliofemoral Stabilization in Femoral Deficiency

The abductor-extensor lurch in patients with femoral deficiency is a significant functional and cosmetic problem. Reconstructive osteotomies of the upper femur should be directed toward restoring the abductor mechanics, and they are appropriate when a reasonable anatomic reconstruction is feasible. These procedures should be done as early as ossification of the fragments permits.

Other stabilization procedures that have been proposed to improve the abductor-extensor lurch are Steel's iliofemoral fusion, Brown's iliofemoral fusion and rotationplasty, and Ilizarov's pelvic support osteotomy. Because little long-term follow-up is available, outcome studies are needed to determine complications and patient function following each of these procedures.

Chapter 11

Lengthening Reconstruction Surgery for Congenital Femoral Deficiency

Dror Paley, MD, FRCSC

Introduction

Congenital femoral deficiency (CFD) is a spectrum of severity of femoral deficiency and deformity. Deficiency implies a lack of integrity, stability, and mobility of the hip and knee joints. Deformity refers to malorientation, malrotation, and soft-tissue contractures of the hip and knee. Both deficiencies and deformities are present at birth, nonprogressive, and of variable degree.

Classification

Existing classifications of congenital short femur and proximal femoral focal deficiency are descriptive but are not helpful in determining treatment. A recent longitudinal follow-up of different classification systems[1] showed that they were inaccurate in predicting the final femoral morphology based on the initial radiograph. Furthermore, previous classification systems were designed with prosthetic replacement surgery (eg, Syme's amputation or rotationplasty) in mind rather than lengthening reconstruction surgery (equalization of limb length with realignment of lower limb and preservation of joints). My classification system (Fig. 1) is based on factors that influence lengthening reconstruction of the congenital short femur.

In type 1, there is an intact femur with mobile hip and knee; ossification of the proximal femur is normal in 1a and delayed in 1b. In type 2, there is a mobile pseudarthrosis with a mobile knee; the femoral head is mobile in the acetabulum in 2a and absent or stiff in the acetabulum in 2b. Type 3 is a diaphyseal deficiency of the femur with knee motion > 45° in 3a and < 45° in 3b.

Knee joint mobility/deficiency, rather than hip joint mobility/deficiency, is the most important factor determining functional outcome and reconstructability of CFD. Previous classifications (such as the Aitken classification) emphasize the extent of hip deficiency. The extent of hip deficiency is used as a guideline to indications for amputation and prosthetic fitting despite the fact that amputation does not improve hip function. Types 1 and 2 are the most reconstructable. A wide spectrum of hip and knee dysplasia and deformity exists in type 1 cases. Because this is the type most amenable to lengthening, it merits a subclassification according to factors that require

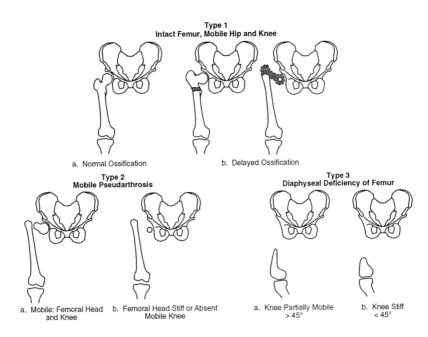

Fig. 1 *Paley classification of congenital short femur syndrome, types 1-3.*

correction before lengthening can be carried out. These factors affect the age at which the lengthening process can begin because multiple corrections will delay the first lengthening. They also affect the number of surgeries that are required prior to starting lengthening and, therefore, may affect the decision of reconstruction versus amputation or rotationplasty.

Type 1 is subclassified as follows: 0, ready for surgery, no factors to correct before lengthening; 1, one factor to correct before lengthening; 2, two factors to correct before lengthening; 3, three factors to correct before lengthening; and so on. (Factors requiring correction prior to lengthening include neck shaft angle < 90° with or without delayed ossification of the proximal femur, center edge angle < 20°, subluxating patella, and/or dislocating knee.)

Neck shaft angle < 90° is corrected by proximal femoral osteotomy; center edge angle < 20° is corrected by pelvic osteotomy. Subluxating patella and/or dislocating knee are corrected by soft-tissue reconstruction.

The strategy of management of all type 1 cases is to convert type 1b into type 1a, and types 1a-1 or worse into 1a-0. Type 1a-0 cases can be treated by one or more lengthenings and/or epiphysiodesis or femoral shortening procedures.

The strategy of management for type 2 cases is to first determine the presence of a mobile pseudarthrosis or the absence of a femoral head. It is important to differentiate between type 1b cases and type 2 cases. In type

2a cases where there is mobility between the femoral head and the acetabulum and between the femoral shaft and the femoral head, union of the pseudarthrosis is an initial goal of treatment, converting type 2a to type 1a. Type 2b cases should not be converted to type 1b because the femoral head has no mobility in the acetabulum. To prevent proximal migration of the femur, the external fixator pins are extended onto the pelvis during lengthening. To stabilize the hip in type 2b cases, a valgus extension proximal femoral osteotomy (pelvic support osteotomy) is performed in conjunction with the final lengthening.

The strategy of management for type 3 cases is determined by preoperative knee and ankle joint motion. If the knee has < 45° of motion (type 3b) and the ankle has a good range of motion, a rotationplasty with prosthetic fitting should be considered. If the ankle has a poor range of motion, a Syme's amputation with prosthetic fitting is preferred. Equalization of limb length by multiple lengthenings is possible but yields the functional outcome of an arthrodesed knee. If there is > 45° of knee motion (type 3a), lengthening can be considered with all efforts made to preserve knee joint function. The goal of surgery in these cases is to convert a type 3a femur to a type 2b femur. The rest of the reconstruction is as for type 2b. This type of reconstruction, while feasible, is very complicated. Prosthetic options may be preferable to minimize the complexity of treatment.

Evaluation of the Infant With CFD

The Hip

Based on the clinical examination and the initial radiograph, the surgeon should try to determine the presence of a femoral head or a pseudarthrosis. If the femoral head is present without a mobile pseudarthrosis, the femur is considered intact. In the intact femur, the neck shaft angle should be evaluated for varus and the acetabulum for dysplasia. A pseudarthrosis, if present, should be examined under anesthesia with an arthrogram and fluoroscopy to determine if it is mobile or stiff. With a stiff pseudarthrosis, the femoral head moves with the rest of the femur; it does not with a mobile pseudarthrosis. If the pseudarthrosis is mobile, then it is important to establish if the femoral head is mobile within the acetabulum. Abduction-adduction, flexion-extension, and internal-external rotation movements under image intensification with the dye in the joint will demonstrate whether the femoral head moves in the acetabulum. The relative movement of the femoral head versus the femoral shaft to the pelvis can be compared on the abduction and adduction radiographs (Fig. 2). Push-pull stress movements with the dye in the joint also help differentiate whether a mobile pseudarthrosis is present. An unossified femoral neck appears like a pseudarthrosis but demonstrates synchronous motion of the femoral head, neck, and shaft. The presence of a well-developed acetabulum is the best clue that the femoral head is present and probably mobile. Magnetic resonance imaging (MRI) and ultrasound may

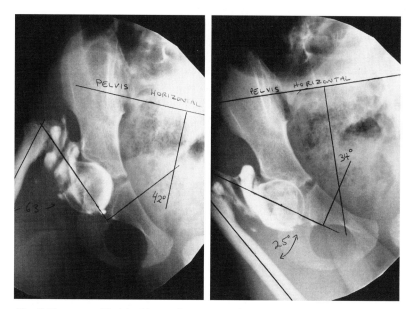

Fig. 2 *Five-year-old girl with type 2a congenital short femur. Arthrogram with abduc-*
*tion (**left**) and adduction (**right**) stress anteroposterior views of the right hip. The*
femoral head and the shaft are both seen to move relative to the acetabulum. There is
more movement between the femoral head and the femoral shaft than between the
femoral head and the acetabulum. This indicates that there is mobile pseudarthrosis
with mobility of the femoral head in the acetabulum.

be helpful but are often difficult to interpret in infants with such abnormal anatomy. The arthrogram performed by the orthopaedic surgeon remains my preferred testing modality.

It is important to examine the range of motion of the hip and identify the presence of fixed adduction, flexion, and external rotation of the hip. Fixed flexion deformity of the hip (Thomas test) should be compared to the other side in infants before walking age. There is normally some fixed flexion deformity for many months after birth. In the absence of fixed flexion deformity of the hip, there is usually an absence of hyperextension of the hip on the short side (measured prone). The Ely test is often positive, indicating a tight rectus femoris tendon. Lack of abduction is a sign of coxa vara rather than contracture or dislocation. External rotation of the limb (hip retroversion) is also typical of all grades of CFD. External rotation of the hip is best measured prone with the pelvis held flat.

The Knee

The initial evaluation of the knee is also performed clinically and radiographically. The range of motion of the knee is a critical feature. Fixed flexion deformity on the affected side greater than on a normal contralateral limb is significant. A stiff knee is rarely found except in patients with severe proximal femoral deficiency. In these patients it may be difficult to assess the range of motion of the knee because of the short, chubby thigh. Examination under anesthesia may be required together with an arthrogram. The arthrogram in patients with a stiff knee may show flattening of the femoral condyles, an absent patellofemoral pouch, and an absent patella.

Mobile knees should also be evaluated for stability of the tibiofemoral joint and tracking of the patella. The tibia may dislocate as it goes into full extension as a result of tight lateral structures (fascia lata and hamstrings), incompetent capsuloligamentous structures, and anterior deficiency of the femoral condyles. There are two patterns of subluxation or dislocation of the tibia on the femur: anterolateral and posterolateral. In the anterolateral pattern, the tibia subluxates or dislocates anteriorly and the foot rotates internally as the knee extends. In the posterolateral pattern the tibia subluxates or dislocates posteriorly and the foot rotates externally as the knee extends. Lateral patellar subluxation or dislocation is associated with both types. Lengthening with the patella laterally subluxated can lead to dislocation or further subluxation of the patella and limitation of knee motion. To identify patellar subluxation, place a thumb over the center of the intercondylar notch of the 90° flexed knee. In a normal knee the thumb will lie over the patella. With patellar subluxation, the thumb will lie medial to the patella and the intercondylar groove can be palpated.

Treatment

Type 1a: Ossified Proximal Femur, Mobile Hip and Knee

This group is the most reconstructable. Lengthening treatment in these patients should not begin until the neck shaft angle is greater than 90°, the center edge angle is greater than 20°, and there is a nonsubluxating patella and nondislocating knee. Each of these prerequisites will be examined separately.

Coxa Vara

If the neck is ossified but the neck shaft angle is less than 90°, a proximal femoral valgus, extension, internal rotation subtrochanteric osteotomy should be performed prior to lengthening. My preference is to perform this osteotomy with external fixation. The hip osteotomy should correct the varus, flexion, and external rotation deformity. If the hip osteotomy is performed with internal fixation, the hardware should be removed prior to lengthening. I prefer to use the Ilizarov device to perform the hip osteotomy to avoid a long scar and hardware removal and to increase the accuracy and magnitude of correction of a complex valgus, lateral translation, extension, and external rotation osteotomy. Following the osteotomy the patient frequently will have an abduction contracture that will stretch out with time.

For neck shaft angles < 90°, especially in infants and young children, I prefer to perform the hip osteotomy separate from the lengthening procedure (Fig. 3) because both acute valgus hip corrections and lengthening

117

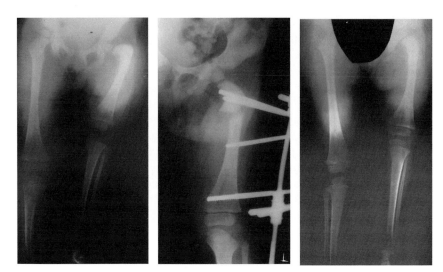

Fig. 3 Left, *Anteroposterior (AP) radiograph of a 2-year-old girl with congenital short femur and coxa vara; neck shaft angle = 80°. The proximal femoral physis is vertically inclined.* **Center,** *Acute correction osteotomy stabilized with four half pins and the Ilizarov apparatus. The correction includes internal rotation, valgus with lateral translation, and extension with posterior translation. The neck shaft angle is restored to normal on the AP view and the femoral head is now anteverted on the lateral view.* **Right,** *AP radiograph 1 year after correction. The neck shaft angle is 124° and the proximal femoral physis is more horizontally inclined.*

of the femur apply significant pressure to the hip joint. When the neck shaft angle is > 90° and/or if diaphyseal varus deformity is present, these can be corrected acutely together with lengthening of the femur (Fig. 4). Small degrees of coxa vara (neck shaft angle 110° to 120°) stabilize the hip in the face of a dysplastic acetabulum and should not be corrected prior to lengthening.

Acetabular Dysplasia

If the center edge angle is < 20°, a pelvic osteotomy should be performed to stabilize the hip before a lengthening procedure.[2] If a proximal femoral osteotomy is necessary to correct a severe hip varus, it should be performed separately prior to the pelvic osteotomy. A three-dimensional (3-D) reconstruction computed tomography (CT) scan of both hips is useful in deciding which pelvic osteotomy to perform. The inferior and posterior 3-D views are the best to assess posterior coverage. If the 3-D scan shows good coverage of the affected hip posteriorly and deficiency anterolaterally, the Millis-Hall modification of the Salter osteotomy for coverage and pelvic lengthening is performed.[3] If the 3-D scan shows decreased coverage posteriorly as a result

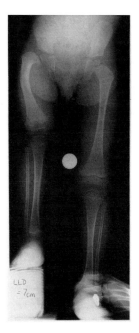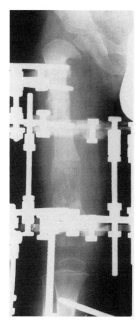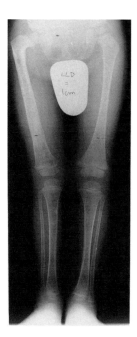

Fig. 4 Left, Two-year-old boy with congenital short femur (leg-length discrepancy = 7 cm) and coxa vara. The neck shaft angle = 95° relative to the proximal shaft of the femur. The proximal femoral physis is relatively horizontally inclined. There is a dia-physeal varus of 20°. **Center,** Treatment by proximal femoral valgus external rotation osteotomy. The proximal coxa vara was not corrected but the diaphyseal varus was corrected. The lengthening is performed through a distal femoral osteotomy. **Right,** Final anteroposterior radiograph after (6 cm) limb lengthening. The residual leg-length discrepancy is 1 cm.

of a hypoplastic posterior lip of the acetabulum, my preference is a Dega osteotomy with anterior shelf augmentation if necessary.

Dislocation of Patella or Tibia

Dislocation of the patella or tibia with flexion or extension, respectively, necessitates a stabilizing procedure prior to lengthening. Isolated anteropos-terior (AP) instability of the tibiofemoral joint without dislocation does not need to be addressed before lengthening. Isolated subluxation or dislocation of the patella should be treated before lengthening. The knee reconstruction that I developed is based on a combination of elements from the Langenskiöld,[4] MacIntosh,[5] and Grammont[6] procedures. This procedure may be performed at the same sitting as a pelvic osteotomy because both need to be in a long leg cast postoperatively.

In the Paley knee construction technique, the knee is exposed through a long S-shaped incision. The anterior margin of the fascia lata and the poste-rior margin where it blends with the intermuscular septum are incised longitudinally. The fascia lata is transected as proximally as possible and reflected distally until its insertion onto the tibia. The biceps tendon is z lengthened if needed.

In the posterolateral tibiofemoral instability pattern, if the patella is subluxated but not dislocating then a lateral release is performed by cutting the capsule laterally without cutting the synovium. The vastus lateralis tendon is released off the patella and attached to the rest of the quadriceps muscle. The patellar tendon is displaced medially by internally rotating the tibia on the femur. If the patella tracks well in this position following the releases noted above, no further patellar stabilization is required. To prevent the tibia from externally rotating on the femur (leading to subluxation of the patella), the fascia lata is routed overtop the patellar tendon and knee joint capsule to insert into the medial femoral condyle. A drill hole is placed in the femoral epiphysis from a medial stab incision. A 6-mm hole is drilled into the condyle through to the lateral side. The fascia lata is anchored on the lateral side after passing through the bony tunnel. The knee is mobilized after 6 weeks in an extension cast.

In the anterolateral tibiofemoral instability pattern, if the subluxation pattern is anterolateral, the fascia lata is looped over itself after passing under the lateral collateral ligament or the lateral capsule (these children often do not have a well defined lateral collateral ligament) and through a subperiosteal tunnel proximal to the growth plate to reattach to Gerdie's tubercle (MacIntosh[5]) (Fig. 5). This procedure tightens the tibia into external rotation, and it can make the patellar subluxation worse by lateralizing the patellar tendon insertion site. The patellar tendon insertion site can be moved medially. The patellar tendon is sharply elevated off the apophyseal cartilage and is left connected to periosteum distally. The patellar tendon can be moved medially as much as needed pivoting on the distal periosteum. The medial side of the tendon is stitched medially (Grammont and associates[6]).

If the patella tracks in a laterally subluxated position even after the lateral releases and medialization of its tendon or if the patella is dislocated to begin with, then a Langenskiöld[4]-type reconstruction is performed. The capsule is separated from the patella and synovium medially and laterally. The synovium is cut from the patella circumferentially. The quadriceps tendon is left attached to the patella proximally and the patellar tendon remains attached to the patella distally. The synovium now has a patella-sized hole in it. A longitudinal incision is made in the synovium more medially. The patella is inserted into this new hole in the synovium and the synovium is sewn to the patella circumferentially. The original synovial hole is closed laterally where the patella was removed. The capsule is stitched overtop the patella on the medial side and left open laterally. After multiple-layer wound closure the knee is put in a cylinder cast for 6 weeks followed by active and passive motion exercises.

The above hip and knee problems must all be addressed before beginning the femoral lengthening. Once they are corrected, the femur is considered a type 1a-0, which is ready for lengthening.

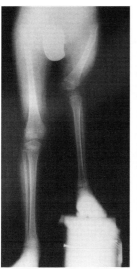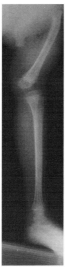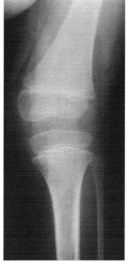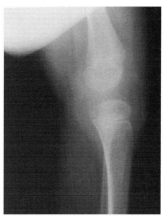

*Fig. 5 Left, Anterolateral dislocation of the knee. **Left center,** The tibia is internally rotated on the femur. **Right center,** After reconstruction; the knee is reduced and stable. **Right,** The fascia lata was looped around the lateral collateral ligament to externally rotate the tibia.*

Type 1b Femora: Delayed Ossification Proximal Femur, Mobile Hip and Knee

The natural history of the intact, unossified femoral neck is usually to eventually ossify. Radiographically, the lack of ossification is often interpreted as a pseudarthrosis. Arthrographic examination reveals that the neck and shaft move as one. The coxa vara associated with these unossified femoral necks probably contributes to the shear forces on the neck that delay its ossification. Therefore, the treatment of the delayed ossification of the femoral neck is a valgus proximal femoral osteotomy, which is performed in the manner described above for the ossified proximal femur.

One particular type of delayed ossification is a stiff nonunion line in the inter- or subtrochanteric region. There is no movement seen at this nonunion line under fluoroscopy or stress radiographs. This type of nonunion always is associated with coxa vara. It can be ignored and the rest of the treatment carried out as for the delayed ossification cases with coxa vara. One alternative treatment I have used in these cases is distraction of the pseudarthrosis to correct deformity and lengthen. Although this method works, the regenerate produced is narrow. An acute correction by osteotomy as previously described is preferable and less complication-ridden.

121

Lengthening of Type 1 Congenital Femoral Deficiency

Choice of Osteotomy Level for Lengthening of the Congenital Short Femur Distal osteotomies have the advantages of a broader cross-sectional diameter for better bone formation and lesser deforming forces from the hamstrings and adductors. Proximal osteotomies have less effect on knee range of motion, but are more prone to poor bone consolidation, and they should be reserved for the technique of lengthening over nails (Fig. 6).

Deformations that require simultaneous correction must also be considered. Derotation and coxa vara correction are performed proximally. Valgus deformity of the knee is corrected distally. If both are needed, a proximal osteotomy is performed for derotation and varus correction, and a distal osteotomy for valgus correction and lengthening (Fig. 4). If the femur is completely straight with only some rotational deformity, the osteotomy can be made in the mid-diaphysis, which has a wider cross-sectional area than the proximal femur and is not in the zone of sclerotic, poorly-healing bone.

In older children with a wider medullary canal (> 7 mm), lengthening over a nail can be performed[7] (Fig. 6). A proximal osteotomy can be used for lengthening with this technique because there is little risk of refracture with a rod in the medullary canal. Intramedullary nailing in children adds the risk of disturbance of growth of the apophysis[8] and osteonecrosis of the femoral head.[9] To avoid the latter, I use a greater trochanteric starting point and a nail with a proximal bend (eg, humeral or tibial). To avoid a coxa valga deformity, I prefer to use this technique in patients with some coxa vara. The apophyseodesis created by the nail can lead to gradual correction of the coxa vara. Fixator-only lengthening is usually used for the first lengthening. Lengthening over a nail is usually the method chosen for the second lengthening if the anatomic dimensions and deformities mentioned above permit.

External Rotation Deformity Most congenital short femora have an external rotation deformity (Figs. 3 and 4). This deformity should not be corrected through a distal femoral osteotomy for fear of subluxation of the patella. If the derotation osteotomy is performed proximally (subtrochanteric), the entire quadriceps mass attached to the shaft of the femur rotates medially, decreasing the Q angle.

Distal Femoral Valgus Deformity The distal femur usually has a nonprogressive valgus deformity resulting from hypoplasia of the lateral femoral condyle. The center of rotation of angulation of this valgus deformity is at the level of the knee joint line. Therefore, any osteotomy to correct the valgus in the supracondylar region needs to angulate into varus and translate laterally to avoid creating a secondary translational deformity. This deformity does not need to be corrected before lengthening but should be corrected at the time of the lengthening. The fascia lata should be transected or lengthened at the time of correction to help prevent recurrence, increased pressure on the lateral compartment of the knee, knee subluxation during lengthening, and loss of knee motion.

Soft-Tissue Releases for Lengthening of the Congenitally Short Femur Patients with congenitally short femur may have a fixed flexion deformity of the hip or knee, have an increased popliteal angle without fixed deformity, a

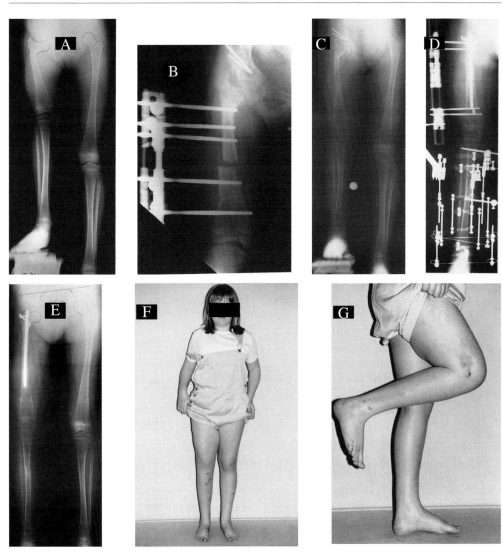

Fig. 6 A, *Preoperative radiograph of 8-year-old girl with congenital short femur with a leg-length discrepancy of 14.5 cm. Predicted leg-length discrepancy at skeletal maturity is 20.8 cm.* **B,** *Due to the dysplastic acetabulum a Millis-Hall modification of the Salter osteotomy was performed prior to lengthening. This procedure gained 2.5 cm of length. At age 9 she underwent her first lengthening and acute derotation through a mid-diaphyseal osteotomy using the Orthofix™ apparatus. The apparatus was not extended across the knee because her knee joint was noted to be stable preoperatively. Note the well-developed tibial spines that imply the presence of cruciate ligaments.* **C,** *Final radiograph following the first lengthening. Note the overgrown greater trochanter and the coxa vara.* **D,** *At age 12 she underwent simultaneous lengthening of her femur and tibia. The femur was lengthened over a nail, and the femur and tibia frame were linked with hinges.* **E,** *Her final result following two lengthenings demonstrates near equalization of limb length (limb-length discrepancy = 1.9 cm) at bone and chronologic age 14. Total length gain = 2.5 cm (pelvis) + 4 cm (femur) + 8 cm (femur) + 5 cm (tibia) = 19.5 cm. The remaining leg-length difference will be made up by valgus osteotomy of the coxa vara which will acutely lengthen the leg by about 2 cm.* **F and G,** *Knee extension and flexion range of motion 3 months after removal of apparatus.*

positive Ely test, and a thick, tight fascia lata. Soft-tissue releases are essential in conjunction with lengthening to prevent subluxation and stiffness of the knee and hip. I always release the rectus femoris tendon at its origin and the fascia lata distally. Through the same distal incision, the anterior fascia of the thigh and the lateral hamstring tendinous portion are cut, leaving the underlying muscle in continuity. If there is a popliteal angle > 10°, a separate incision is made to fractionally lengthen the semimembranosus and gracilis tendons. The semitendinosis tendon is transected. The adductor muscles are also released. For distal femoral lengthenings, a percutaneous release is sufficient. For proximal femoral lengthenings, I prefer an open more extensive adductor release.

Botulinum toxin injected at the time of surgery is useful to temporarily weaken or paralyze some of the hamstrings and adductors and the rectus femoris. It seems to reduce muscle spasm and pain and may increase knee range of motion.

The timing of soft-tissue release may be important. Although I usually perform the release at the time of application of fixator and lengthening osteotomy, I have recently observed that in a few cases where the soft-tissue release was performed as a planned second-stage procedure (4 to 6 weeks after the lengthening began), I was able to achieve greater lengthening because the knee motion was better maintained for a longer period of time. Delayed soft-tissue release cuts the soft tissues when they are under tension and prevents them from healing before the distraction is over.

Knee Instability Consideration Almost all congenitally short femurs can be assumed to have hypoplastic or absent cruciate ligaments with mild to moderate anteroposterior (AP) instability. Some also have mediolateral (ML) and torsional instability. Nevertheless, the knee tracks normally preoperatively and there is no indication to do a ligamentous reconstruction in most cases. The significance of the knee instability to lengthening is the tendency to subluxation of the knee with lengthening (Fig. 6). Knee subluxation with lengthening is usually posterior or posterior plus external rotation, but can also be anterior. Posterior subluxation can only occur with knee flexion. Therefore, to prevent posterior subluxation some people recommend splinting the knee in extension throughout the distraction phase.[10] Splinting promotes knees stiffness while protecting the knee from subluxation. I prefer to protect the knee by extending the fixation to the tibia with hinges. The hinges permit knee motion while preventing posterior as well as anterior subluxation. Fixation can be extended easily with the Ilizarov circular fixator but not as readily with the monolateral fixators.

A less common knee instability is anterior dislocation of the tibia on the femur (Fig. 5). This type of dislocation occurs as the knee goes into extension. It is important to document at which angle of flexion the knee relocates (conversely at which angle short of full extension the knee dislocates). The dislocation is caused by an anterior deficiency of the distal femur (the lateral radiograph of the knee shows a lack of the anterior protruberance of the femoral condyles). One treatment of this instability is extension osteotomy of the knee. The distal femur is extended by the number of degrees of flexion required to relocate the knee, but I prefer the soft-tissue reconstruction procedures described, because knee extension osteotomy leads to loss of knee flexion.

Rehabilitation and Follow-up During Lengthening

Femoral lengthening requires close follow-up and intensive rehabilitation in order to identify problems and maintain a functional extremity. Follow-up is usually every 2 weeks for radiographic and clinical assessment. Clinically the patient is assessed for hip and knee range of motion, knee subluxation, nerve function, and pin-site problems. The distraction gap length, regenerate bone quality, limb alignment, and joint location are assessed radiographically.

Knee flexion should be maintained at > 45°. If knee flexion is 40° or less, the lengthening should be stopped and the knee rehabilitated more. If after a few days knee flexion > 45° is regained, lengthening may resume. Never sacrifice function for length; an additional lengthening can provide more length but surgeons cannot recreate a knee joint. A flexion contracture may develop during lengthening. To prevent this, a knee-extension bar may be used at night and for 1 or 2 hours during the day. A fixed flexion deformity of the knee places it at risk of posterior subluxation. Subluxation of the knee can be suspected clinically based on a change in shape of the front of the tibia relative to the kneecap. Posterior subluxation of the tibia presents with a very prominent kneecap and a depression of the tibia relative to the kneecap (skihill sign). Extension of the external fixation across the knee with hinges prevents posterior subluxation.[11,12]

Hip motion may become more limited with lengthening. Adduction and flexion contractures are the most significant because they lead to hip subluxation and dislocation. Rerelease of the adductors and the rectus, sartorius, and the tensor fascia lata during lengthening may need to be considered to allow further lengthening.

The deep peroneal nerve is the nerve at greatest risk with femoral lengthening. Pain referred to the anterior distal leg or dorsum of the foot should be considered peroneal nerve related until proven otherwise. Hyper- or hypoesthesia in the distribution of the peroneal nerve or weakness of the extensor hallucis longus muscle are corroborative evidence of nerve entrapment. A nerve conduction study (my preference is near nerve conduction using very fine needle technique at the level of the fibular neck) may show evidence of nerve injury. Quantitative sensory testing, if available, is the most sensitive test to assess for nerve involvement. With quantitative sensory evidence and sensory signs only, the distraction is slowed to see if the referred pain goes away. If the referred pain does not dissipate or if motor signs or positive nerve conduction evidence of nerve injury are present, nerve decompression at the neck of the fibula is carried out. Lengthening may continue after the decompression at 0.75 or 0.5 mm/day.

Hypotrophic regenerate formation requires slowing of the distraction rate. Overabundant bone formation may lead to premature consolidation and requires increasing the distraction rate for a few days. A mismatch between the increase in the distraction gap from one visit to the next and the number of millimeters of distraction carried out in the same time period is a sign of an impending premature consolidation. Radiographs are also used to assess joint location. A break in Shenton's line or increased medial-lateral head-teardrop distance indicates subluxation of the hip. In the knee, posterior or anterior subluxation can be monitored on the lateral full knee extension radiograph.[12] Limb-length equalization should be based on full-length standing radiographs. If there is a knee flexion deformity, a scanogram with the knees equally flexed and the hip, knee, and ankle equally positioned to the radiographic plate is used instead. Limb alignment is assessed for femur and tibia separately and in combination. The joint orientation of the knee should be measured separately using the malalignment test.[13] Axial deviation from lengthening (procurvatum and valgus for distal femoral lengthening and procurvatum and varus for proximal lengthening) is identified and corrected at the end of the distraction phase when the regenerate bone is still malleable. When there is malalignment of the femur and tibia, the femoral malalignment is corrected to a normal distal femoral joint orientation. The femur is not over- or undercorrected to compensate for the tibial deformity. The tibia should be corrected separately either during the same or at a later treatment.

Physical therapy starts within 1 or 2 days from surgery and should continue daily throughout the distraction and consolidation phase. It stops briefly after removal of the external fixator to avoid a fracture through the regenerate bone or a pin hole. Once the bone is strong enough, it continues. During the distraction phase, one to two formal sessions each day (45 to 60 minutes each) with a therapist are required. In addition, at least two home sessions per day (30 minutes each) are recommended. The more therapy the better the potential functional result and the faster the rehabilitation following removal. Inpatient rehabilitation is often the only practical method of achieving this quantity of therapy. The philosophy of therapy for lengthening is very different than for other orthopaedic surgical procedures. Following most orthopaedic procedures the patient is at his or her worst after surgery and gradually recovers. One week following surgery, lengthening patients are at their best. Thereafter, because of the distraction, the muscles become tighter and range of motion of joints more limited. It is not until the consolidation phase that the usual pattern of rehabilitation and recovery occurs. The lengthening surgery can be thought of as ending at the end of the distraction phase: a surgical procedure that can be measured in months rather than hours. In the absence of a therapy program, I will not even consider femoral lengthening.

The majority of the therapy time should be spent obtaining knee flexion and maintaining knee extension. Passive exercises are the most important during the distraction phase and passive plus active exercises during the consolidation phase. Hip abduction and extension are the two important hip exercises. Strengthening exercises should be focused on the hip abductors and the quadriceps. Electric muscle stimulation is used on the quadriceps. Upper extremity strengthening is helpful for use of walking aids and transfers. Weightbearing is encouraged and allowed as tolerated.

Type 2a Femora: Femoral Head Mobile in Acetabulum, Mobile Pseudarthrosis and Knee

The goal of treatment in this group is to convert the femur into a type 1. This requires obtaining union of the pseudarthrosis. To classify this group into type 2a it is necessary to do an arthrogram and fluoroscopic examination to demonstrate differential motion of the mobile nonunion and mobile femoral head.

In order to obtain union of the head to the femur it is necessary to open the pseudarthrosis, bone graft it, and reorient it. A proximal femur valgus osteotomy is performed to reorient the nonunion and the coxa vara. If the femur is proximally migrated, it may be necessary to pull down the femur relative to the pelvis as a first stage. If this is not possible acutely, it should be done gradually. It is important to extend the fixation to the pelvis in order to neutralize the forces at the pseudarthrosis site. Once the pseudarthrosis is united the rest of the treatment is as per type 1.

Type 2b Femora: Femoral Head Stiff or Absent in Acetabulum, Mobile Pseudarthrosis and Knee

If the femoral head is stiff or absent but the knee is mobile, reconstruction can still be performed combined with lengthening. Motion of the hip in these patients comes from the mobile pseudarthrosis. The proximal femoral shaft should not be fixed to the femoral head because this will result in a stiff hip. To preserve hip motion but create stability for lengthening and gait, the proximal femur should be osteotomized into valgus under the femoral head and acetabulum (pelvic support osteotomy) between 10 and 16 years of age (Fig. 7).

Prior to this age, the femur can be lengthened once or twice. Frequently the femur is so short that it cannot be lengthened together with hinging of the knee. In these cases, the knee can be locked in extension for the first lengthening. Either femoral lengthening alone or simultaneous femur and tibial lengthening may be performed. Fixation must extend to the pelvis to prevent proximal migration of the femur.

If there is a major deficiency of the proximal femoral diaphysis, the first lengthening is performed to grow the femoral shaft. Obviously the more deficient the proximal femur the more complicated the lengthening program becomes. The risk of losing knee motion in this group is very high. Knee flexion deformity is very common in this group. An arthrogram should be done to determine if the femoral condyles are round. If the femoral condyles are round, the knee can be extended by soft-tissue releases and distraction. If the femoral condyles are flat, the knee should be extended by osteotomy. As the degree of deficiency increases, the appeal of a prosthetic option of treatment increases. This issue will be addressed later.

Type 3a: Diaphyseal Deficiency of Femur, Knee Motion > 45°

Deficiency of the proximal femur with absent femoral head, greater trochanter, and proximal femoral metaphysis results in a mobile pseudarthrosis and a very short femoral remnant. Some cases have a mobile knee with > 45°

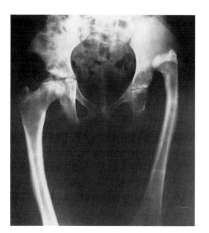
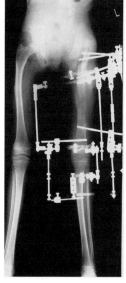
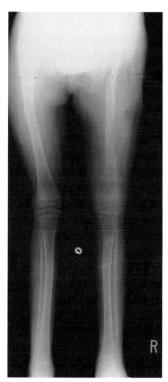

Fig. 7 Left, *Radiograph of a 12-year-old girl with type 2b congenital short femur. There is no acetabu-lum or femoral head and the proximal femur is proximally dislocated.* **Center,** *A valgus-extension proxi-mal femoral pelvic support osteotomy was peformed with distal femoral varus realignment. No fixation to the pelvis was used during the 13-cm femoral lengthening. Note that fixation is extended with hinges across the knee to the tibia.* **Right,** *Final standing anteroposterior radiograph shortly after removal of the fixator.*

of motion, usually with a 45° knee flexion deformity. The treatment option in these cases includes lengthening or prosthetic reconstruction (van Nes or Syme's). To lengthen a type 3a femur deficiency, the femur should be con-verted to a type 2b. After that, treatment is as described for type 2b. The knee flexion deformity in these cases can be addressed by extension osteotomy of the distal femur. Because of the severe discrepancy from this type of defi-ciency, a combined femur and tibia lengthening can be carried out. The frame is extended across the knee joint without hinges. The fixator is also extended across the hip to the pelvis to prevent proximal migration of the femur.

Type 3b Femora: Diaphyseal Deficiency, Knee Motion < 45°

Reduction of knee motion to < 45° is due to malformation of the lower end of the femur and abnormalities and deficiencies of some of the soft tissues. The femoral condyles are flat and the tibia articulates in flexion with the squared-off end of the femur. There is an absence of the suprapatellar pouch. The quadriceps muscle and tendon are usually present although the patella is usually absent. Complete rigidity of the knee is frequently related to an abnormal ligament running from the insertion site of the anterior cruciate to the anterior surface of the distal femoral condyles. Resection of this ligament frequently results in 45° or more of knee flexion. Because the femur is so short, it is very difficult to exercise the knee; there is no proximal lever to stabilize. The best result that can be hoped for in these limbs with a lengthening program is equalization of limb length, a mobile hip, a mobile ankle, and a stiff knee with at the most 45° of motion. Functionally this is probably not as good as a van Nes rotationplasty or Syme's amputation and prosthetic fitting. With either of these procedures the hip is still deficient and unstable. Ilizarov hip reconstruction to minimize limp and give better pelvic support can be considered. A lengthening program requires multiple procedures to achieve limb length equality, and should only be considered in patients who absolutely refuse a prosthetic option, have bilateral disease, or have phocomelia affecting the upper extremities.

Age Strategies

The majority of type 1 congenital short femurs require at least two lengthenings. As the expected discrepancy at skeletal maturity increases, the number of lengthenings required to equalize limb length discrepancy increases (Table 1). The amount of lengthening that can be performed in the femur at any one stage depends on the initial length of the femur. Generally 4 to 6 cm can be performed safely in toddler (age 2 to 4 years) femurs. In children older than age 6 years, at least 6 to 8 cm is usually possible. In adolescents and young adults, 8 to 12 cm may be possible. Combined femur and tibia lengthenings allow greater lengthening amounts. Tibial lengthening of up to 5 cm can be combined with the above femoral lengthening amounts. Toddler lengthening should be considered only in children with a well developed hip joint including an ossified femoral neck. Toddler lengthening is usually limited to 4 to 6 cm although I have safely performed up to 8 cm in the older toddlers if knee motion is well maintained. The two main advantages of toddler lengthening are growth stimulation and reduction of prosthetic needs. Growth stimulation was seen consistently in my toddler femoral lengthenings. It is a progressive stimulation in some cases, whereas in others it returns to the previous growth rate. With a reduction of the leg length difference, toddlers are able to reduce one level of prosthetic/orthotic need. This means going from a long leg prosthesis to an ankle-foot orthosis (AFO) and shoe lift, from an AFO and shoe lift to only a shoe lift, or from a shoe lift to no lift. The complication rate in this group is no higher than in older children in my experience.

Table 1 Treatment strategies and timing of reconstructive stages in management of congenital short femur

Discrepancy at Maturity	Treatment Strategy Options	Timing
≤ 6 cm	1 lengthening	over age 6
7–12 cm	2 lengthenings	toddler (< 5 cm) + age 8–10 (< 8 cm)
	1 lengthening	toddler (< 5 cm) or age 6 (< 8 cm) + epiphhyseodeisis (< 5 cm)
12–16 cm	2 lengthenings	toddler (< 5 cm) or age 6–8 (<8 cm) + age 10–12 (8–10 cm)
16–20 cm	2 lengthenings	toddler (< 5 cm) or age 6 –8 (< 8 cm) + age 10–12 (8–10 cm) + tibial (< 5 cm) during one of the femoral lengthenings
	3 lengthenings	toddler (< 5 cm) + age 8–10 (6–8 cm) + age 10–14 (8–10 cm)
	2 lengthenings	toddler (< 5 cm) or age 6–8 (< 8 cm) + age 10–12 (8–10 cm) + epiphyseodeisis (< 5 cm)
21–25 cm	3 lengthenings	toddler (< 5 cm) + age 8–10 (6–8 cm) + age 12–16 (10–12 cm)
	3 lengthenings	age 6–8 (< 8 cm) + age 10–12 (8–10 cm) + age 12–16 (8–12 cm) + tibia (< 5 cm) during one of the femoral lengthenings
	2 lengthenings + epiphyseodesis	age 6–8 (< 8 cm) + age 10–12 (8–10 cm) + epiphyseodesis (< 5 cm), tibial lengthening (< 5 cm) with one of the femoral lengthenings > 25 cm
	3 lengthenings + epiphyseodesis	
	4 lengthenings	

Lengthening Reconstruction Surgery Versus Prosthetic Replacement Surgery

My results in 54 patients to date with congenital short femur syndrome are given in Table 2. Many of these patients have completed only one lengthening, whereas others have completed as many as three lengthenings. In a separate study of 70 Ilizarov femoral lengthenings, clinical and radiographic results were compared between congenital, posttraumatic, and developmental cases undergoing lengthening (unpublished data, 1996). There was no significant difference in results based on etiology.

Because of the improvements in results of lengthening with the introduction of Ilizarov's techniques, more authors are recommending limb reconstructive surgery. However, currently the presence of a pseudarthrosis and the status of the hip are used as the primary deciding factors for limb reconstructive surgery versus amputation and prosthetic fitting. It should be emphasized that the hip status does not change after amputation and prosthetic fitting. I argue, therefore, that the status of the hip should not be a

Table 2 Results of lengthening

Type	No.	Results*			
		Excellent	Good	Fair	Poor
1a	45	32	10	3	0
1b	2	0	1	1	0
2a	1	0	1	0	0
2b	3	1	1	1	0
3a	1	0	1	0	0
3b	2	0	2	0	0

* Result score is based on clinical subjective, clinical objective, and radiographic criteria

major deciding factor for amputation and prosthetic fitting. In fact, hip procedures used for limb reconstructive surgery are useful to stabilize the hip and improve gait even after amputation and prosthetic fitting. For me, the status of the knee is the deciding factor to recommend limb reconstructive surgery versus amputation and prosthetic fitting. Therefore, my absolute indications for amputation and prosthetic fitting are primarily in type 3 cases. In type 2 cases it should also be considered depending on how functional the knee is and on the magnitude of the predicted discrepancy. Type 1a and b should rarely be considered for amputation and prosthetic fitting, unless there is an associated stiff knee. Finally, in type 1 congenital femoral deficiency, limb reconstructive surgery is so reliable in my hands that amputation and prosthetic fitting should be considered only when psychologic or socioeconomic reasons prevail.

One of the arguments for amputation and prosthetic fitting is the contention that limb reconstructive surgery leads to psychologic scarring and loss of childhood. In my experience, limb reconstructive surgery if properly conducted with an appropriate rehabilitation program and surgeries strategically spaced apart does not lead to obvious psychological scarring to the child. It can truly be a 'growing experience.' Limb reconstructive surgery is an investment. The child invests part of his or her childhood in order to live the majority of life as an adult with as near normal an extremity as possible. I try to complete the limb reconstructive surgery before the child enters high school whenever possible so that the formative years of body image at the time when the children are most self-conscious occur with both limbs of equal length and near normal function. In this manner, most go through a normal adolescence. The psychologic stress of wearing a prosthesis during adolescence is not well quantified by psychologic profiles performed on these individuals as adults. Therefore, it is difficult to compare limb reconstructive surgery versus amputation and prosthetic fitting.

Psychosocioeconomic stresses can play a major role in deciding between limb reconstructive surgery and amputation and prosthetic fitting. Single parents, marital difficulties, financial difficulties, drug problems, behavioral problems, learning disabilities, mental capacity, and other problems may interfere with compliance, maturity, and home stability required to undergo limb reconstructive surgery. Amputation and prosthetic fitting is easier, more painless, and requires far less treatment assistance by the family. In situations where the family would find it difficult to comply or too stressful for the other family members, amputation and prosthetic fitting is the preferable option. Finally, successful limb reconstructive surgery requires a team dedicated to this type of treatment. It is not a procedure that should be performed casually or by surgeons inexperienced in the treatment of these patients. Experience in limb lengthening for other conditions is not sufficient to know how to successfully perform lengthening in children with congenital femoral deficiency. It requires a long commitment of time on the surgeon's part and on the part of the surgeon's team. It requires appropriate rehabilitation services. If all of these facilities are not available, limb reconstructive surgery should not be considered at that venue. The latter is perhaps the main limiting factor today in the availability of limb reconstructive surgery.

References

1. Sanpera I Jr, Sparks LT: Proximal femoral focal deficiency: Does a radiologic classification exist? *J Pediatr Orthop* 1994;14:34–38.

2. Suzuki S, Kasahara Y, Seto Y, Futami T, Furukawa K, Nishino Y: Dislocation and subluxation during femoral lengthening. *J Pediatr Orthop* 1994;14:343–346.

3. Millis MB, Hall JE: Transiliac lengthening of the lower extremity: A modified innominate osteotomy for the treatment of postural imbalance. *J Bone Joint Surg* 1979;61A:1182–1194.

4. Langenskiöld A, Ritsila V: Congenital dislocation of the patella and its operative treatment. *J Pediatr Orthop* 1992;12:315–323.

5. Sisk TD: Knee injuries, in Crenshaw AH (ed): *Campbell's Operative Orthopaedics*, ed 7. St. Louis, MO, CV Mosby, 1987, vol 3, pp 2283–2496.

6. Grammont PM, Latune D, Lammaire IP: Treatment of subluxation and dislocation of the patella in the child: Elmslie technic with moveable soft tissue pedicle (8 year review). *Orthopade* 1985;14:229–238.

7. Paley D, Herzenberg JE, Paremain G, Bhave A: Femoral lengthening on an intramedullary nail: A matched-case comparison with Ilizarov femoral lengthening. *J Bone Joint Surg* 1997;79A:1464–1480.

8. Gonzalez-Herranz P, Burgos-Flores J, Rapariz JM, Lopez-Mondejar JA, Ocete JG, Amaya S: Intramedullary nailing of the femur in children: Effects on its proximal end. *J Bone Joint Surg* 1995;77B:262–266.

9. Astion DJ, Wilber JH, Scoles PV: Avascular necrosis of the capital femoral epiphysis after intramedullary nailing for a fracture of the femoral shaft: A case report. *J Bone Joint Surg* 1995;77A:1092–1094.

10. Pouliquen JC, Gorodischer S, Verneret C, Richard L: Femur lengthening in children and adolescents: A comparative study of a seires of 82 cases. *Rev Chir Orthop* 1989;75:239–251.

11. Hollister AM, Jatana S, Singh AK, Sullivan WW, Lupichuk AG: The axes of rotation of the knee. *Clin Orthop* 1993;290:259–268.

12. Paley D: Problems, obstacles, and complications of limb lengthening by the Ilizarov technique. *Clin Orthop* 1990;250:81–104.

13. Paley D, Tetsworth K: Mechanical axis deviation of the lower limbs: Preoperative planning of uniapical angular deformities of the tibia or femur. *Clin Orthop* 1992;280:48–64.

Chapter 12
Femoral Lengthening With Monolateral Half-Pin Devices

Charles T. Price, MD
Kenneth J. Noonan, MD

Introduction

Treatment of patients with longitudinal deficiency of the femur can be challenging because of the potential presence of axial malalignment; pseudarthrosis; associated abnormalities of the hip, knee, leg, and foot; and significant limb length discrepancy. The femur usually is retroverted with occasional varus alignment in the femoral neck, subtrochanteric region, or diaphysis.[1] Genu valgum may also be present as a result of hypoplasia of the lateral femoral condyle.[1-6] Pseudarthroses often are detected in the femoral neck or the subtrochanteric region; differences in healing rates and prognosis exist between these types.[7] Associated abnormalities of the affected extremity have been noted in up to 75% of cases;[8-12] and compared to the contralateral femur, the affected bone may be shortened from 10% to 100% (complete femoral aplasia).

Successful reconstruction requires production and maintenance of normal limb alignment, preservation of normal joint function, and correction of limb length inequality. It is important to diminish the psychological impact on young patients by using techniques that minimize the number of procedures, complications, and total treatment time. Lengthening with methods such as the Wagner technique produced high rates of infection, poor bone healing, and the need for multiple operations. Contemporary external fixators and distraction osteogenesis represent significant advances in the treatment of congenital abnormalities of the femur. Different types of external fixation that can be used for distraction osteogenesis include ring fixation with or without transfixing wires and monolateral fixation with half pins. Use of either system requires significant experience and has different indications, with advantages and disadvantages to each system. It could be argued that ring fixation may be used in all cases of femoral dysplasia that merit lengthening; however, in many cases, monolateral fixation is preferable because of ease of application and greater patient acceptance.[13-15] This chapter outlines the indications, use, results, and complications of femoral lengthening with monolateral fixation in the treatment of congenital longitudinal deficiencies of the femur.

Indications for Lengthening

There have been many attempts to classify congenital femoral dysplasias.[1,4,8,10,16,17] In many respects these classification systems are limited only by the number of available cases. Gillespie and Torode[1] classified these deformities as either type 1, congenital hypoplasia of the femur with fairly normal hip and knee relationships, or type 2, proximal femoral focal deficiency. We consider each case of longitudinal femoral deficiency to represent a point on a continuum from complete congenital femoral aplasia to mild femoral shortening with normal anatomic relationships. Therefore, we currently characterize congenital deficiencies of the femur using the classification system proposed by Pappas[4] (Fig. 1).

Although some examples may be difficult to neatly place into one of the nine different classes, this system encompasses the complete spectrum of congenital femoral dysplasia and is useful in guiding treatment. In 1983, Pappas[4] recommended surgical treatment to facilitate prosthetic fitting in classes I through VI. He suggested individualization of treatment for patients with femoral deformity in classes VII through IX, reasoning that available lengthening techniques may be useful in patients with mild to moderate length discrepancy and normal joint function. These recommendations were made prior to wide implementation of distraction osteogenesis. With current reconstructive techniques, other authors have extended the indications for lengthening.[12,18] In these patients, several operations may be needed to correct proximal femoral varus, femoral instability, and pseudarthrosis prior to femoral lengthening.

We presently use monolateral fixation in femoral lengthenings for congenital femoral dysplasias that closely fit into Pappas classes VI through IX. The decision to proceed with femoral lengthening in unilateral femoral hypoplasia depends greatly on projected discrepancy, associated abnormalities in the affected limb, and the status and stability of the ipsilateral knee and hip. In predicting ultimate femoral discrepancy, several authors have pointed out that the limb length inequality is proportional throughout growth.[1,4,11] Therefore, the final discrepancy can be calculated on the basis of two or three data points using the Moseley growth chart.[19] We concur with those authors[2,11] who consider staged lengthening a viable alternative in patients with stable joints and projected discrepancies of 15 to 17 cm.

Many associated malformations may be present; the most common is fibular deficiency with residual leg deformity and mild to moderate shortening or ankle instability.[9–12] It is important to recognize concurrent lower leg shortening, which accentuates femoral shortening. In these instances, staged ipsilateral femoral and tibial lengthenings will reduce the rate of associated complications, especially in the presence of abnormal joints or instability.

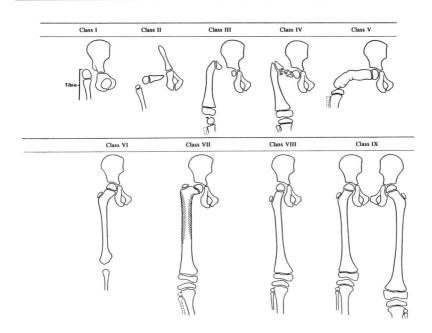

Fig. 1 Classification of congenital short femur. Approximate discrepancies for each class are: I, agenesis; II, 70% to 90%; III, 45% to 80%; IV, 40% to 67%; V, 48% to 85%; VI, 30% to 60%; VII, 10% to 50%; VIII, 10% to 41%; and IX, 6% to 20%. (Reproduced with permission from Pappas AM: Congenital abnormalities of the femur and related lower extremity malformations: Classification and treatment. J Pediatr Orthop *1983;3:45–60.)*

Effects and Complications of Lengthening

Forces Generated During Lengthening

During distraction osteogenesis, forces are required to overcome the friction inherent to the external fixator as well as the incremental tension produced in skin, muscles, tendons, nerves, vessels, periosteum, and regenerated bone. Typically, incremental distraction produces a peak tension that diminishes with soft-tissue relaxation and creep.[20,21] It may be important to maintain the same frequency of distraction even when faced with evidence of excessive soft-tissue tension.[20] Decreasing the distance obtained at each interval rather than decreasing the number of lengthening cycles per day may be preferable because with this alteration, peak tension is decreased and typical stress-relaxation patterns are maintained.[20]

In general, greater forces are required for lengthening of the femur than of the tibia, probably as a result of bone and soft-tissue differences.[22] In a series of patients undergoing limb lengthening for a variety of diagnoses, Pouliquen and associates[21] discovered that 50 to 140 kg of force are required to produce between 1 and 5 cm of distraction. Most of the force required was needed to overcome friction in the fixator; these values were less with slide lengtheners than with telescopic lengtheners. Simpson and associates[23] noted gradual force rise for lengthening of acquired discrepancies, but very high peak forces developed early in the course of lengthening for congenital deformities, to as much as 1,000 N in some instances.

Effect of Distraction on Muscle

The most significant obstruction to large lengthenings is the tension and associated effects on muscle, tendons, and neurovascular structures.[24] Increased strain in these tissues may affect physiologic, histologic, and clinical results.

Citing experimental animal work from the Soviet Union, Paley[25] reports that lengthening less than 10% leads to stretch without tissue neogenesis. Lengthening greater than 10% produces fibrogenesis and myogenesis along the whole muscle. These processes occur predominately at the level of the osteotomy in lengthenings greater than 20%.[25,26] Lengthening of muscle produces histologic changes that include myofibril loss, nuclei centralization, and production of type 2 myofibrils.[27–29] In a recent study using a rabbit model, Simpson and associates[29] have demonstrated increased fibrosis and diminished muscle compliance in lengthenings at rates greater than 1 mm per day. They found fibrosis to be the limiting factor to lengthening and recommended distraction at rates less than 1 mm per day.[29]

Retrospective evaluation up to 20 years after lengthening has demonstrated gait abnormalities and decreased strength in patients whose legs were lengthened via techniques other than distraction osteogenesis.[30,31] Kaljumae and associates[32] presented electromyographic studies of patients who underwent one-stage lengthenings of the femur. They documented diminished motor unit recruitment and greater fatigability after limb lengthening. The extent of neuromuscular tissue damage correlated with the percentage of length gained. However, a recent prospective study of distraction osteogenesis in seven patients with congenital short femur revealed a return to preoperative function at 18 months.[33] Holm and associates,[34] in their study of pre- and postoperative limb performance in nine short-statured patients who underwent bilateral femoral lengthenings via distraction osteogenesis, found no decreases in Cybex muscle testing at 2 year's follow-up.

Although experimental evidence clearly supports physiologic and histologic changes in muscle with lengthening, it is not clear what the long-term clinical effects of these changes may be. Some evidence suggests that a minimal clinical effect of muscle weakness is present after distraction osteogenesis.[33,34] However, extensive lengthenings of abnormal muscle, such as seen in congenital cases, might be expected to produce clinical effects that may be long lasting.

Effect of Distraction on Nerve

Distraction likely affects peripheral nerves by diminishing intraneural blood flow and axoplasmic function; these effects have been shown in nerves acutely stretched more than 10% of their length.[23,26] Other papers have documented decreases in nerve conduction velocities and motor action potentials after limb lengthening in both animals and humans.[26,35,36] However, nerves that are stretched gradually (1 mm/day) still appear to have good capacity for function.[23,27] Green[24] believes that it is possible to distract limbs up to 2 mm per day without adversely effecting clinical function. Gradual distraction, at a rate of 1 mm per day, usually will not produce clinically evident decreased function or weakness that is long lasting. However, poor placement of transfixing wires with ring fixation may directly damage nerves in 10% of cases[37] or may tether them during distraction.

Effect of Femoral Distraction on Joint Function

Hip

In congenital femoral deficiency, preexisting proximal femoral valgus or acetabular dysplasia may be present. Excessive lengthening of the femur may result in soft-tissue tension, producing hip joint contracture, usually of adduction and flexion. Such contracture may result in hip subluxation and dislocation, particularly in hips with preexisting dysplasia. Suzuki and associates[38] demonstrated that femoral subluxation is more common in hips with a center edge angle less than 20°. In cases of possible acetabular instability, some authors recommend prophylactic acetabular osteotomies[2,12,38] or soft-tissue releases[39] prior to femoral lengthening.

During lengthening, it is critical to regularly examine patients for contracture and obtain anteroposterior pelvic radiographs to detect hip subluxation. When faced with subluxation of the hip, the distraction process must be halted and tenotomies of the rectus femoris and adductors performed. If needed, the iliotibial band should be sectioned. Extension of the fixator to the pelvis is also possible. In cases of hip dislocation, the lengthening process is stopped and external fixation is placed across the hip.[38] With this technique, the hip can be gradually distracted and then openly reduced with or without pelvic osteotomy.

Knee

Knee stiffness frequently results from femoral lengthening as a result of increased muscle tension and tethering of muscle, ligaments, and fascia by half pins or transfixing wires.[40] Herzenberg and associates[41] documented peak loss of knee motion at the end of distraction, but the majority of motion was restored after fixator removal. Age, diagnosis, amount of lengthening, and the duration of fixation had no statistical effect on final motion in their retrospective study of patients lengthened with ring fixation.

Knee subluxation can occur during femoral lengthening, particularly in patients with congenital femoral shortening.[3,42–45] Anteroposterior instability in cases of congenital femoral shortening caused by the absence of the anterior or both cruciate ligaments has been noted by several authors.[10,46] The lack of these ligaments may be suspected by radiographic evidence of hypoplastic tibial spines or narrowing of the intracondylar notch.[3,46] Distal femoral valgus and patella alta may also be present. These deformities may predispose to lateral patellar subluxation during lengthening.[5,6] Prevention and early detection is the best treatment of posterior knee subluxation. In cases of excessive anteroposterior instability it may be desirable to place distal external fixation pins close to the knee joint to tether the iliotibial band and prevent posterior subluxation (J Canadell, Pamplona, Spain, personal communication). We recommend maintaining the knee in full extension during lengthening including the use of nighttime extension splinting.[42] During the lengthening we periodically obtain lateral knee films to detect posterior subluxation. If subluxation occurs, we halt distraction and perform distal hamstring lengthening. Other options include spanning the knee with external fixation or Quengel type casts. Lateral patellar subluxation may be treated with lateral parapatellar release or may require distal femoral varus osteotomy.[3]

Other Complications and Problems in Congenital Femoral Deficiency

Other complications include fracture, poor bone formation, malalignment, and residual limb length inequality due to subsequent growth disturbance caused by lengthening. Pappas[4] originally felt that new bone formation during lengthening of congenital femoral abnormalities might be poorer than in other conditions. Our review of the literature documented high rates of fracture following all types of femoral lengthening for congenital short femur.[9,47] Glorion and associates[42] reported a predominance of fractures and other bone problems in femurs lengthened for congenital shortening compared to femurs lengthened for other reasons. Grill and associates[9] noted relatively poorer bone formation when osteotomy for lengthening is performed proximally. They and others recommend osteotomy of the distal diaphysis or metaphysis for lengthening, and we concur. Patients who require staged lengthenings should have subsequent lengthening osteotomies in bone that has not been lengthened or previously traumatized.[18,40] We advocate intramedullary stabilization with or without bone grafting[9] in cases of poor bone formation.

Axial malalignment during limb lengthening has been attributed to failure to correct preexisting initial malalignment, excessive soft-tissue tension, fixator or pin instability, asymmetric callus formation, premature consolidation, and improper placement of the fixator on the limb.[48] The axis of the fixator should be placed parallel to the mechanical axis of the femur. Placement of the fixator axis parallel to the anatomic axis (usually 7° convergent to the mechanical axis) may result in medialization of the knee and accentuation of valgus deformity. Axial malalignment occurring during femoral lengthening, however, is more often varus. When we hope to achieve lengthening greater than 15% we believe the femur should be preset in 5° of valgus to compensate for this expected varus angulation. After fixator application and before the onset of distraction, we routinely obtain standing alignment films to detect immediate malalignment. This malalignment usually can be rectified under light sedation prior to the lengthening stage. If progressive malalignment is noted during the distraction phase, we recommend continuing until the required length is gained. The fixator and bone can then be manipulated under anesthesia prior to the consolidation of the distraction site.

Subsequent limb growth may be favorably or unfavorably affected by femoral lengthening. Several authors have reported satisfactory resumption of growth following femoral lengthening with the Wagner technique.[49,50] However, reports of growth following Wagner lengthening may not be comparable to current techniques. The Wagner method uses circumferential division of the periosteum, which may spare the physis. With callotasis techniques, an intact periosteum is necessary for good bone formation but probably increases tension across the physis. Sharma and asssociates[51] reported severe tibial growth retardation following tibial lengthening and a 22% reduction in growth rate of the femur as a result of femoral lengthening for discrepancy associated with fibular deficiency (Pappas class VII) using callotasis techniques. Two of our ten cases have developed partial or complete growth arrest.[52] We believe that growth retardation has not been adequately assessed for femoral lengthenings using current methods.

In cases of extreme length discrepancy (15 or 17 cm), we will normally plan two (or three) lengthenings. Staged lengthenings allow time for soft-tissue recuperation. In cases of two planned lengthenings the first procedure ideally is performed when the child is between 7 and 9 years of age. If a relatively small discrepancy (5 cm) remains after the first procedure, we will plan the second prior to skeletal maturity. If a length discrepancy of 7 or more cm remains, we will recommend the second lengthening earlier to allow for remaining correction with contralateral epiphysiodesis. In patients with fibular deficiency, undergoing tibial lengthening, we recommend "overlengthening" of the ipsilateral tibia. We believe that unequal knee height is an acceptable compromise for equalization of limb-length discrepancy.

Published Results of Lengthening

It is difficult to compare the published results of lengthenings in congenital femoral hypoplasia because most papers do not include objective parameters, such as neuromuscular testing, strength testing, or gait analysis, to document restoration of length and maintenance of normal joint function and muscular strength. Furthermore, the technique used and patient severity vary in these reports. Few reports of femoral lengthening with monolateral external fixation and distraction osteogenesis include more than four or five cases of congenital femoral dysplasia. We believe that correction of a 15-cm discrepancy should not be considered successful treatment if multiple procedures were required, or knee and hip contracture and potentially irreversible muscle weakness resulted. In addition to the amount of length gained, lengthening in congenital femoral hypoplasia may be best judged by associated complication rates.

Bowen and associates[40] reported their results of femoral lengthening monolateral fixation in 23 patients, 17 of whom had congenital short femur. Patients were grouped according to distal fixation pattern and osteotomy level (metaphyseal osteotomy with transfixing wires or diaphyseal osteotomy with distal half pin fixation). Both groups were lengthened 10 cm. Worse final knee range of motion in the group with distal wire fixation was believed to result from multiple adhesions. Better bone formation was noted in the segments that had metaphyseal osteotomies.

Glorion and associates[42] reported the results for 22 patients with congenital femoral shortening. These femurs were lengthened an average of 5.3 cm (24%). The total complication rate was substantially higher in the congenital group (64%) than in the acquired femoral discrepancy group (23%). Renzi-Brivio and associates[53] reviewed 35 cases of congenital short femur treated with distraction callotasis or distraction epiphysiolyses. Seventeen patients had distraction of the growth plate, with only one instance of diminished knee range of motion. The remaining 18 were treated with distraction callotasis. Three patients had premature consolidation, two had fractures, and there was one case of hip subluxation. These authors recommend callotasis in younger patients and chondrodiastasis for small discrepancies in patients close to maturity.[53]

Grill and Dungl[18] report the results of femoral lengthening procedures in 51 patients with congenital femoral dysplasia (Pappas classes III, IV, VII, VIII, and IX). In classes III and IV, hip instability and pseudarthrosis were corrected before lengthening. Fixation across the hip was used during femoral lengthening. These classes were lengthened over 90% with high rates of knee subluxation and femur fractures. The remaining classes were lengthened 16% to 25% and had lower rates of knee subluxation and fracture. The authors concluded that a stable hip is a prerequisite to femoral lengthening. This approach is similar to that reported by Saleh and Goonatillake,[12] who outlined a treatment protocol that emphasizes early (2 or 3 years of age) correction of hip varus, retroversion, and any pseudarthrosis. In cases with predicted discrepancy less than 8 cm, they recommended lengthening in one stage, while greater discrepancies required two lengthenings.

Our Rationale for Monolateral Fixators in Femoral Lengthening

We believe that most complications of lengthening for congenital short femur are related to soft-tissue tension and joint instability rather than fixator design. When these biologic issues are addressed, the choice of fixator usually depends on the experience and preference of the surgeon. We also believe that monolateral fixators can be used effectively for the majority of patients with congenital short femurs that are suitable for lengthening.

Monolateral fixation of the thigh is better tolerated by patients than is ring fixation with transfixion wires.[13–15,40] High levels of pain over several months have been reported with the Ilizarov device for lengthenings,[54] but pain during lengthening is unusual with monolateral fixation.

Most reports demonstrate that regenerate bone formation is the same regardless of the fixator used.[55,56] However, Grill and Dungl[18] observed that the Ilizarov device yielded better regenerate bone formation than the Orthofix device for patients with congenital short femur. However, all of their lengthenings using the Ilizarov apparatus were distal, whereas all but one of the lengthenings using the Orthofix device were proximal. The location of the osteotomy may have affected the bone formation more than the type of device.[57] We believe that most lengthenings for congenital short femur should avoid the proximal femur regardless of the device used.

A major concern of monolateral fixation is the inability to span the knee joint to prevent posterior subluxation of the knee during lengthening. However, this method is cumbersome, time consuming, and unnecessary in the majority of patients. We encountered posterior knee subluxation in two of ten congenital short femurs lengthened with monolateral fixators. Early recognition allows such cases to be treated by soft-tissue release and cast immobilization with the knee in extension without resorting to extension of the fixator beyond the knee[12] (R Aldegheri, Verona, Italy, personal communication).

Spanning the knee prophylactically may prevent articular cartilage damage during major lengthenings. Stanitski[58] has shown that 30% femoral lengthening in dogs causes cartilage changes. When lengthenings of this magnitude are planned, it may be advisable to span the knee.[59] However, we prefer to stage lengthenings and limit each stage to 20% in most cases.

Varus deformity during lengthening can occur with any device if it is improperly applied. Galpin and associates[60] demonstrated that monolateral and ring devices are strong enough to resist bending forces during lengthening. Under cantilever testing, the unilateral fixators were considerably stronger than the ring devices. The problem occurs at the pin-bone interface. This problem can be overcome by using more rigid constructs and performing appropriate soft-tissue releases. Varus has occurred in only one of our ten patients and was not serious enough to need correction. Glorion and associates[42] reported two angular deviations in 22 monolateral lengthenings for congenital short femur. We believe that varus during lengthening is avoidable with proper attention to technical details.

Our Treatment Principles

Lengthening with a monolateral fixator is appropriate for congenital short femur with projected discrepancy of less than 17 cm in the presence of a stable hip and a knee that has an intact posterior cruciate ligament. Hip stability should be obtained prior to lengthening by appropriate surgery as early in life as reasonable.

Multiple, staged lengthenings should be planned for projected discrepancy greater than 7 cm. The goal of each stage should be a 15% to 20% gain in length. More may be achieved at each stage if the postoperative course is exceptionally benign. Patients should be advised that more than 20% gain per stage is unlikely.

Avoid bilevel lengthenings. Bilevel lengthenings may shorten the total time required for osteogenesis but experimental evidence indicates muscles and nerves respond more favorably to slower rates of distraction.[23,29,61] Similarly, ipsilateral lengthening of the femur and tibia should be avoided in most cases because neurovascular structures are lengthened at a rate of 2 mm per day. Nerves, arteries, and veins demonstrate degenerative changes and fibrous metaplasia when lengthened more than 20% of their original length.[62] Ipsilateral femoral and tibial lengthenings may exceed this limit in addition to being more cumbersome and difficult for the patient.

Rigid monolateral constructs should be used with multiple large diameter pins. Fixator alignment should be parallel to the mechanical axis to avoid translation during lengthening. Pins in each cluster should be inserted parallel in all planes to avoid stress at the pin-bone interface. Osteotomies for lengthening should usually be made distal to the midshaft of the femur to avoid abnormal bone in the proximal segment.

The iliotibial band should be released distally at the time of distal pin insertion. Additional soft-tissue releases can be planned as soon as contracture begins to develop.[42] If the adductor magnus is tight, consideration may be given to releasing it at the adductor hiatus.

Knee subluxation should be avoided by distal pin placement, avoidance of knee flexion exercises, and splinting in extension for a minimum of 12 hours a day. Early detection of knee subluxation is essential and should be treated by hamstring lengthening or traction and immobilization in extension. Hip subluxation or dislocation requires treatment by appropriate soft-tissue releases, femoral shortening, extension of fixation across the hip joint, open reduction, or a combination of these treatments.

Establish realistic goals for each stage and abandon lengthening in the presence of complications that do not respond promptly to management. It is safer to try a different approach at a later time than to proceed in the presence of serious difficulty.

References

1. Gillespie R, Torode IP: Classification and management of congenital abnormalities of the femur. *J Bone Joint Surg* 1983;65B:557–568.

2. Damsin JP, Pous JG, Ghanem I: Therapeutic approach to severe congenital lower limb length discrepancies: Surgical treatment versus prosthetic management. *J Pediatr Orthop* 1995;4B:164–170.

3. Jones DC, Moseley CF: Subluxation of the knee as a complication of femoral lengthening by the Wagner technique. *J Bone Joint Surg* 1985;67B:33–35.

4. Pappas AM: Congenital abnormalities of the femur and related lower extremity malformations: Classification and treatment. *J Pediatr Orthop* 1983;3:45–60.

5. Ring PA: Congenital short femur: Simple femoral hypoplasia. *J Bone Joint Surg* 1959;41B:73–79.

6. Sanpera I Jr, Fixsen JA, Sparks LT, Hill RA: Knee in congenital short femur. *J Pediatr Orthop* 1995;4B:159–163.

7. Goddard NJ, Hashemi-Nejad A, Fixsen JA: Natural history and treatment of instability of the hip in proximal femoral focal deficiency. *J Pediatr Orthop* 1995; 4B:145–149.

8. Aitken GT: Proximal femoral focal deficiency: Definition, classification and management, in Aitken GT (ed): *Proximal Femoral Focal Deficiency: A Congenital Anomaly.* Washington, DC, National Academy of Sciences, 1969, pp 1–22.

9. Grill F, Dungl P, Steinwender G, Hosny G: Congenital short femur. *J Pediatr Orthop* 1993;2B:35–41.

10. Hamanishi C: Congenital short femur: Clinical, genetic and epidemiological comparison of the naturally occurring condition with that caused by thalidomide. *J Bone Joint Surg* 1980;62B:307–320.

11. Koman LA, Meyer LC, Warren FH: Proximal femoral focal deficiency: Natural history and treatment. *Clin Orthop* 1982;162:135–143.

12. Saleh M, Goonatillake HD: Management of congenital leg length inequality: Value of early axis correction. *J Pediatr Orthop* 1995;4B:150–158.

13. Grill F: Correction of complicated extremity deformities by external fixation. *Clin Orthop* 1989;241:166–176.

14. Markbreiter LA, Cannon RM, Dick HM: Complications of femoral circular fixators. *Orthop Trans* 1993;16:698–699.

15. Pouliquen JC, Gorodischer S, Verneret C, Richard L: Femoral lengthening in children and adolescents. *Fr J Orthop Surg* 1989;3:162–173.

16. Fixsen JA, Lloyd-Roberts GC: The natural history and early treatment of proximal femoral dysplasia. *J Bone Joint Surg* 1974;56B:86–95.

17. Kalamchi A, Cowell HR, Kim KI: Congenital deficiency of the femur. *J Pediatr Orthop* 1985;5:129–134.

18. Grill F, Dungl P: Lengthening for congenital short femur: Results of different methods. *J Bone Joint Surg* 1991;73B:439–447.

19. Moseley CFA: A straight-line graph for leg-length discrepancies. *J Bone Joint Surg* 1977;59A:174–179.

20. Leong JC, Ma RY, Clark JA, Cornish LS, Yaau AC: Viscoelastic behavior of tissue in leg lengthening by distraction. *Clin Orthop* 1979;139:102–109.

21. Pouliquen JC, Pauthier F, Ucla B, Kassis B, Ceolin JL, Langlais J: Tension measurements during lengthening of the lower limbs in children and adolescents. *J Pediatr Orthop* 1994;3B:107–113.

22. Younger AS, Mackenzie WG, Morrison JB: Femoral forces during limb lengthening in children. *Clin Orthop* 1994;301:55–63.

23. Simpson AH, Cunningham JL, Kenwright J: The forces which develop in the tissues during leg lengthening: A clinical study. *J Bone Joint Surg* 1996;78B:979–983.

24. Green SA: Postoperative management during limb lengthening. *Orthop Clin North Am* 1991;22:723–734.

25. Paley D: Current techniques of limb lengthening. *J Pediatr Orthop* 1988;8:73–92.

26. Galardi G, Comi G, Lozza L, et al: Peripheral nerve damage during limb lengthening: Neurophysiology in five cases of bilateral tibial lengthening. *J Bone Joint Surg* 1990;72B:121–124.

27. Carroll NC, Grant CG, Hudson R, Gilbert J, Mubarak SJ, Warren R: Experimental observations on the effects of leg lengthening by the Wagner Method. *Clin Orthop* 1981;160:250–257.

28. Lindboe CF, Fjeld TO, Steen H: Morphological changes in continuously stretched skeletal muscles in sheep. *Eur J Appl Physiol* 1985;54:184–190.

29. Simpson AH, Williams PE, Kyberd P, Goldspink G, Kenwrigh TJ: The response of muscle to leg lengthening. *J Bone Joint Surg* 1995;77B:630–636.

30. Kawamura B, Hosono S, Takahashi T, et al: Limb lengthening by means of subcutaneous osteotomy: Experimental and clinical studies. *J Bone Joint Surg* 1968;50A:851–878.

31. Sofield HA, Blair SJ, Millar EA: Leg lengthening: A personal follow-up of forty patients some twenty years after the operation. *J Bone Joint Surg* 1958;40A: 311–322.

32. Kaljumae U, Martson A, Haviko T, Hanninen O: The effect of lengthening of the femur on the extensors of the knee: An electromyographic study. *J Bone Joint Surg* 1995;77A:247–250.

33. Maffulli N, Fixsen JA: Muscular strength after callotasis limb lengthening. *J Pediatr Orthop* 1995;15:212–216.

34. Holm I, Steen H, Ludvigsen P, Bjerkreim I: Unchanged muscle function after bilateral femoral lengthening: A prospective study of 9 patients with 2-year follow-up. *Acta Orthop Scand* 1995;66:258–260.

35. Chuang TY, Chan R-C, Chin L-S, Hsu TC: Neuromuscular injury during limb lengthening: A longitudinal follow-up by rabbit tibial model. *Arch Phys Med Rehabil* 1995;76:467–470.

36. Young NL, Davis RJ, Bell DF, Redmond DMA: Electromyographic and nerve conduction changes after tibial lengthening by the Ilizarov method. *J Pediatr Orthop* 1993;13:473–473.

37. Makarov MR, Delgado MR, Birch JG, Samchukov ML: Intraoperative SSEP monitoring during external fixation procedures in the lower extremities. *J Pediatr Orthop* 1996;16:155–160.

38. Suzuki S, Kasahara Y, Seto Y, Futami T, Furukawa K, Nishino Y: Dislocation and subluxation during femoral lengthening. *J Pediatr Orthop* 1994;14:343–346.

39. Salai M, Chechick A, Ganel A, Blankstein A, Horoszowski H: Subluxation of the hip joint during femoral lengthening. *J Pediatr Orthop* 1985;5:642–644.

40. Bowen JR, Levy EJ, Donohue M: Comparison of knee motion and callus formation in femoral lengthening with the Wagner or monolateral-ring device. *J Pediatr Orthop* 1993;13:467–472.

41. Herzenberg JE, Scheufele LL, Paley D, Bechtel T, Tepper S: Knee range of motion in isolated femoral lengthening. *Clin Orthop* 1994;301:49–54.

42. Glorion C, Pouliquen JC, Langlais J, Ceolin JL, Kassis B: Femoral lengthening using the callotasis method: Study of the complications in a series of 70 cases in children and adolescents. *J Pediatr Orthop* 1996;16:161–167.

43. Guidera KJ, Hess WF, Highhouse KP, Ogden JA: Extremity lengthening: Results and complications with the Orthofix system. *J Pediatr Orthop* 1991;11:90–94.

44. Stanitski Df, Bullard M, Armstrong P, Stanitski CL: Results of femoral lengthening using the Ilizarov technique. *J Pediatr Orthop* 1995;15: 224–231.

45. Stephens DC: Femoral and tibial lengthening. *J Pediatr Orthop* 1983; 3:424–430.

46. Johansson E, Aparisi T: Missing cruciate ligament in congenital short femur. *J Bone Joint Surg* 1983;65A:1109–1115.

47. Danziger MB, Kumar A, DeWeese J: Fractures after femoral lengthening using the Ilizarov method. *J Pediatr Orthop* 1995;15:220–223.

48. Paley D: Problems, obstacles, and complications of limb lengthening by the Ilizarov technique. *Clin Orthop* 1990;250:81–104.

49. Hope PG, Crawfurd EJ, Catterall A: Bone growth following lengthening for congenital shortening of the lower limb. *J Pediatr Orthop* 1994;14:339–342.

50. Shapiro F: Longitudinal growth of the femur and tibia after diaphyseal lengthening. *J Bone Joint Surg* 1987;69A:684–690.

51. Sharma M, MacKenzie WG, Bowen JR: Severe tibial growth retardation in total fibular hemimelia after limb lengthening: *J Pediatr Orthop* 1996;16:438–444.

52. Price CT, Carantzas AC: Severe growth retardation following limb lengthening: A case report. *Iowa Orthop J* 1996;16:139–146.

53. Renzi-Brivio L, Lavini F, de Bastiani G: Lengthening in the congenital short femur. *Clin Orthop* 1990;250:112–116.

54. Young N, Bell DF, Anthony A: Pediatric pain patterns during Ilizarov treatment of limb length discrepancy and angular deformity. *J Pediatr Orthop* 1994;14:352–357.

55. Hamdy RC, Walsh WR, Ehrlich MG, et al: Is there any difference in bone lengthening by Orthofix and Ilizarov fixators? *Orthop Trans* 1995;19:653.

56. Lokietek W, Legaye J, Lokietek JC: Contributing factors for osteogenesis in children's limb lengthening. *J Pediatr Orthop* 1991;11:452–458.

57. Boden SD, Fallon MD, Davidson R, Mennuti MT, Kaplan FS: Proximal femoral focal deficiency: Evidence for a defect in proliferation and maturation of chondrocytes. *J Bone Joint Surg* 1989;71A:1119–1129.

58. Stanitski DF: The effect of limb lengthening on articular cartilage: An experimental study. *Clin Orthop* 1994;301:68–72.

59. Stanitski DF, Rossman K, Torosian M: The effect of femoral lengthening on knee articular cartilage: The role of apparatus extension across the joint. *J Pediatr Orthop* 1996;16:151–154.

60. Galpin RD, Willis RB, McLaren AC, et al: Biomechanical evaluation of four limb lengthening devices and the effects of distraction. *Orthop Trans* 1990;14:287.

61. Saleh M, Hamer AJ: Bifocal limb lengthening: A preliminary report. *J Pediatr Orthop* 1993;2B:42–48.

62. Ippolito E, Peretti G, Bellocci M, et al: Histology and ultrastructure of arteries, veins, and peripheral nerves during limb lengthening. *Clin Orthop* 1994;308:54–62.

63. Eyring EJ: Staged femoral lengthening. *Clin Orthop* 1978;136:83–91.

Consensus

Limb Lengthening of the Congenital Short Femur

Limb lengthening has a prominent role in management of the congenital short femur. The procedures are difficult because of the tendency for knee and hip subluxation. When there is a risk of hip subluxation, the hip should be stabilized prior to lengthening the femur. Coxa vara and retroversion should be corrected early when possible. Knee subluxation may be prevented by fixation frames or other support that crosses the knee. Technology is improving, and indications for this type of surgery will expand. Current techniques for limb lengthening include use of ring fixators, use of unilateral frame fixators, and lengthening over intramedullary rods.

Hip stability, knee stability, and overall discrepancy are major considerations in limb lengthening. Patients and parents should be well informed about the procedures and their complications. Current indications for lengthening include a femur that is predicted to be at least half as long as the normal femur at maturity, a predicted discrepancy of less than 17 to 20 cm, and one that can be correccted with no more than three separate equalization procedures.

An ongoing physical therapy program is essential and ideally should be arranged preoperatively. The program should include monitoring of knee extension, and weightbearing should be stressed. Early return to school and participation in normal activities should also be encouraged. Functional outcome studies are needed for proper evaluation of surgical and physical therapy techniques.

Section 3
Fibular Deficiency

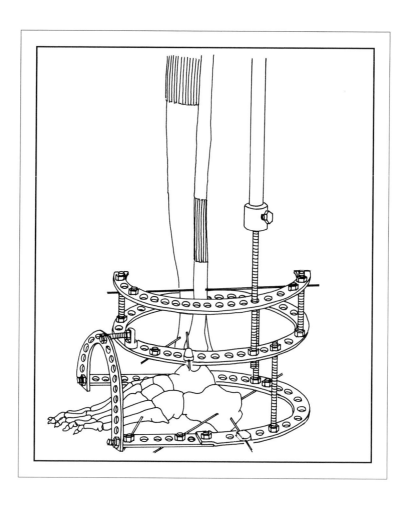

Chapter 13
Fibula Deficiencies

Leon M. Kruger, MD

History and Incidence

Fibula deficiency is described as the most frequent long bone absence. Froster and Baird[1] state that the incidence of absent fibula is 1.07 per 10,000 live births or, in other terms, one instance in 9,337 live births. Haudek,[2] in 1896, reported a single case of absent fibula and stated that he had found 96 others described in the European literature. Harmon and Fahey[3] in 1937 found 296 cases of absent fibula described in the literature prior to 1935. Although Aitken and Frantz[4] in 1953 described 103 patients with amputations, they did not mention absent fibula. Experience in the Shriners Hospital for Children in Springfield, Massachusetts, includes 163 patients with longitudinal deficiency of the fibula, which develops to an incidence of 1 in 200 new patients seen in the past 70 years. A computer printout of the Shriners Hospital System indicates that over 2,200 cases of fibula deficiency have been reported in the 19 orthopaedic hospitals.

Although there are many reports of syndromes in which fibula deficiency is a part, there has been no evidence of genetic transmission of isolated fibula deficiency.[5] Gupta and associates[6] did report four siblings who had bilateral fibula deficiency, but also had normal parents and normal chromosomes. There was no history of consanguinity, and they referred to this as an autosomal recessive nonsyndromic fibula agenesis. At the Shriners Hospital in Springfield, Massachusetts, there was no family history of fibula deficiency in the 163 patients, nor have there been any siblings or offspring with fibula deficiency. In fact, there have been at least two cases in which one twin had a fibula deficiency with the other twin normal.

Terminology

Coventry and Johnson[7] were the first to present a classification and terminology for congenital absence of the fibula. Subsequently, O'Rahilly,[8] and Frantz and O'Rahilly[9] introduced a terminology that is still in use in many areas. Later, under the auspices of the International Society for Prosthetics/Orthotics (ISPO), a new, more descriptive terminology was presented.[10] The most recent classification of fibula deficiency was that of Achterman and Kalamchi.[11] They described their type I, including IA and IB, as a hypoplasia with a portion of the fibula present; and type II as complete absence of the fibula.

Clinical Description

Longitudinal deficiency of the fibula has been described extensively by Coventry and Johnson,[7] Farmer and Laurin,[12] Kruger and Talbott,[13] and Wood and associates.[14] Many other authors recognize that there are several characteristic features of longitudinal deficiency of the fibula.[5] Most important is to recognize that this is a limb deficiency and not simply the absence of a long bone. There is involvement of other tissues including the femur, the knee joint, the tarsals, the metatarsals, and the phalanges, which may be absent, and the skin is characterized by a dimple over the anterior bow of the tibia. The tibia itself may be straight or bowed and shortened, and the distal tibial epiphysis usually is involved, with a deficiency in its lateral portion. According to the classification by Achterman and Kalamchi,[11] a partial absence of the fibula may take several forms. It may involve only a hypoplasia of the involved fibula as compared with the normal limb. In the more severe involvement, and particularly in those with distal involvement of the fibula, there is an ankle valgus, which may be stable or unstable, and an associated tarsal coalition that will eventuate in a ball and socket ankle joint. As a rule, with partial deficiency there is not a bow in the tibia. Valgus of the knee may occur, and limb-length discrepancy is frequent.

Total Deficiencies

Total longitudinal deficiency of the fibula is much more severe and should be recognized as a total limb deficiency, and not simply the absence of a long bone.[13] The limb is short, and there is involvement of the hip, which usually has retroversion (limited internal rotation at the hip joint). Knee involvement has been well described by Torode and Gillespie;[15] it is characterized by anterior/posterior shuck or cruciate insufficiency and valgus of the knee. The femur may be completely normal in length and equal to the contralateral side in the patient with unilateral involvement, or it may be minimally shortened and considered as normal. On the other hand, there may be a proximal femoral focal deficiency (PFFD), in which case the patient must be treated as having a PFFD with the fibula deficiency as a secondary problem. The tibia may be straight, but it may also have a severe anterior bow. This bowing is not associated with pseudarthrosis should osteotomy be undertaken. The ankle is in valgus, which may be extreme with subluxation or very mild; the ankle may be stable or unstable. The tarsal bones are usually involved, with partial absence and/or tarsal coalitions. Amstutz[16] and others[5,13] have shown that the growth of the affected limb remains proportional to the normal limb. The ability to predict the length discrepancy at maturity is probably the most important factor in planning treatment.

Radiographic examination of the limb will usually show, in addition to the total absence of the fibula, underdevelopment of the lateral femoral condyle. The intercondylar notch is shallow, and the tibial spine may be flattened; valgus is usually present and may be progressive. The anterior bow of the tibia, when present, is easily demonstrable radiographically, and the thickening of the posterior cortex at the bow is also noted. The distal tibial epiphysis and growth plate are abnormal. The tarsal coalition will not be identifiable at birth, but will be recognized as ossification progresses. Absent rays are readily evident on radiographic examination, and there may be an osseous synostosis of the metatarsals.

It is now possible to diagnose fibula deficiency antepartum.[17-19] Hirose and associates[18] reported ultrasound examination of a patient at 28-week gestation without mention of the fibula. At 35 weeks, the right fibula "could not be identified." At 38 weeks, the child was delivered by cesarean section and diagnosed as having a femur-fibula-ulna syndrome. Sepulveda and associates[19] diagnosed an absent fibula by ultrasonography at 16 weeks' gestation.

Tarsal coalitions associated with the ball and socket ankle joint have been reported in 50% of patients by Achterman and Kalamchi,[11] while Bohne and Root[20] reported no instance of ball and socket ankle. The progressive length discrepancy and foot deformity should be recognized as determining factors in definitive treatment.

Treatment

Management of the child with a limb deficiency is best carried out in a clinic setting. Here the parents of a newborn not only have the chance to talk to parents of other children with the same or similar deformity, but they can also see the result of treatment. Under these circumstances, it is much easier for the parent to make the decision that amputation and prosthetic restoration, when indicated, is the procedure of choice, rather than to be encouraged by the surgeon. For this reason, it is recommended that all children with limb deficiencies be seen in a limb deficiency clinic rather than in a one-on-one examination room.

The major goal in the treatment of fibula deficiency, whether partial or complete, is functional restoration. Functional restoration implies a plantigrade functional foot and appropriate length equalization. Accomplishment of these goals is paramount in all patients. Although cosmesis is a secondary consideration, it is important to recognize the implications of severe foot deformity. In the small child, management of a foot deformity with shoe inserts or build-up is no problem. However, this solution usually becomes intolerable, especially to females after puberty, a fact that should be taken into account in the early management of the patient. Although correction of the deformity and an equalization of leg length may take place, the severe foot deformity may be sufficient indication for ablation and prosthetic restoration.[5,13,21]

The clinical description of partial fibula deficiencies has been well reported.[5,11,20] Treatment of the partial deficiencies of the fibula has been outlined by Achterman and Kalamchi.[11] According to their classification, in types IA and B, no treatment may be indicated when the limb is only minimally short. If there is a progressive shortening, the patient may require an epiphysiodesis for limb-length equalization. Only three of their patients required a leg lengthening. Two ultimately ended up with ablation of the foot. It should be reemphasized that foot deformity in and of itself may be an indication for ablation.

Total Longitudinal Deficiency of the Fibula

Oppenheim[5] has summarized the history and philosophy of treatment in fibula deficiencies. Early descriptions of treatment protocols[5,13] included manipulations of the foot and casting. When these methods failed, correction of foot deformity by soft-tissue surgical procedures followed. On failure of maintenance of correction by manipulation and bracing, further surgeries with bony procedures, including arthrodesis, were described.

In spite of all efforts at correction of the foot deformity, leg-length discrepancy remained the major problem. Epiphysiodesis and early leg lengthening procedures usually failed to equalize leg length. Prior to 1960, there were few reports of recommended amputation except in the unusual case. Coventry and Johnson[7] and Farmer and Laurin[12] suggested that amputation was a last resort. However, later reports from Kruger and Talbott,[13] and Wood and associates[14] suggested that amputation and prosthetic restoration as a primary treatment was indicated. Boyd and Syme amputation procedures are advised.[5,11,13,14,21] The Syme procedure has been well documented.[22] Fulp and associates[23] preferred the modified Boyd procedure. Primary amputation is advised by numerous others.[5,11,21]

Our[13] indications in 1961 were leg-length discrepancy, foot deformity, psychological aspect, and economic considerations. In 1991, Oppenheim[5] gave as indications foot deformity and leg-length discrepancy, but concluded that a Syme amputation is "compatible with athletic and psychological function closely approaching that of a nonhandicapped child of the same age." Herring and associates[24] also noted the psychological benefits of primary amputation when compared to amputation after multiple reconstructive procedures. There have been recommendations that 2 in (5 cm)[21] or up to 3 in (7.5 cm) of discrepancy at birth[5,25] suggest that the leg-length discrepancy at maturity will be excessive; and, therefore, that efforts at reconstruction are contraindicated. Instead, primary amputation early in life has been the treatment of choice for such patients. Our[13] own experience showed the progression of leg-length discrepancy in patients occurred according to the chart. In spite of this, there have been numerous efforts at reconstruction of the ankle joint.[5,26–28] Exner and Rüttimann[26] had one patient followed up for 18 years, but the patient was able to walk for only 1.5 hours a day. It would appear that their patients ended up with a poor foot and a short leg requiring brace treatment and a lift, and that some patients reconstructed in this way ultimately did come to amputation.

Leg lengthening, even through the period in which the technique of Wagner was in use, was not frequently advised for these children.[29] Choi and associates[30] reported on their experience with the Wagner lengthening technique and its complications. With the institution of distraction osteogenesis, lengthening of limb deficiencies became very popular.[31] There are many recent reports in the literature of successful lengthening of the limbs of children with total fibula deficiency.[31-34] All of these, however, are only short-term reports; not a great deal of attention is paid to the condition of the foot or definitive function, only to the equalization of leg length.

There is certainly good evidence that these limbs can be lengthened sufficiently to attain length equalization. However, Price[35] indicates that there is need for additional study regarding current lengthening treatment options because complications are frequent. Gibbons and Bradish[36] reported complications in nine of ten limbs and subluxation of the knee in two of eight patients. They also found knee stiffness in two additional patients. Mean follow-up was only 26.7 months. If necessary, multiple lengthenings have been carried out. The experience of Miller and Bell[34] with 11 patients was that there was a high rate of complication, but no knee or ankle dislocation. They did not mention functional capacity, and the follow-up was very short. Catagni and associates,[32] likewise, did not have any long-term follow-ups, nor did Gibbons and Bradish.[36] It will probably be some years before long-term follow-up on these patients is available.

When leg lengthening is to be undertaken, the surgeon should take into consideration the amount of time the child will spend with the apparatus or protective bracing if this treatment is instituted. If a child has an initial lengthening at 3 or 4 years of age and then a second lengthening 4 or 5 years later, a good deal of that child's active childhood years are taken up by the surgical interventions. Ghoneem and associates[37] pointed out the importance of considering the psychological impact of prolonged treatment required by the Ilizarov method. They noted that "psychological changes can be extreme;" however, based on information from questionnaires, these problems were found to be transient, and most of their patients were without permanent functional or psychological disturbance. In their review, Maffuli and Fixsen[31] found that "significant psychological morbidity is experienced." Herring and associates[24] have pointed out the adverse psychological reaction of children who have had multiple surgical procedures prior to amputation. When discussing with the parents of children with fibula deficiency the option for lengthening and retention of the foot, they must be made aware of these facts. Damsin and associates,[38] in discussing limb lengthening, conclude that "surgeons should remain humble and wise during decision making," and "not yield to the temptation offered by a brilliant equalization procedure."

Consideration must also be given to the problems of the knee in total fibula deficiency. Valgus of the knee must be dealt with. Thompson and associates[39] suggested that excision of the lateral band (the anlage of the fibula) might prevent progressive valgus of the knee. Fulp and associates[23] have reported excision of the lateral band in a large number of patients, but did not note whether it made a difference in the progression or recurrence of valgus. With progression of the valgus, the decision on osteotomy is necessary. Because the valgus occurs from the hypoplasia of the lateral femoral condyle and underdevelopment laterally, the approach should be above the knee. Supracondylar osteotomy or, more recently, stapling of the medial femoral growth plate have been the procedures used in these patients. Boakes and associates[40] reported on 28 patients and concluded that tibial osteotomy and femoral stapling were the best approach. They also noted either patella dislocation or frequent subluxation. The latter is a very difficult problem to deal with, and prevention of dislocation or subluxation is important.

Discussion

Although treatment must be individualized for all patients with fibula deficiencies, there is general agreement that amputation and prosthetic restoration is the treatment of choice for most patients with longitudinal total deficiency of the fibula, with excessive and progressive length discrepancy, or with foot deformity. Since 1987 and the advent of the technique of distraction osteogenesis, many children have been managed with tibial or femoral and tibial lengthenings and retention of the foot.

More recently, planned repeat lengthenings have been carried out where the anticipated leg-length discrepancy is too great to equalize at one sitting. To date there are no long-term follow-up studies among patients who have had such lengthenings, although Choi and associates[30] reported their findings after Wagner-type lengthening and discussed the option of amputation versus leg lengthening. Initial correction of length discrepancy as well as angular deformity and maintenance of a plantigrade foot have been reported. It is important, however, to consider the time that a child must spend with instrumentation on the limb and the recovery period following lengthening.

This consideration is even more important when staged lengthenings are planned. Herring and associates[24] have reported psychological problems in children with multiple surgical procedures, and parents of these patients must be made aware of this possibility when discussing definitive treatment. Recent reports of antenatal diagnosis of fibula deficiency by ultrasound have permitted discussions regarding treatment options even before the child is born. However, following the birth of the child, it is important to have the parents and the child seen in a limb deficiency clinic setting where they have the opportunity to see other childen with similar problems in the later stages of life after treatment. This approach also provides parents with the opportunity to discuss the problem with other parents. No effort should be made to persuade the parents to consider any one treatment option.

As time goes on, there will certainly be further reports of long-term follow-up on those patients who have been treated by lengthening and retention of the foot. These reports will indicate whether there are problems with the ankle in late follow-up, and whether the persistence of a severe foot deformity precludes good shoe wear in adult life. In females particularly, shoe wear is an important consideration. Definitive long-term function should be the goal of treatment in all of these patients.

At the Shriners Hospital for Children in Springfield, Massachusetts, we have found 28 patients with fibula deficiency who were 25 years or older at the most recent evaluation. Five had no amputation. Six patients were below-knee amputees. This procedure was carried out before the era of modern Syme prosthesis. Of the six below-knee amputations, five were done prior to

1955, and the sixth was done in 1959. No below-knee amputations have been performed on a child with fibula deficiency since 1959. The main concern of patients, particularly in these early years, was the appearance of the carved willow wood Syme socket with lacer. Current Syme prosthetic sockets are much improved, and the cosmetic appearance of the Syme or Boyd prosthesis is very acceptable.

There were 17 patients with either Syme or Boyd amputations. Nine were 40 years of age or older; the oldest patient was 66, and he had a Syme amputation in 1934. He had worked all of his life, earlier as a wood cutter in the forest and later as a mechanic. He had had no further surgical procedure, and was married with grown children. No patient with Syme or Boyd amputation required revision or other surgery of the amputation stump.

Two patients of the 28 had symptomatic patellofemoral problems. The first was a 31-year-old male with a Boyd amputation who had a lateral dislocation of his patella, which had remained asymptomatic until about age 29 years. He had been employed until that time, but ceased working with increasing symptoms in his knee, and has not considered any intervention since then. The second patient was a 37-year-old female with bilateral longitudinal deficiency of the total fibula, who did not have an amputation. Her feet remain plantigrade, and her ankles are asymptomatic though limited in motion. She does have a recurrent dislocation of the patella, which on occasion becomes symptomatic. In spite of this, she continues to work full time as a nurse. She has not considered any further surgical intervention.

None of the patients with retained feet had significant ankle symptoms. One patient with severe valgus of the right ankle was fully active, even riding a motorcycle. He was considering surgery for cosmetic reasons even though he had only minor complaint of pain in the ankle joint.

Summary

Longitudinal partial deficiency of the fibula may take many forms, and treatment must be individualized. Whereas a shoe lift may be indicated with minimal length discrepancy, it may also be necessary to consider a length-equalization procedure. In the severe distal form with involvement of the distal tibia, surgical intervention is usually necessary.

For the patient with total longitudinal deficiency of the fibula, length discrepancy and foot deformity are the major indications for surgical intervention. Multiple surgical procedures for correction of the foot deformity may eventuate in amputation if unacceptable length discrepancy or persistent foot deformity are still present later in life; the psychological implications of multiple surgical interventions have been well discussed. Lastly, the economic impact of multiple hospitalizations may be weighed against the cost of a single surgical procedure and replacement prostheses. Because most patients with reconstructive procedures require orthoses, this last economic consideration may not be of significance.

References

1. Froster UG, Baird PA: Congenital defects of lower limbs and associated malformations: A population based study. *Am J Med Genet* 1993;45:60–64.

2. Haudek M: Über congenitalen Defect der Fibula und dessen Verhalten zur sogenannten intrauterinen Fractur der Tibia. *Ztschr f Orthop Chir* 1895;4:326–401.

3. Harmon PH, Fahey JJ: The syndrome of congenital absence of the fibula: Report of 3 cases with special reference to pathogenesis and treatment. *Surg Gynecol Obstet* 1937;64:876–887.

4. Aitken GT, Frantz CH: The juvenile amputee. *J Bone Joint Surg* 1953;35A:659–664.

5. Oppenheim WL: Fibular deficiency and the indications for Syme's amputation. *Prosthet Orthot Int* 1991;15:131–136.

6. Gupta AK, Berry M, Verma IC: Congenital absence of both fibulae in four siblings. *Pediatr Radiol* 1994;24:220–221.

7. Coventry MB, Johnson EW Jr: Congenital absence of the fibula. *J Bone Joint Surg* 1952;34A:941–955.

8. O'Rahilly R: Morphological patterns in limb deficiencies and duplications. *Am J Anat* 1951;89:135–193.

9. Frantz CH, O'Rahilly R: Congenital skeletal limb deficiencies. *J Bone Joint Surg* 1961;43A:1202–1224.

10. Kay HW, Day HJ, Henkel HL, et al: The proposed international terminology for the classification of congenital limb deficiencies. *Dev Med Child Neurol* 1975;34(suppl):1–12.

11. Achterman C, Kalamchi A: Congenital deficiency of the fibula. *J Bone Joint Surg* 1979;61B:133–137.

12. Farmer AW, Laurin CA: Congenital absence of the fibula. *J Bone Joint Surg* 1960;42A:1–12.

13. Kruger LM, Talbott RD: Amputation and prosthesis as definitive treatment in congenital absence of the fibula. *J Bone Joint Surg* 1961;43A:625–642.

14. Wood WL, Zlotsky N, Westin GW: Congenital absence of the fibula: Treatment by Syme amputation. Indications and technique. *J Bone Joint Surg* 1965;47A:1159–1169.

15. Torode IP, Gillespie R: Anteroposterior instability of the knee: A sign of congenital limb deficiency. *J Pediatr Orthop* 1983;3:467–470.

16. Amstutz HC: Abstract: Natural history and treatment of congenital absence of the fibula. *J Bone Joint Surg* 1972;54A:1349.

17. Capece G, Fasolino A, Della Monica M, et al: Prenatal diagnosis of femur-fibula-ulna complex by ultrasonography in a male fetus at 24 weeks of gestation. *Prenat Diagn* 1994;14:502–505.

18. Hirose K, Koyanagi T, Hara K, Inoue M, Nakano H: Antenatal ultrasound diagnosis of the femur-fibula-ulna syndrome. *J Clin Ultrasound* 1988;16:199–203.

19. Sepulveda W, Weiner E, Bridger JE, Fisk NM: Prenatal diagnosis of congenital absence of the fibula. *J Ultrasound Med* 1994;13:655–657.

20. Bohne WH, Root L: Hypoplasia of the fibula. *Clin Orthop* 1977;125:107–112.

21. Kruger LM: Fibular hemimelia, in Aitken GT (ed): *Selected Lower Limb Anomalies: Surgical and Prosthetic Management.* Washington, DC, National Academy of Sciences, 1971, pp 49–71.

22. Herring JA: Symes amputation for fibular hemimelia: A second look in the Ilizarov era, in Eilert RE (ed): *Instructional Course Lectures XLI.* Park Ridge, IL, American Academy of Orthopaedic Surgeons, 1992, pp 435–436.

23. Fulp T, Davids JR, Meyer LC, Blackhurst DW: Longitudinal deficiency of the fibula: Operative treatment. *J Bone Joint Surg* 1996;78A:674–682.

24. Herring JA, Barnhill B, Gaffney C: Syme amputation: An evaluation of the physical and psychological function in young patients. *J Bone Joint Surg* 1986;68A:573–578.

25. Pappas AM, Hanawalt BJ, Anderson M: Congenital defects of the fibula. *Orthop Clin North Am* 1972;3:187–199.

26. Exner GU, Rüttimann B: Fibular aplasia: Early surgical correction in two cases. *Int Orthop* 1991;15:229–232.

27. Serafin J: A new operation for congenital absence of the fibula: Preliminary report. *J Bone Joint Surg* 1967;49B:59–65.

28. Shatilov OE, Rozkov AV, Cheminova TV: Reconstructive surgery for fibular deficiency. *Prosthet Orthot Int* 1991;15:137–139.

29. Hood RW, Riseborough EJ: Lengthening of the lower extremity by the Wagner method: A review of the Boston Children's Hospital Experience. *J Bone Joint Surg* 1981;63A:1122–1131.

30. Choi IH, Kumar SJ, Bowen JR: Amputation or limb-lengthening for partial or total absence of the fibula. *J Bone Joint Surg* 1990;72A:1391–1399.

31. Maffuli N, Fixsen JA: Distraction osteogenesis in congenital limb length discrepancy: A review. *J R Coll Surg Edinb* 1996;41:258–264.

32. Catagni MA, Bolano L, Cattaneo R: Management of fibular hemimelia using the Ilizarov method. *Orthop Clin North Am* 1991;22:715–722.

33. Catagni M, Villa A: Video: *Lengthening of the Tibia by the Ilizarov Method.* Milan, Italy, ASAMI, Milan Surgical Video, 1988.

34. Miller LS, Bell DF: Management of congenital fibular deficiency by Ilizarov technique. *J Pediatr Orthop* 1992;12:651–657.

35. Price CT: Editorial: Are we there yet? Management of limb-length inequality. *J Pediatr Orthop* 1996;16:141–143.

36. Gibbons PJ, Bradish CF: Fibular hemimelia: A preliminary report on management of the severe abnormality. *J Pediatr Orthop* 1996;5:20–26.

37. Ghoneem HF, Wright JG, Cole WG, Rang M: The Ilizarov method for correction of complex deformities: Psychological and functional outcomes. *J Bone Joint Surg* 1996;78:1480–1485.

38. Damsin JP, Pous JG, Ghanem I: Therapeutic approach to severe congenital lower limb length discrepancies: Surgical treatment versus prosthetic management. *J Pediatr Orthop* 1995;4:164–170.

39. Thompson TC, Straub LR, Arnold WD: Congenital absence of the fibula. *J Bone Joint Surg* 1957;39A:1229–1237.

40. Boakes JL, Stevens PM, Moseley RF: Treatment of genu valgus deformity in congenital absence of the fibula. *J Pediatr Orthop* 1991;11:721–724.

Chapter 14

Functional Classification of Fibular Deficiency

John G. Birch, MD
Todd L. Lincoln, MD
Philip William Mack, MD

Introduction

Fibular deficiency is a longitudinal deficiency of the lower extremity characterized by a combination of foot deformity, partial or complete absence of the fibula, and variable shortening of the tibia.[1-5] The elements of the deformity are quite variable. The fibula may be absent, rudimentary, or shortened. In the mildest cases, fibular shortening may only be confirmed by a careful comparison with the normal limb.[6-8] The foot may be normal clinically, with normal movement and a full complement of rays, or, at the other extreme, consist only of a rudimentary single digit and hindfoot locked into a severe equinovalgus position. The limb-length discrepancy associated with the disorder varies from clinically insignificant to greater than 30% overall shortening. Many subtle cases likely escape clinical detection, whereas extreme cases of limb shortening and foot deformity have been treated with amputation and prosthetic fitting.[9-15] The classification of fibular deficiency is made more difficult by the frequent association of this disorder with other deformities. The most common of these are femoral deficiency, varying from mild shortening and distal femoral valgus to the more severe forms of congenital femoral deficiency, and upper extremity limb deficiency.

Technically, according to the International Standards Organization (ISO) terminology,[16] this limb deficiency is a longitudinal deficiency of the fibula, partial or complete, depending on whether the fibula is partially or wholly absent. However, when the above described deformity dominates the clinical picture, the terms "fibular deficiency (or hemimelia)" or "partial fibular deficiency (or hemimelia)" appear to be firmly rooted in the orthopaedic literature, so we have elected to refer to this disorder in the familiar terms. For the purposes of brevity and simplification, in this manuscript, we refer to all varieties of this deficiency simply as "fibular deficiency."

For many years in North America, the more severe forms of this disorder have been treated by a combination of amputation at walking age (Syme's or Boyd) and prosthetic fitting.[9-15,17] Such treatment negates the need for management of limb-length inequality by anything more complex than adjusting the length of the prosthesis, and, in patients with severe foot deformity provides a more functional (albeit prosthetic) foot and ankle. With the introduction of more complex and more successful reconstructive procedures, particularly limb lengthening by the Ilizarov method,[18-21] we have witnessed in our patient population a rejuvenated interest in limb salvage. There has long been a resistance to amputation in the management of fibular deficiency in Europe, and a number of reconstructive techniques have been developed[22-24] (Chapter 16).

As these reconstructive techniques have evolved, we have noted that the existing classifications of this disorder have not helped us make treatment decisions or aided in the evaluation of the results of our management. We therefore embarked on an effort to devise a more functional classification of fibular deficiency.

What Is Wrong With Fibular Deficiency Classifications

The purpose of any classification scheme in orthopaedics should be to provide insight into the likely outcome or functional disability associated with a particular disorder, and, ideally, to provide treatment guidelines related to the various categories of the condition. Commonly cited classifications for fibular deficiency include those of Coventry and Johnson,[3] Dal Monte, as described by Catagni and associates,[22] Achterman and Kalamchi,[25] Choi and associates,[26] and Letts and Vincent.[27] Coventry and Johnson[3] classified fibular deficiency as type I (partial, unilateral absence of the fibula), type II (complete, or nearly complete, unilateral absence of the fibula), and type III (type I or II with other congenital deformities, or bilateral).

Achterman and Kalamchi[25] also classified fibular deficiency based on the extent of fibular preservation. Type I has some portion of fibula preserved. It is subdivided into two groups: IA, in which the proximal fibular epiphysis is distal to the level of the tibial growth plate and the distal fibular growth plate is proximal to the dome of the talus, and IB, in which the proximal fibula is 30% to 50% absent, and the distal fibula does not support the ankle. Type II represents limbs in which the fibula was absent or had only a vestigial fragment. The extent of shortening and the function of the foot are not directly addressed by this scheme, although increasing severity with greater hypoplasia or absence of the fibula is implied.

Dal Monte's three-grade classification as described by Catagni and associates[22] is based on the degree of preservation of the fibula, from mildly hypoplastic (grade I) to absent (grade III). He implies that increasing foot deformity, shortening, and femoral deformity parallel increasing hypoplasia of the fibula. Neither Dal Monte's nor Achterman and Kalamchi's classifications include a specific category for bilateral deficiency.

Choi and associates[26] proposed a classification based solely on the percentage of shortening of the limb. Group I has shortening of 15% or less and the foot is at the level of the lower one third of the opposite limb; group II has 16% to 25% shortening with the foot at the level of the middle one third of the opposite limb; and group III has shortening of greater than 25% with the foot at the level of the upper one third of the opposite limb. This classification does not take into consideration the function of the foot, and their review included some patients with congenital femoral deficiency.

More recently, Letts and Vincent[27] proposed a classification based on predicted absolute shortening and foot deformity. Type A includes unilateral deformities with predicted final discrepancy of less than 6 cm, minimal foot deformity, and femoral shortening; type B includes unilateral deformities with 6 to 10 cm of shortening, minimal foot deformity, and femoral shortening; type C includes unilateral deformities with greater than 10 cm of shortening and major foot and femoral deformities; and type D are bilateral cases.

We have noticed in the patients we have treated at Texas Scottish Rite Hospital for Children (TSRH) that none of these classifications specifically helps us make treatment decisions. For example, we have encountered patients with an absent fibula without major shortening or foot deformity. Therefore, we have found that the classifications of Coventry and Johnson,[3] Achterman and Kalamchi,[25] and Dal Monte by Catagni and associates[22] are not helpful in determining the best treatment for these patients. In addition, some femoral deformity is almost invariably present, contributing to the overall shortening encountered, but is not considered in these three classifications.

The classification of Choi and associates[26] considers overall percentage shortening but does not consider foot function. Their review included patients with congenital femoral deficiency. We believe that such patients present quite different management problems related not only to the more severe shortening but also to hip and often knee dysfunction, and thus should not be included in a classification of fibular deficiency.

The classification scheme proposed by Letts and Vincent[27] is similar to that which we propose here with some exceptions. We believe that percentage shortening is the more appropriate method for quantifying limb-length inequality whenever lengthening procedures are considered. In addition, we place more emphasis on the function of the foot, and do not believe that patients with bilateral deficiency should be considered in a separate category from patients with unilateral deficiency. We, therefore, decided to review our experience to determine if a more satisfactory classification scheme, aimed at aiding clinical decision-making, could be devised.

Review of the TSRH Patient Population

We reviewed the records and radiographs of all patients with the diagnosis of fibular deficiency treated at Texas Scottish Rite Hospital for Children between 1957 and 1996. We excluded patients who did not have radiographs of both lower extremities adequate to qualify the extent of deformity. We also excluded patients whose predominant deformity was congenital femoral deficiency variants, such as Pappas types I-V[28] or Gillespie types B and C (Chapter 6), in whom dysfunction of the hip and major femoral shortening were the major deficiency, and patients with one of the generalized short-stature syndromes associated with variants of fibular deficiency (Chapter 4).

Radiographs were assessed for femoral shortening and deformity, fibular length, level of the distal fibular physis relative to the ankle mortise, ankle shape, foot position, and number of metatarsals present. Absolute and relative percentage measurements of the femur, tibia, and overall length were taken from plain radiographs or serial scanograms when available. Clinical photographs of the deformity were assessed when available. The medical chart was reviewed, with particular emphasis on the description of the deformity (especially the foot), all treatment rendered, and the functional status of the patient.

A total of 146 extremities in 122 patients with adequate records and radiographs met the criteria for inclusion in this study. Definitive management has been completed in 82 limbs (65 patients) at the time of this review, 52 patients are skeletally immature and/or undergoing treatment, and five patients were lost to follow-up prior to definitive management. A review of our observations in these patients confirmed our initial premises, ie, there were many instances where the severity of fibular hypoplasia did not correlate with the severity of limb shortening or foot deformity, and shortening and its management were determined by the combination of femoral and tibial shortening, rather than that of the tibia only. Therefore, we were motivated to attempt to devise a more clinically relevant classification scheme for the limb deficiency characterized as "fibular deficiency."

Outline of New Classification Scheme of Fibular Deficiency

The classification scheme can be thought of as the process of asking two fundamental questions for each limb. No specific consideration is given as to whether the deformity is bilateral or unilateral or to the degree of fibular hypoplasia, because they are not relevant to the classification scheme or clinical management. First, is the foot functional? We define a functional foot as one with three or more rays (metatarsals) that is plantigrade or has a correctable contracture. If the foot is functional, the second question is, what is the overall extent of limb-length discrepancy (irrespective of unilateral or bilateral deficiency). If the foot is not functional, ablation will be considered unless there are upper extremity deficiencies requiring foot use to replace hand function.

The division of type I (functional foot) into subgroups is based on overall limb-length discrepancy expressed as a percentage of the opposite side. There are four divisions, based on current probable treatment requirements to equalize limb-length inequality. Type IA has shortening of 5% or less. Patients in this group usually require no treatment, shoelift, or epiphysiodesis, depending on absolute shortening and functional implication in individual patients. Type IB patients have 6% to 10% shortening and require equalization of limb length by epiphysiodesis or a single lengthening. Type IC patients have shortening of 10% to 30%, which requires a minimum of two staged lengthenings with or without contralateral epiphysiodesis. In selected patients, depending on surgeon and parental wishes, early amputation might be appropriate. Type ID patients have shortening greater than 30%. These patients require "heroic" reconstruction with multiple lengthenings; early amputation is a strong alternative consideration.

Type II patients (nonfunctional foot) are subdivided into two groups. Type IIA patients have functional upper extremities and do not require the use of a foot remnant for prehension. In these patients, early amputation is advised. Type IIB patients also have a rudimentary foot, but associated upper extremity deficiencies require, or potentially require the use of the foot remnant for prehension. In such patients, recommendation for amputation is deferred until the pattern of foot use is established. The proposed functional classification scheme with treatment guidelines is summarized in Table 1.

Analysis of TSRH Patient Population Using the Proposed Classification Scheme

The total number of cases identified as meeting the radiographic and clinical criteria for inclusion in the study was 146 limbs in 122 patients. Based on the presence or absence of a functional foot, 117 limbs were classified as type I (functional foot) and 29 as type II (nonfunctional foot). Based on radiographic measurements of the 117 type I extremities, 53 were type IA, 32 were type IB, 29 were type IC, and one was type ID. Of the 29 type II extremities, 28 were type IIA (functional upper extremities) and one was type IIB (nonfunctional upper extremities).

Twenty-four patients had bilateral lower extremity involvement. Twenty of 48 feet in this group were considered nonfunctional and underwent early amputation. Most of the remainder of patients with bilateral involvement were classified as type IA, ie, with clinically insignificant limb-length inequality. They were, however, relatively short by virtue of the bilateral shortening.

Fibular length measured greater than 50% of expected length in 76 extremities and less than 50% in six; the fibula was entirely absent in 63, and could not be accurately measured in one. Seventy-four of the 76 extremities with fibular length greater than 50%, five of six with fibular length less than 50%, and 36 of 63 with absent fibula had functional feet (type I).

Overall limb-length inequality correlated with the extent of fibula present. Of the 76 extremities with fibular length greater than 50%, 42 were type IA, 28 type IB, and three type IC. In contrast, of the 36 type I extremities with no fibula, 11 were type IA, three type IB, 21 type IC, and one type ID.

The number of rays present in the foot correlated directly with foot salvage in this group. There were 42 feet with five rays, 46 with four rays, 44 with three rays, and ten with two rays or less. One hundred percent of feet with five rays, 90% of those with four rays, and 64% of those with three rays

Table 1 Functional classification of fibular deficiency with treatment guidelines for each group

Classification	Treatment
Type I: Functional foot	
IA 0 to 5% inequality	Orthosis/epiphysiodesis
IB 6% to 10% inequality	Epiphysiodesis ± lengthening
IC 11% to 30% inequality	1 to 2 lengthenings (or amputation)
ID > 30% inequality	> 2 lengthenings versus amputation
Type II: Nonfunctional foot	
IIA Functional upper extremity	Early amputation
IIB Nonfunctional upper extremity	Consider salvage

were salvaged as functional feet. No foot with two rays or less was salvaged in this group. All feet with less than three rays were associated with an absent fibula.

Femoral shortening was noted in 50% of cases. As could be expected, there was a direct correlation between the extent of femoral shortening and the overall shortening of the extremity. There was no correlation between the extent of femoral shortening and the likelihood of a nonfunctional foot. Furthermore, the ratio of femoral-to-tibial shortening had no impact on treatment decisions.

Definitive Management in the TSRH Population

Sixty-five patients with 82 affected extremities from the above-discussed group have completed definitive management at our institution. Forty-three extremities were treated by foot salvage, and 39 by Syme's amputation. In general, definitive treatment correlated well with our proposed guidelines.

Of 30 type IA limbs (shortening 5% or less), nine extremities required no treatment, seven required surgery to improve foot position, 13 required contralateral epiphysiodesis, and one underwent Syme's amputation. Of 11 type IB limbs (6% to 10% shortening) one had no treatment, seven had contralateral epiphysiodesis, two had lengthening, and one had a Syme's amputation. There were 12 type IC limbs (10% to 30% shortening). Three had lengthening, and nine had Syme's amputation. The single patient with a type ID limb (> 30% shortening) had a Syme's amputation.

All 27 type IIA extremities (nonfunctional foot with functional upper extremities) had Syme's amputations. The single type IIB extremity (nonfunctional foot required for prehension) underwent tibial osteotomy to improve position; the foot was preserved.

Other Findings From TSRH Patient Population Review

In the entire group of patients, the male:female ratio was 1.6:1. There was no appreciable difference in this distribution within the classification groups.

Twenty-seven of the 122 patients had some associated upper extremity anomaly, ranging from simple syndactyly to amelia. Upper extremity involvement was seen with equal frequency in unilateral and bilateral lower extremity cases and did not correlate with the extent of foot deformity. Whenever there was unilateral upper and lower extremity involvement, the ipsilateral limbs were affected.

Feet were typically in a plantigrade, valgus, or equinovalgus position. However, there were 12 feet with equinovarus deformity, ie, these cases represented fibular deficiency with a clubfoot. Clubfeet were seen in all classification groups and did not confer prognostic significance.

Discussion

The spectrum of severity of deformity associated with the term "fibular deficiency" is broad, varying from clinically insignificant to cases with severe deformity and shortening that render the affected extremity nonfunctional without treatment. In addition, there are many subtle and not-so-subtle deformities associated with this condition that impact treatment decisions. These deformities include size and position of the foot, femoral shortening, proximal and distal femoral deformity, and upper extremity deficiency. While these associated deformities impact treatment of patients with fibular deficiency, they largely have not been taken into consideration in previous classification schemes in which fibular deficiency is the predominant deformity.

The role of early Syme's or Boyd amputation in cases of severe shortening or foot deformity has been clearly established by previous studies.[9–15] Patients so treated spend a minimum of time hospitalized, require no more than prosthetic adjustment to compensate for limb-length inequality, and lead functional, well-adjusted lifestyles as children.[13–15] Whether they will continue to do so as adults, and whether attempts to salvage more severely-affected limbs with multiple lengthenings and reconstructions can provide comparable, cost-effective results remains to be determined. Nevertheless, parental resistance to early amputation, always present and the norm in Europe, appears to be increasing as the lay press and early published series[18–24] suggest that limb salvage by staged lengthenings is feasible.

Clearly, with the appreciation of the Ilizarov method of limb lengthening, more limbs affected with fibular deficiency can and perhaps should be subjected to reconstruction rather than foot ablation. The boundary between these two extraordinarily different treatments is difficult to define, but our proposed classification (Table 1) is designed to aid in that definition. Most publications regard lengthening of the lower extremity as regularly achievable when the discrepancy is 15% to 20%, whereas lengthening becomes progressively more difficult as the surgeon attempts to correct 30% shortening or more. This experience forms the basis for our subdivision of type I patients (Table 1).

We began this work because we found that the exisiting classifications of fibular deficiency did not help us make decisions about managing the patient's deformities. A major problem with the current classifications is that they do not address overall shortening of the limb, which is one of the most important factors to consider in management. Half of our group of patients had shortening of the femur, which added to the limb-length discrepancy. In addition, these classifications imply a relationship between the length of the fibula and the severity of the deformity, and in our cases the fibular length did not predict the severity of the deformity. For example, more than half of our patients with a completely absent fibula had a salvageable lower extremity with a functional foot.

In this retrospective study, 82 extremities have completed definitive treatment. Of these, one of 30 type IA and one of 11 type IB extremities were treated by Syme's amputation. We consider it likely that, in the current era of limb lengthening, these extremities would have had treatment other than amputation. Furthermore, nine of 12 type IC extremities underwent Syme's amputation. We believe that the patients with a type IC deformity (shortening between 10% and 30%) still represent a gray area, and that in some of these patients, amputation is preferable to a prolonged course of reconstruction.

This proposed classification scheme has many shortcomings. First, and perhaps foremost, it does not strictly adhere to ISO-recommended nomenclature for limb deficiency. However, the term "fibular deficiency," despite encompassing a wide spectrum of deformity, is also vividly recognized and understood within the orthopaedic community, with little, if any, confusion as to what type of deformity the term implies (except as to severity in individual cases). Therefore, we have not discarded it.

Perhaps more difficult is defining a "functional foot." For our purposes, we defined that as a foot which was or could be made plantigrade, with three or more rays. In fact, this definition served us well in that there was a direct correlation between the number of rays and the likelihood of foot preservation in this patient population, with 100% of five-rayed feet, and 0% of feet two-rayed or less being preserved.

The most difficult problem, however, is to determine whether limb salvage through multiple stages of lengthening and/or deformity correction or early foot ablation with prosthetic fitting is the appropriate management for individual patients. Patients with less than 10% shortening may choose a lengthening as the method to correct limb length inequality, but are not obligated to, and are most unlikely to require more than one stage of such treatment. Patients with between 10% and 30% shortening will require lengthening, and as the deformity becomes more severe, multiple stages of such treatment become more likely. We have, based on our own experience and that of others, labeled limb preservation in the presence of > 30% shortening as "heroic," implying that many (perhaps up to three to five) stages of lengthening and deformity correction would be required. In our institution, we prefer to recommend early amputation instead.

Defining the boundary between staged reconstructive procedures and early amputation in patients with more severe deformity is likely to remain a matter of philosophy and debate. That boundary is also likely to change as techniques of limb lengthening improve and become more certain in outcome and less onerous on the patient and family. It would be helpful to have some "tool" to guide the physician and family as to which course to follow, avoiding an ambitious multistage treatment failure or an unnecessary foot ablation.

Conclusion

We propose a new functional classification of fibular hemimelia based on a review of experience in patients with the disorder treated at Texas Scottish Rite Hospital for Children between 1957 and 1996. The classification is based on two questions. Is the foot functional? If the foot is functional, what is the extent of shortening compared to the contralateral limb, expressed as a percentage?

If the foot is not functional, is there concomitant upper extremity deficiency that prevents prehension? If not, then early foot ablation is recommended. If upper extremity deformity prevents prehension, a decision to amputate must be deferred. While such a condition is rare in our experience (one case in 122), the point is well worth making, because the need for prehension supersedes all other considerations in lower extremity function and reconstruction.

References

1. Arnold WD: Congenital absence of the fibula. *Clin Orthop* 1959;14:20–29.

2. Farmer AW, Laurin CA: Congenital absence of the fibula. *J Bone Joint Surg* 1960;42A:1–12.

3. Coventry MB, Johnson EW Jr: Congenital absence of the fibula. *J Bone Joint Surg* 1952;34A:941–956.

4. Amstutz HC: Abstract: Natural history and treatment of congenital absence of the fibula. *J Bone Joint Surg* 1972;54A:1349.

5. Hootnick D, Boyd NA, Fixsen JA, Lloyd-Roberts GC: The natural history and management of congenital short tibia with dysplasia or absence of the fibula. *J Bone Joint Surg* 1977;59B:267–271.

6. Bohne WH, Root L: Hypoplasia of the fibula. *Clin Orthop* 1977;125:107–112.

7. Maffulli N, Fixsen JA: Fibular hypoplasia with absent lateral rays of the foot. *J Bone Joint Surg* 1991;73B:1002–1004.

8. Maffulli N, Fixsen JA: Management of forme fruste fibular hemimelia. *J Pediatr Orthop* 1996;5B:17–19.

9. Kruger LM, Talbott RD: Amputation and prosthesis as definitive treatment in congenital absence of the fibula. *J Bone Joint Surg* 1961;43A:625–642.

10. Eilert RE, Jayakumar SS: Boyd and Syme ankle amputations in children. *J Bone Joint Surg* 1976;58A:1138–1141.

11. Westin GW, Sakai DN, Wood WL: Congenital longitudinal deficiency of the fibula: Follow-up of treatment by Syme amputation. *J Bone Joint Surg* 1976;58A:492–496.

12. Anderson L, Westin GW, Oppenheim WL: Syme amputation in children: Indications, results, and long-term follow-up. *J Pediatr Orthop* 1984;4:550–554.

13. Herring JA, Barnhill B, Gaffney C: Syme amputation: An evaluation of the physical and psychological function in young patients. *J Bone Joint Surg* 1986;68A:573–578.

14. Epps CH Jr, Schneider PL: Treatment of hemimelias of the lower extremity: Long-term results. *J Bone Joint Surg* 1989;71A:273–277.

15. Herring JA: Symes amputation for fibular hemimelia: A second look in the Ilizarov era, in Eilert RE (ed): *Instructional Course Lectures XLI*. Park Ridge, IL, American Academy of Orthopaedic Surgeons, 1992, pp 435–436.

16. Schuch CM, Pritham CH: International standards organization terminology: Application to prosthetics and orthotics. *J Prosthet Orthot* 1994;6:29–33.

17. Naudie D, Hamdy RC, Fassier F, Morin B, Duhaime M: Management of fibular hemimelia: Amputation or limb lengthening. *J Bone Joint Surg* 1997;79B:58–65.

18. Dal Monte A, Donzelli O: Tibial lengthening according to Ilizarov in congenital hypoplasia of the leg. *J Pediatr Orthop* 1987;7:135–138.

19. Miller LS, Bell DF: Management of congenital fibular deficiency by Ilizarov technique. *J Pediatr Orthop* 1992;12:651–657.

20. Gibbons PJ, Bradish CF: Fibular hemimelia: A preliminary report on management of the severe abnormality. *J Pediatr Orthop* 1996;5B:20–26.

21. Stanitski DF, Shahcheraghi H, Nicker DA, Armstrong PF: Results of tibial lengthening with the Ilizarov technique. *J Pediatr Orthop* 1996;16:168–172.

22. Catagni MA, Bolano L, Cattaneo R: Management of fibular hemimelia using the Ilizarov method. *Orthop Clin North Am* 1991;22:715–722.

23. Catagni MA: Management of fibular hemimelia using the Ilizarov method, in Eilert RE (ed): *Instructional Course Lectures XLI*. Park Ridge, IL, American Academy of Orthopaedic Surgeons, 1992, pp 431–434.

24. Boakes JL, Stevens PM, Moseley RF: Treatment of genu valgus deformity in congenital absence of the fibula. *J Pediatr Orthop* 1991;11:721–724.

25. Achterman C, Kalamchi A: Congential deficiency of the fibula. *J Bone Joint Surg* 1979;61B;133–137.

26. Choi IH, Kumar SJ, Bowen JR: Amputation or limb-lengthening for partial or total absence of the fibula. *J Bone Joint Surg* 1990;72A:1391–1399.

27. Letts M, Vincent N: Congenital longitudinal deficiency of the fibula (fibular hemimelia): Parental refusal of amputation. *Clin Orthop* 1993;287:160–166.

28. Pappas AM: Congenital abnormalities of the femur and related lower extremity malformations: Classification and treatment. *J Pediatr Orthop* 1983;3:45–60.

Consensus

Classification of Fibular Deficiency

Current classifications are inadequate because there is (1) too much emphasis on the presence or absence of the fibula, (2) not enough emphasis on the anatomy and function of the foot and ankle, (3) not enough emphasis on limb-length inequality, and (4) no consideration of the upper limbs. International terminology is descriptive, but it is not oriented toward treatment.

A new classification oriented toward management should consider the parameters listed in Outline 1. Function should include both childhood and adult function, and an overall score would be useful.

Outline 1 Parameters for management-oriented classification

A. Percentage of limb-length discrepancy in childhood and the predicted segmental and total discrepancy at maturity
   1. < 5%
   2. 6% to 10%
   3. 11% to 20%
   4. 21% to 30%
   5. > 30%
B. The deformity of the tibia
   1. Angulation < 30°
   2. Angulation > 30°
D. The orientation and stability of the ankle
   1. Ball and socket with > 20° of motion
   2. Stiff ball and socket
   3. Severe equinovalgus deformity
E. The ray* deformity of the foot
   1. 4, 5 rays
   2. 3 rays
   3. < 3 rays
F. An upper extremity absence that may require foot prehension contraindicates amputation

* Ray = at least a metatarsal or most of a metatarsal

Chapter 15

Comparison of Functional Outcome in Fibular Deficiency Treated by Limb Salvage Versus Syme's Amputation

Charles E. Johnston II, MD
Nasreen F. Haideri, ME

The case for Syme's amputation in the treatment of moderate to severe fibular deficiency is well known and widely accepted. Ablation of the foot and prosthetic management is attractive from a treatment perspective for its simplicity, lack of morbidity, and its definitiveness with infrequent need for revision or further surgery.

Herring and Birch (unpublished data, 1997) have reported excellent functional and psychological outcomes over a long follow-up of children with Syme's ankle disarticulation. They believe that amputation with prosthetic fitting just prior to normal walking age is important for this approach to be successful, because normal ambulatory milestones are achieved with the prosthesis.

Surgical reconstruction and lengthening of fibular deficiency of equivalent severity often involves several surgical procedures that involve frequent and sometimes long hospitalizations with functional and psychological outcomes yet to be determined by any long-term study. Nevertheless, in patients with a unilateral, predominantly lower-segment deformity, a functional foot, and predicted shortening of less than 20%, surgical reconstruction is not only possible but generally attempted, because it is more desirable to both parents and surgeon.

Guidelines are needed to offer optimal management for patients with "gray zone" deficiencies, who are possible candidates for either amputation or reconstruction because of an extremity with, for example, 30% shortening, a three-rayed foot that has "mild" valgus and equinus positioning, and no other significant orthopaedic deformities. In an attempt to objectively evaluate the functional outcome of these two radically different treatment options, we compared the gait and muscle strength of patients who had undergone tibial lengthening and reconstruction for fibular deficiency to those of patients who had been treated by Syme's amputation.

Materials and Methods

Ten patients, six with Syme's amputations and four with limb salvage/lengthening, were evaluated in the Texas Scottish Rite Hospital Movement Science Laboratory, where they underwent gait analysis and Cybex muscle testing. All six patients with amputations had severe tibial shortening (> 30% shorter than the contralateral segment) and three-rayed feet in "fixed" equinovalgus. All underwent ablation at 11 months of age or younger. They were fitted with standard Syme's prostheses at walking age. Four of the six had undergone further surgery (osteotomy, hemiepiphysiodesis, or hemiepiphyseal stapling) for either progressive anterior bowing or valgus that was affecting prosthetic function. At the time of gait study, the patients ranged from 5 years 10 months to 14 years 7 months old, and were from 5 to 13.5 years postamputation.

Four patients underwent tibial lengthening. One patient had two lengthening sessions, one with additional angular correction, for an Achterman I-B[1]/Birch I-D (chapter 14) deformity, eventually achieving 11 cm of lengthening. The other three patients, all with Achterman I-A/Birch I-B or I-C deformities, had a single lengthening of 5 to 9 cm. At the time of study, these patients ranged from 15 to 27 years of age, and were 1 to 11 years post-treatment.

Results

Isokinetic Testing

Muscle strength determination for the knee and ankle were adjusted for age and body weight. The affected limb was more than 50% weaker (21 versus 45 ft/lbs, $p = 0.006$) in plantarflexion (PF) compared to the normal limb in the patients with tibial lengthening. For obvious reasons, no PF strength determinations were possible in the patients with Syme's amputation. At the knee, extension strength in the normal limb was significantly greater compared to the affected limb in both patients with Syme's amputation ($p = 0.003$) and lengthening ($p = 0.015$). Flexion strength in the normal limb was also significantly greater than in the affected limb in patients with Syme's amputation ($p = 0.014$) and patients with lengthening ($p = 0.002$). When comparing the affected limbs of the two groups, lengthened limbs had greater knee flexion strength than limbs with Syme's amputation ($p = 0.006$), while there was no difference in extension strength.

Kinematics

Patients with tibial lengthening demonstrated foot drops in their affected limbs, combined with loss of dorsiflexion (DF) during stance phase (Fig. 1). At the knee, patients with lengthening showed mild hyperextension in stance, secondary to this lack of DF. No unusual sagittal plane kinematics were seen in the affected limbs of patients with Syme's amputation, but they

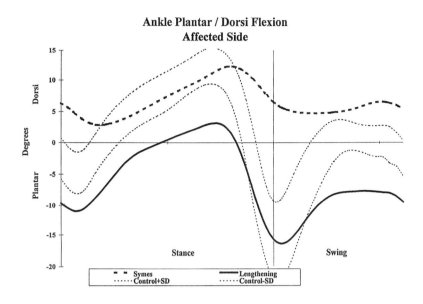

Fig. 1 *Ankle kinematics (sagittal plane) for affected limbs.*

had increased PF at toe-off on the normal side, presumably to compensate for the lack of ankle power on the prosthetic side. Both groups demonstrated a mild increase in stance phase pelvic obliquity, caused by residual shortening, on the affected side.

The main kinematic problem noted for patients with Syme's amputation was increased knee valgus on the affected side (Fig. 2), often in spite of treatment. Persistent tibia valga or lateral knee instability resulting from hypoplasia of the lateral femoral condyle are probable explanations. Angular deformity was not seen in patients with lengthening ($p = 0.05$). The normal limbs in both groups were without deformity.

Kinetics

Power generation (ankle push-off, Fig. 3) on the affected side was significantly less than on the normal side in Syme's limbs ($p = 0.001$), whereas in lengthened limbs there was less ($p = 0.09$) difference. The affected ankle in patients with lengthened limbs also did significantly more work than the ankles in patients with Syme's ($p = 0.003$). Because of the lack of ankle power in limbs with Syme's amputation, the affected hip performed more work than the normal hip ($p = 0.012$), presumably to compensate. The normal hips in patients with lengthened limbs, on the other hand, produced more power and performed more work than the hip on the affected side ($p = 0.048$).

175

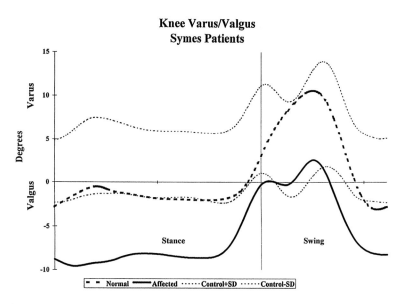

Fig. 2 *Knee kinematics (frontal plane) in patients with Syme's amputation.*

Discussion

Kinematic and kinetic comparison of limb function in these two treatment groups must be cautiously interpreted because of the small number of patients and the difference in severity of the limb deficiency before treatment. The patients with Syme's amputation uniformly had severe shortening and nonfunctional feet, while three of four patients who underwent limb lengthening had much less severe involvement. It appears, however, that while lengthened limbs are significantly less strong than their normal contralateral counterparts, they are at least as strong as or stronger than limbs having foot ablation. Even though lengthened limbs showed stiffness (loss of DF in stance) and foot-drop (tibialis anterior weakness secondary to lengthening), these ankles still produced sufficient power so that they were not significantly different from those of the normal limb, and clearly were more functional than a prosthetic "ankle" for push-off. It should be noted that the total power generation of the entire Syme's limb was no different than the total power of the lengthened limbs, because the hip on the extremity with a Syme's amputation made up for the lack of ankle push-off by producing significantly more power than the normal hip. This probably explains, in conjunction with good knee extension function, why patients with Syme's amputation qualitatively have little or no functional problems.[2]

The significant valgus deformity of the tibia in patients with Syme's amputation is of uncertain functional implication. It frequently can affect prosthetic function and fit and then must be treated. This deformity was not

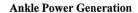

Ankle Power Generation

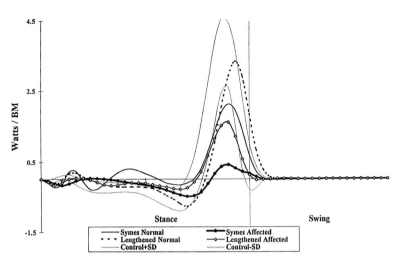

Fig. 3 *Ankle power generation (BW = body weight) during gait. Peak power generation, beginning at heel-off, was significantly reduced in both groups when comparing affected versus normal limbs.*

seen in lengthened tibias, because the frontal plane alignment was corrected simultaneously with lengthening by the external fixator.

It would appear that functional outcome for patients with milder degrees of fibular deficiency treated with limb salvage and lengthening/reconstruction is at least as good, if not better, than that of patients treated with amputation and prosthetic fitting. Considering the total cost of all the Syme's prostheses that a child fitted at age 1 year would go through by age 18 (approximately $81,000) (D Cummings, CP, personal communication), and the estimated cost of surgical reconstruction per treatment session ($40,000 to $50,000), there is ample justification from a cost analysis alone to pursue limb salvage procedures if the reconstruction can be completed in no more than two treatment sessions.

References

1. Achterman C, Kalamchi A: Congenital deficiency of the fibula. *J Bone Joint Surg* 1979;61B:133–137.
2. Herring JA: Symes amputation for fibular hemimelia: A second look in the Ilizarov era, in Eilert RE (ed): *Instructional Course Lectures XLI*. Park Ridge, IL, American Academy of Orthopaedic Surgeons, 1992, pp 435–436.

Chapter 16

Management of Fibular Hemimelia Using the Ilizarov Method

Maurizio A. Catagni, MD
Francesco Guerreschi, MD

Introduction

The term fibular hemimelia encompasses a broad spectrum of congenital limb deficiency, characterized in all cases by variable limb shortening, fibular hypoplasia or absence, and foot deficiency and deformity.[1–4] The more severe varieties can be successfully treated with foot ablation by Syme's or Boyd amputation combined with prosthetic fitting.[5–10] Traditionally there has been cultural resistance to amputation in Italy, however, and this treatment is rarely accepted in our country.[11,12] The introduction to Italy in 1981 of Ilizarov's external fixator, and more importantly, his method of limb lengthening has greatly changed management of fibular hemimelia, particularly for the more severe forms of this congenital anomaly.[13–18] This chapter presents a classification of this disorder modified from that of Dal Monte and Donzelli,[19] outlines my treatment program for the management of this severe congenital limb deficiency, and presents results of treatment to date using the Ilizarov method.

Characteristics of Fibular Hemimelia Deformity

Fibular hemimelia often is associated with many other anomalies of the same and other limbs. For example, patients with proximal femoral focal deficiency frequently have fibular hemimelia as well. However, a distinction is made between patients with predominantly proximal femoral focal deficiency and those with predominantly fibular hemimelia because the clinical problems requiring reconstruction are different in these two groups. Patients with predominantly congenital short femur deformity with severe acetabular dysplasia or proximal femoral focal deficiency represent a therapeutic challenge and functional deficit distinct from those patients in whom the features of fibular hemimelia predominate. The management of such patients is not within the scope of this chapter, and the reader is referred to the chapters by Gillespie, Brown, Steel, and Paley.

Fibular hemimelia has many components contributing to the overall deformity. When treatment is aimed at reconstruction, particularly when lengthening is required, the presence, severity, and functional impact of all of these deformities must be considered. Potential deformities are listed in Outline 1.

Acetabular dysplasia in patients with fibular hemimelia is usually not as severe as in patients with predominantly congenital short femur or proximal femoral focal deficiency. However, hip range of motion, stability, and radiographic acetabular dysplasia must be carefully assessed in patients who will require femoral lengthening as part of their reconstruction, because patients with hip abnormalities are at greater risk for hip subluxation as a complication of femoral lengthening. Patients with more severe acetabular dysplasia may require a preliminary acetabular reconstruction prior to femoral lengthening. Proximal femoral valgus, with or without shortening of the femoral neck, usually does not require reconstruction. Occasionally, patients will have proximal femoral varus with or without associated acetabular dysplasia. We believe that correction of proximal femoral varus should be deferred until the final stage of deformity correction and lengthening of the femur, because the proximal varus may help prevent the complication of hip subluxation.

The amount of ipsilateral femoral shortening varies from minimal to being responsible for a significant amount of the overall limb shortening. In the latter circumstance, one or more femoral lengthenings may be a required component of the limb reconstruction plan.

Distal femoral valgus secondary to lateral femoral condylar hypoplasia is virtually universally present in patients with fibular hemimelia. Only in the mildest cases of femoral deformity can this be ignored, because subsequent tibial lengthening will aggravate the valgus appearance, or alternatively, valgus deformity corrected at the level of the proximal tibia will result in knee joint obliquity. The valgus deformity can be corrected simultaneously with lengthening of the femur.

Typically, the femur has excessive external rotation as well. This deformity, particularly when combined with distal femoral valgus, can result in patellar instability that may require correction by a combination of valgus and rotational deformity correction and patellar stabilization procedures. The more common clinically significant instability of the knee, however, is anteroposterior femorotibial instability due to hypoplastic or absence cruciate ligaments, particularly the anterior cruciate ligament. Radiographically, this is evidenced by hypoplasia of the tibial eminence. Clinically, in the untreated child and adolescent, instability at the knee is only a rare complaint. However, this instability places the knee at risk for subluxation (usually posteriorly) with lengthening, particularly of the femur. The risk of knee subluxation during lengthening must carefully be assessed by the treating surgeon preoperatively and during the course of lengthening. Prophylactic stabilization of the knee joint by extension of the apparatus across it is sometimes advisable, and reduction of the knee joint by extension of the apparatus and correction of the deformity is required if subluxation occurs during lengthening.

The predominant shortening of the limb in patients with fibular hemimelia is typically in the tibia. The extent of such shortening is a sig-

Outline 1 Potential deformities in fibular hemimelia

Femur:	Acetabular dysplasia
	Proximal femoral valgus, or occasionally, varus
	Femoral shortening
	Distal femoral valgus (lateral femoral condyle hypoplasia)
Knee:	Ligamentous laxity with potential patellofemoral or femoral–tibial instability
Tibia:	Shortening
	Proximal, diaphyseal, and/or distal valgus deformity
Fibula:	Hypoplasia
	Absence
Ankle:	Lateral malleolar absence or extreme hypoplasia with potential instability
	Ball-and-socket ankle joint
Foot:	Equinovalgus deformity
	Valgus hindfoot
	Absence of one or more lateral rays of the foot

nificant component of the overall deformity and will, in large part, dictate the extent of reconstructive procedures required to normalize the affected limb. Thus, anywhere from one to four lengthenings over many years will be required. Proximal, diaphyseal, and/or distal tibial valgus deformity often is present along with shortening, but these deformities usually are managed easily by appropriately planned corticotomies (low energy percutaneous osteotomy) that allow simultaneous lengthening and deformity correction.

By definition, the fibula in fibular hemimelia or deficiency is hypoplastic, rudimentary, or completely absent. The hypoplastic or rudimentary fibula often is associated with the development of a ball-and-socket ankle joint (Fig. 1). If stable and asymptomatic, these deformities usually do not require reconstruction. In a young patient with an unstable ankle however, the fibula may be lengthened distally to provide a more normal ankle mortise (Figs. 2 and 3). This reconstruction can be combined with tibial lengthening or performed as a separate reconstructive procedure.

Patients with a completely absent fibula usually have a flat distal tibial articular surface, which may point in a posterolateral direction. These patients are at risk for joint subluxation or aggravation of the deformity during tibial lengthening, and they almost always require foot and ankle stabilization during tibial lengthening to prevent such subluxation from occurring. Occasionally, tibiotalar fusion may be required as a final stage of reconstruction for stiffness or deformity associated with pain in the ankle.

In fibular hemimelia, the foot invariably is involved in the overall deformity, including shortening, except in the mildest cases. In most cases, one or two lateral rays are missing, and the foot has a mild valgus. In severe cases, there may be only one or two rays present, and the foot will appear dislocat-

181

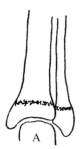 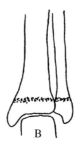 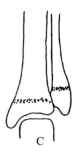

Fig. 1 *Different stages of ball-and-socket ankle joints. Type C is indicated for distal translation of the fibular remnant. (Reproduced with permission from Catagni MA: Management of fibular hemimelia using the Ilizarov method, in Eilert RE (ed):* Instructional Course Lectures XLI. *Park Ridge, IL, American Academy of Orthopaedic Surgeons, 1992, pp 431–434.)*

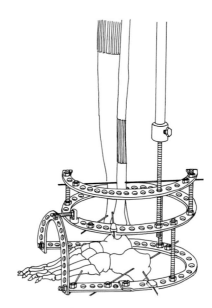

Fig. 2 *Scheme for reconstruction and stabilization of the ankle joint mortise in partial fibular hemimelia during distal fibula translation. The fibula is translated distally using the anteroposterior wire on the half ring.*

ed because of the severe associated distal tibial deformity in an equinovalgus position, aggravated by soft-tissue contracture of the posterior and peroneal muscle compartments. Milder cases may require distal tibial angular defor-

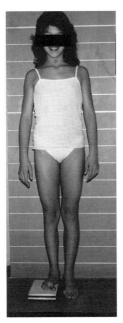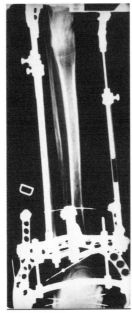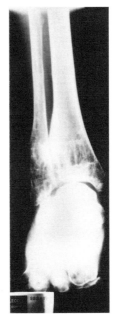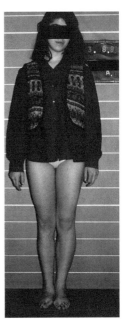

*Fig. 3 A, Preoperative clinical photograph of patient with type C fibular remnant. **B,** Anteroposterior (AP) radiograph of tibia during lengthening and distal fibular remnant transfer. **C,** AP radiograph of ankle after reconstruction. **D,** Postoperative clinical appearance.*

mity correction or calcaneal osteotomy. Severe cases may require early soft-tissue release with or without tibial osteotomy to bring the foot into a plantigrade position. Such feet will require stabilization in the Ilizarov apparatus during subsequent tibial lengthenings. We do not, as a rule, attempt to increase the volume of the foot by longitudinal or transverse lengthenings of the foot remnant, but instead prefer to use a shoe filler if the patient encounters difficulty with shoe wear.

All of the above deformities can be present in patients with fibular hemimelia to different degrees and in variable combinations. Those combinations dictate the overall severity of the deformity and the reconstructive treatment course to be undertaken. We find Dal Monte's and Donzelli's[19] division into three grades of severity to be a useful descriptive classification scheme on which to base a reconstructive treatment outline.

Modified Dal Monte Classification of Fibular Hemimelia

Grade I Fibular Hemimelia

Grade I fibular hemimelia (Fig. 4, *A*) is the mildest form characterized by mild shortening of the fibula and tibia. Usually, angular tibial deformity, femoral deformity, and joint instability (knee and ankle) are mild or absent. Lower extremity shortening is also mild, typically 3 to 5 cm at skeletal maturity. The ankle may be ball-and-socket shaped but is stable. A lateral ray may be absent, but this is not functionally significant.

Grade II Fibular Hemimelia

Grade II fibular hemimelia (Fig. 4, *B*) is a more severe deformity than grade I; it consists of severe fibular hypoplasia and more severe tibial shortening. Typically, there is no functional lateral malleolus. The foot often is deformed with equinovalgus of the ankle and absence of one or two lateral rays. The tibia frequently has proximal and/or distal valgus with some anterior bow (procurvatum). The femur frequently is involved with shortening and/or hypoplasia of the lateral condyle.

Grade III Fibular Hemimelia

Grade III fibular hemimelia (Fig. 4, *C*) represents the most severe form of this disorder. The fibula is rudimentary or completely absent; the tibia is extremely short, and typically is severely deformed as well. The foot is in severe equinovalgus, often accentuated by the anteromedial angular deformity of the tibia, or frankly dislocated from the ankle mortise. The femur is typically shortened with a variable amount of distal valgus and lateral femoral condylar hypoplasia. There may be mediolateral and anteroposterior knee instability, and external rotational deformity of the thigh, femoral neck deformity, and acetabular dysplasia.

Reconstructive Treatment Schemes for Fibular Hemimelia

There are many reasons why we prefer to use the Ilizarov apparatus for reconstructive procedures involving angular deformity correction and/or lengthening for the management of patients with fibular hemimelia. The most important of these reasons include the ability to construct the apparatus so as to imitate the complex, multilevel deformity typically present in these patients as the first step in deformity correction, and the ability to stabilize joints during the lengthening/deformity correction period as necessary. For example, complex proximal and distal deformity of the tibia can be accommodated and corrected using Ilizarov's apparatus and corticotomy at multiple levels (Fig. 5) in a way that is difficult or impossible with other external fixation devices. Furthermore, prophylactic stabilization of the knee or ankle joints frequently is desirable during reconstruction for fibular hemimelia because of the coexisting joint deformity or instability, and this stabilization is relatively easily accomplished with Ilizarov's apparatus.

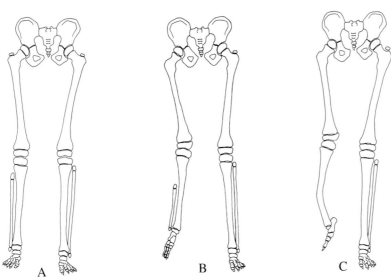

Fig. 4 *Classification of fibular hemimelia, modified from Dal Monte.* **A,** *Grade I fibular hemimelia. There is mild shortening of the tibia, hypoplasia of the fibula.* **B,** *Grade II fibular hemimelia. There is more severe tibial shortening and angular deformity, distal femoral valgus deformity, markedly hypoplastic fibula, and absence of the lateral rays of the foot.* **C,** *Grade III fibular hemimelia. There is severe shortening of the leg, distal femoral valgus deformity with femoral shortening, only a small remnant of fibula or none at all, and absence of the lateral rays of the foot. (Reproduced with permission from Catagni MA: Management of fibular hemimelia using the Ilizarov method, in Eilert RE (ed):* Instructional Course Lectures XLI. *Park Ridge, IL, American Academy of Orthopaedic Surgeons, 1992, pp 431–434.)*

Grade I Fibular Hemimelia

Grade I fibular hemimelia usually can be treated by a single lengthening of the tibia, because the total functional discrepancy is usually 8 cm or less. Because the ankle usually is stable without clinically significant deformity, it is usually unnecessary to include the foot in the apparatus. This is the only deformity where less complex external fixation devices may reasonably used in place of Ilizarov's apparatus. We prefer, however, to use the apparatus for all cases, because foot and ankle deformity or tibial deformity may result during the lengthening period, and either of these problems is managed relatively easily by extension or redirection of the apparatus. The ideal time for lengthening of the tibia in patients with grade I fibular hemimelia is at or near the end of growth. At this stage, the total final discrepancy resulting from femoral, tibial, and foot shortening easily is determined, and the patient is young enough that a relatively uneventful course can be expected.

In addition to the amount of tibial shortening, the surgeon must ascertain the presence and amount of femoral shortening, distal femoral valgus, and tibial valgus and level, in order to plan accurate, satisfactory reconstruction. The need for femoral lengthening or valgus correction is a function of the

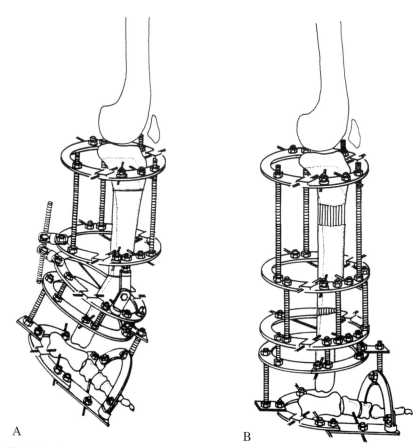

A   B

Fig. 5 A, Complex proximal AND distal tibia deformity and shortening in a grade III fibular hemimelia treated with multiple osteotomies and Ilizarov apparatus. B, Final result at the end of this stage of treatment. The ankle and foot are stabilized in the apparatus with each tibial lengthening and deformity correction. The hindfoot may be translated medially as necessary to correct valgus deformity, and/or a distal fibular transport performed with this apparatus. (Reproduced with permission from Catagni MA: Management of fibular hemimelia using the Ilizarov method, in Eilert RE (ed): Instructional Course Lectures XLI. Park Ridge, IL, American Academy of Orthopaedic Surgeons, 1992, pp 431–434.)

severity of these deformities and individual preference. As previously mentioned, most patients with grade I fibular hemimelia will require only a single tibial lengthening, with or without tibial valgus correction.

Grade II Fibular Hemimelia

For grade II fibular hemimelia, we recommend the Ilizarov apparatus for limb reconstruction in all patients for the reasons mentioned above. The program for these patients involves several steps. Patients are fit with a walking extension orthosis as necessary to facilitate walking prior to reconstructive surgery. At 10 to 12 years of age, the first tibial lengthening is performed along with tibial angular deformity correction if needed, and ankle joint stabilization, if needed. The ankle can be stabilized by pulling the calcaneus into varus (either acutely or gradually) with olive wires inserted from the lateral side and drawing the lateral malleolar remnant distally either through the epiphysis or via a fibular metaphyseal osteotomy. The fibular remnant is translated distally with the use of an anteroposterior wire, independent of the tibia.

The tibial frame is used to lengthen the tibia and correct any associated angular deformity. The more severe the angular and foot deformity to be corrected at this stage, the less tibial lengthening should be attempted.

The second stage is to repeat the tibial lengthening and/or perform femoral deformity correction and lengthening, as needed. This stage typically is performed at skeletal maturity. The need for this stage and the deformities that require correction are quite variable, and often are not predicable after the first lengthening and deformity correction. Some patients, for example, maintain their deformity correction and lengthening after the first stage and do not require further reconstruction. Others will have enough femoral deformity and shortening to require correction. In addition, some patients will have or develop residual tibial shortening requiring the second lengthening. If combined femoral deformity correction/lengthening and repeat tibial lengthening are performed simultaneously, we use the femorotibial frame as routinely used for grade III deformities described below. If the tibia is lengthened or corrected, the foot usually should be incorporated in the apparatus.

Grade III Fibular Hemimelia

Reconstruction of grade III fibular hemimelia is a challenging, complex, multistage process. The treatment program is divided into several stages throughout growth. These staged reconstructions are as outlined as follows.

Because the foot is typically in a nonfunctional, severe equinovalgus position, the first step is to perform a soft-tissue release of the foot and ankle to bring the foot into a more plantigrade position. This step typically is carried out between the ages of 3 and 6 months. An orthosis is then used for walking until the first lengthening stage.

The first tibial angular deformity/lengthening reconstruction is carried out at age 5 to 6 years. The foot will always need to be stabilized in the apparatus in grade III deformities (Fig. 5). This stage is directed primarily to ankle and tibial deformity correction (typically anteromedial angular deformity accentuating the equinovalgus position of the foot and ankle). The amount of lengthening that should be attempted at this stage is inversely proportional to the extent of angular deformity present: the more severe the angular deformity, the less lengthening to be attempted.

A second tibial lengthening is performed, usually between the ages of 8 and 10 years, with simultaneous correction of the femoral valgus and femoral lengthening. A femoral-tibial-foot apparatus is applied at this stage (Fig. 6). The correction of these many deformities with stabilization of the

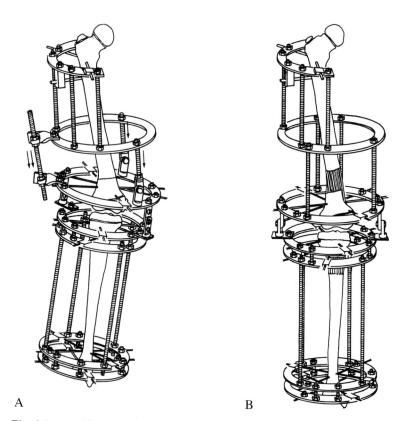

A   B

Fig. 6 *A typical femoral–tibial apparatus for simultaneous distal femoral valgus deformity correction and femoral lengthening, knee joint stabilization in extension, and tibial
lengthening.* **A,** *Immediately after surgery.* **B,** *At the end of axial correction and lengthening. (Adapted with permission from Catagni MA: Management of fibular hemimelia
using the Ilizarov method, in Eilert RE (ed):* Instructional Course Lectures XLI. *Park
Ridge, IL, American Academy of Orthopaedic Surgeons, 1992, pp 431–434.)*

knee and foot is not possible without the use of the Ilizarov apparatus. We
use the Lecco proximal femoral arch modification with 4- or 5-mm half pins,
with full rings distally for both the femur and tibia, and a combination of
wires and half pins for distal fixation.

Further treatment sessions using a femoral-tibial-foot apparatus are repeated as necessary, based on the severity of the original deformity and the development of recurrent deformity. Typically, two further treatment sessions are
required, one at age 12 to 13 years, and a final one at skeletal maturity.

Patients with grade III fibular hemimelia, therefore, are expected to
require as many as four treatment stages involving tibial or femoral-tibial
apparatus, in addition to the soft-tissue release of the foot prior to walking
age. If the ankle is painful or unstable at the time of the final treatment session, or subsequently, tibiotalar arthrodesis is performed.

Results

We report here the results of 161 patients treated between 1981 and 1996 at L'Ospedale di Lecco with the Ilizarov apparatus to reconstruct deformities associated with fibular hemimelia. Thirty-two of the patients were classified as Dal Monte grade I, 61 as grade II, and 68 as grade III. Four patients had bilateral fibular hemimelia. The youngest patient treated with the apparatus for correction of bony deformity was 3 years of age.

Of the four patients with bilateral fibular hemimelia, one underwent bilateral tibial lengthening and correction of unilateral femoral valgus deformity, while three underwent angular deformity correction and lengthening only to the extent necessary to eliminate deformity compared to the opposite, less severely affected side.

One patient presented at age 18 with 30 cm of shortening and deformity. This patient underwent angular deformity correction and Syme's amputation to allow better prosthetic fitting. All other patients have, to date, been treated with preservation of the foot.

Grade I

All 32 patients with grade I fibular hemimelia in this patient population have completed their reconstructive treatment. Thirty-one patients required only one lengthening; one patient required a second lengthening to complete the limb-length inequality and angular deformity corrections. Equal leg lengths were achieved in all patients with maintenance of a plantigrade foot. There were no long-term knee complications. Some patients had mild muscle atrophy on follow-up evaluation, but no other significant long-term sequelae developed in this group.

Grade II

There are 61 patients in this series with grade II fibular hemimelia. Thirty-seven of the 61 have completed treatment. Five of the 37 required three treatment sessions (all including at least one femoral angular deformity correction and lengthening), nine required two treatment sessions, and 23 required only one treatment session.

Two of these 37 patients have developed significant knee stiffness, with an arc of motion averaging from full extension to 40° of flexion as the result of knee dislocation from prior treatment with the Wagner apparatus. One further patient has knee flexion limited to 60° after treatment with the Ilizarov apparatus.

Thirty-five of the patients have ended reconstruction with a plantigrade, functional foot. Two patients have foot pronation requiring an orthotic in the shoe. No patients in this group has required a tibiotalar arthrodesis to date.

Thirty-two of the 37 patients participate in recreational sports. Five patients limit athletic activities to swimming as a result of knee stiffness or preexisting knee instability.

Grade III

Twenty-one limbs in 20 of the 61 patients undergoing reconstructive treatment for grade III fibular hemimelia have completed treatment. Two of the 21 required six stages of reconstruction, four required five stages, six required four stages, three required three stages, and four patients required two stages. In addition, one patient with bilateral grade III fibular hemimelia had bilateral angular deformity correction and lengthening of the shorter side at one treatment session. Eight of these 20 patients underwent foot deformity correction before age 3 years as the initial stage of reconstruction.

Two patients in this group have symptomatic restriction of knee motion, with a range of motion of approximately full extension to 45° of flexion. No patient suffered a permanent knee subluxation.

Sixteen of the 21 preserved feet in the patients who have completed treatment are plantigrade, stable, and asymptomatic (Fig. 7). Five patients have residual foot pronation that, in combination with stiffness, requires the use of a foot orthotic to alleviate symptoms.

Athletic pursuits are more severely limited in this group than they are in the patients with grade I or II fibular hemimelia, primarily because of persistent knee instability or stiffness. Most can bike or swim.

There were no permanent sequelae of knee subluxation, hip subluxation, peripheral neuropathy, nonunion, or osteomyelitis in any patient who has completed treatment. Patients as a whole are quite satisfied and functional with their reconstruction.

Of the 71 patients who have not yet completed reconstruction, ten have had one reconstructive procedure, 31 have had two, and 30 have had three staged reconstructive procedures to date.

Conclusion

The treatment of fibular hemimelia traditionally involves the use of orthotics for mild deformities; leg lengthening, epiphysiodesis, or both for mild to moderate leg-length discrepancy; and Syme's or Boyd amputation and prosthetic fitting for patients with moderate to severe deformities and length discrepancies. In Italy, the management of fibular hemimelia has long been influenced by parental and patient refusal of amputation. More recently, experience with techniques of limb lengthening and deformity correction introduced by Ilizarov have been applied to the spectrum of deformities associated with fibular hemimelia. The application of these techniques has significantly facilitated management of these difficult cases.

The modified Dal Monte classification scheme provides a guideline to the extent and nature of reconstructive procedures that will be required to restore the affected limb. Any reconstructive treatment plan must address the combined and complex problems of limb length inequality, angular deformity, joint deformity, and potential joint instability. The external fixation method used to perform reconstruction in these patients must be able to address these problems, as well as be sufficiently adaptable to be useful for the treat-

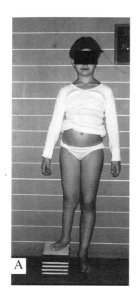
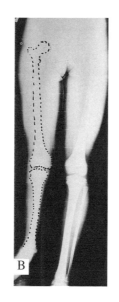
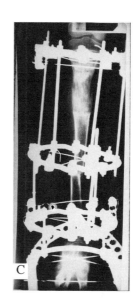

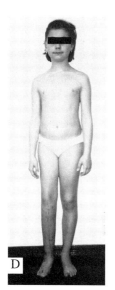
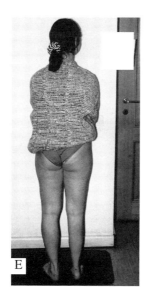
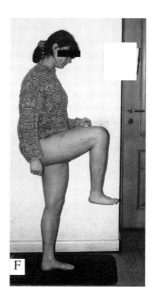

Fig. 7 A, *Eight-year-old girl with grade III fibular hemimelia.* *B,* *Anteroposterior (AP) radiograph of lower extremities prior to lengthening.* *C,* *AP radiograph during first tibial lengthening and deformity correction. Note immobilization of foot in the apparatus.* *D,* *Postoperative clinical appearance after first tibial lengthening.* *E,* *Clinical appearance at age 17 years, after two further tibial and femoral reconstructions.* *F,* *Demonstration of patient's knee flexion and ankle dorsiflexion at the end of reconstruction.*

ment of complications such as joint subluxation when they occur. I believe that the Ilizarov apparatus is the ideal external fixation method for the management of these severe, complex deformities, and it has served me well to date. I have found it wise to divide reconstructions into several stages depending on the severity of the deformity.

It will be many years before enough patients treated in this manner will have reached skeletal maturity to make possible a full accounting of this management. Results to date have been very encouraging in that treatment goals have been met in most cases, even when severe, complex deformities have required multiple stages of reconstruction.

References

1. Hootnick D, Boyd NA, Fixsen JA, Lloyd-Roberts GC: The natural history and management of congenital short tibia with dysplasia or absence of the fibula. *J Bone Joint Surg* 1977;59B:267–271.

2. Coventry MB, Johnson EW Jr: Congenital absence of the fibula. *J Bone Joint Surg* 1952;34A:941–955.

3. Achterman C, Kalamchi A: Congenital deficiency of the fibula. *J Bone Joint Surg* 1979;61B:133–137.

4. Amstutz HC: Abstract: Natural history and treatment of congenital absence of the fibula. *J Bone Joint Surg* 1972;54A:1349.

5. Westin GW, Sakai DN, Wood WL: Congenital longitudinal deficiency of the fibula: Follow-up of treatment by Syme amputation. *J Bone Joint Surg* 1976; 58A:492–496.

6. Kruger LM, Talbott RD: Amputation and prosthesis as definitive treatment in congenital absence of the fibula. *J Bone Joint Surg* 1961;43A:625–642.

7. Wood WL, Zlotsky N, Westin GW: Congenital absence of the fibula: Treatment by Syme amputation. Indications and technique. *J Bone Joint Surg* 1965;47A: 1159–1169.

8. Herring JA, Barnhill B, Gaffney C: Syme amputation: An evaluation of the physical and psychological function in young patients. *J Bone Joint Surg* 1986;68A: 573–578.

9. Choi IH, Kumar SJ, Bowen JR: Amputation or limb-lengthening for partial or total absence of the fibula. *J Bone Joint Surg* 1990;72A:1391–1399.

10. Damsin JP, Pous JG, Ghanem I: Therapeutic approach to severe congenital lower limb length discrepancies: Surgical treatment versus prosthetic management. *J Pediatr Orthop* 1995;4B:164–170.

11. Letts M, Vincent N: Congenital longitudinal deficiency of the fibula (fibular hemimelia): Parental refusal of amputation. *Clin Orthop* 1993;287:160–166.

12. Catagni MA, Bolano L, Cattaneo R: Management of fibular hemimelia using the Ilizarov method. *Orthop Clin North Am* 1991;22:715–722.

13. Dal Monte A, Donzelli O: Tibial lengthening according to Ilizarov in congenital hypoplasia of the leg. *J Pediatr Orthop* 1987;7:135–138.

14. Stanitski DF, Shahcheraghi H, Nicker DA, Armstrong PF: Results of tibial lengthening with the Ilizarov technique. *J Pediatr Orthop* 1996;16:168–172.

15. Miller LS, Bell CF: Management of congenital fibular deficiency by Ilizarov technique. *J Pediatr Orthop* 1992;12:651–657.

16. Gibbons PJ, Bradish CF: Fibular hemimelia: A preliminary report on management of the severe abnormality. *J Pediatr Orthop* 1996;5B:20–26.

17. Ghoneem HF, Wright JG, Cole WG, Rang M: The Ilizarov method for correction of complex deformities: Psychological and functional outcomes. *J Bone Joint Surg* 1996;78A:1480–1485.

18. Fulp T, Davids JR, Meyer LC, Blackhurst DW: Longitudinal deficiency of the fibula: Operative treatment. *J Bone Joint Surg* 1996;78A:674–682.

19. Catagni MA: Management of fibular hemimelia using the Ilizarov method, in Eilert RE (ed): *Instructional Course Lectures XLI*. Park Ridge, IL, American Academy of Orthopaedic Surgeons, 1992, pp 431–434.

Chapter 17

Psychological Considerations in the Planning of Staged Reconstruction in Limb Deficiencies

Anne A. Morton, PhD

Introduction

In the treatment of both congenital and acquired limb deficiencies, the application of external fixators has become increasingly common, particularly with the advancement in the technology of the Ilizarov device. Staged reconstruction presents the patient and family with a lengthy, often stressful, procedure. This may especially be the case with multiple lengthenings with deformity correction. Herring and associates[1] have reported greater psychological problems occurring in children being subjected to multiple surgical procedures. It has already been documented that children with physical handicaps are at an increased risk for behavioral and emotional problems.[2] Adjusting to an external fixator is a psychologically demanding and complex experience for many patients and their families.[3–5] The possible risk for serious psychological sequelae is apparent, particularly in those who are already at some risk from a psychological standpoint.

Hrutkay and Eilert[3] found that, of 22 pediatric patients who underwent femoral or tibial lengthening with the Wagner technique, 64% experienced psychological difficulties, including depression, anxiety, noncompliance, dependence, anorexia, suicidal ideation, self-destructive behavior, and regression. None of the patients experienced long-term sequelae. Preoperative psychological testing was not done, and only eight patients were formally seen by a psychologist both before and during the lengthening procedures. Patients who had longer hospitalizations were found to have greater psychological difficulties.

Ghoneem and associates,[5] in a retrospective study of 45 children treated with the Ilizarov technique (average follow-up, 36 months), found that all of the patients were functioning within normal limits on two psychometric instruments. Forty-two of the patients had no limitations in daily functioning, and 37 were satisfied with the result. Mental status and psychological functioning prior to and during the procedure were not reported.

While reconstruction with an external fixator is prone to a variety of medical complications,[4,6] numerous psychosocial complications,[3,7] including problems with pain, sleep, appetite, and depression, have also been noted. Although there is evidence that this type of procedure exacts a psychological cost for patients, little or nothing has been written regarding the psychosocial cost to the family. In addition, the cost to the institution and the health care system for needed ancillary services needs to be considered, although some have reported that psychological interventions actually reduce overall medical costs.[8]

The purpose of this study was threefold: (1) to examine the psychological and behavioral reactions experienced with the Ilizarov external fixator; (2) to use preoperative evaluation and other means to identify patients who may be at increased risk for treatment failure; and (3) to determine if multiple staged reconstruction leads to increased risk for psychological or behavioral problems. The nature of the psychological support given to these patients will be described.

Subjects and Methodology

Subjects

Psychological records were reviewed for 77 patients referred to the Psychology Department of Texas Scottish Rite Hospital for Children, between 1989 and 1996, for preoperative evaluation or postoperative intervention related to application of an Ilizarov external fixator. Of these, 56 patients have completed the Ilizarov application; 28 were seen both pre- and postoperatively, and 28 were seen only in some phase of the postoperative process.

Preoperative Screening

This screening was performed to provide the patient, family, and physician with pertinent psychosocial information regarding whether to proceed with Ilizarov application at that time, as well as to assist in making recommendations for preoperative preparation of the patient and family and for postoperative support.

Several of the following formal psychometric instruments were used, depending upon the age of the child and clinical indications: The Minnesota Multiphasic Personality Inventory-Adolescent (MMPI-A) and the MMPI-2, measure levels of psychopathology and personality factors in adolescents and adults, respectively.[9,10] The Children's Depression Inventory (CDI) measures the intensity and magnitude of depressive symptoms in children and adolescents.[11] The Revised Children's Manifest Anxiety Scale (RCMAS) measures physiological, social, and overall anxiety in children.[12] The Piers-Harris Children's Self-Concept Scale measures self-concept in children and adolescents.[13] The Family Environment Scale (FES) measures various dimensions of family life.[14] The Child Behavior Checklist (CBC) assesses parent perceptions of child problem behaviors.[15] The Parenting Stress Inventory (PSI) measures three separate sources of parental stress.[16]

Issues that were examined for patient/family, as appropriate, using one or more of these instruments in addition to a clinical interview include: (1) overall adjustment, including psychiatric diagnosis; (2) family psychiatric history; (3) ability to cope with stress; (4) motivations and expectations for the procedure; (5) body image/self-esteem; (6) understanding of the procedure, complications, and so forth; (7) pain tolerance; (8) potential for cooperation and compliance with treatment; (9) level of cognitive and academic functioning; (10) support system; and (11) patient's level of socialization.

Preoperative Preparation

For patients seen preoperatively, pain management training (including biofeedback and breathing exercises), coping skills training, individual and family therapy, and education regarding the procedure were undertaken by a member of the Psychology Staff. In addition, clinic staff provided a video of the procedure for most patients (English or Spanish version), as well as written handouts. Patients and families were also allowed to meet with or talk to at least one other patient who had had a similar procedure.

Postoperative Support

All of the 28 patients seen preoperatively were also followed postoperatively by the Psychology Department. The purpose was to monitor mental status, provide pain management, provide counseling to increase patients' coping skills in dealing with the fixator, and provide family therapy to support the family. The other 28 patients were seen during some phase of the reconstruction process; typically, after being referred for inability to cope.

Results

Subjects

Average age of the 56 patients (35 boys, 21 girls) was 12 years (range, 1 to 19 years) at the time of first Ilizarov. Three patients were younger than 5 years of age, 25 were 6 to 12 years of age, and 28 were adolescents. There were a total of 75 Ilizarov and two Ortho-Fix applications on these 56 patients. Fourteen patients have had more than one application, with nine patients having two, three patients having three, and two patients having four applications. Thirteen applications were for angular correction, 20 were for lengthening, and 44 were for both correction and lengthening. Seventeen patients had an acquired deformity caused by trauma or infection, 17 had congenital anomalies, five had Blounts' Disease, seven had skeletal dysplasia, four had enchondromatosis, one had residual clubfoot deformity, and five had miscellaneous diagnoses.

The mean number of hospitalizations related to the Ilizarov procedure was four (range 1 to 12). The average number of days of hospitalization was 60 (range, 5 to 508). The average number of days patients were in the fixator was

207 (range, 55 to 1,117). One patient had four total applications and lengthy hospital stays. Excluding his data, the average number of hospitalizations was 3.9, average total days of hospitalization was 51.9, and average days in fixator was 199.6 days. One patient had had two prior Ilizarov applications in another country and these data were not available.

Preoperative Evaluations

The most commonly used tests were the MMPI-A (13), the RCMAS (14), the CDI (14), and the Piers-Harris (14). For the parents, the most frequently used tests were the CBC (19 mothers, 12 fathers), MMPI-2 (19 mothers, 13 fathers), the FES (8 mothers, 6 fathers), and the PSI (9 mothers, 6 fathers).

The mean total score on the CDI was 42.9 (range, 36 to 69), with 50 being the normative mean, indicating below average levels of depression in patients tested preoperatively ($p < 0.02$). The RCMAS total anxiety score was 42.8 (range, 26 to 61), with 50 also being the normative mean, indicating below average levels of anxiety in this group ($p < 0.02$). All of the clinical scales on the MMPI-A were below the mean, although there was some evidence of defensiveness in the sample, with three of the validity scales significantly above the mean (THIN, 61.2; range, 51 to 79, $p < 0.001$; Lie Scale, 62.9; range, 42-90, $p < 0.001$; and K Scale, 59; range, 42 to 76, $p < 0.01$). On the Piers-Harris, the total self-concept score was 64.1 (range, 37 to 85), indicating significantly higher self-concept than the normative mean ($p < 0.001$). However, six (21.4%) patients were found to have a psychiatric diagnosis, including attention deficit hyperactivity disorder, depression, or anxiety. Therefore, the patients referred for preoperative evaluation, as a group, scored average or below in anxiety, depression, or other psychopathology, and above average in total self-concept, although approximately one fourth had a psychiatric diagnosis, and the MMPI-A scores indicated a tendency to underreport symptoms or pathology.

On the CBC, total scores were not significantly different from the normative mean, although individual scales often showed statistical, but not clinical, significance. On the MMPI-2, all the means of the clinical scales were not of clinical significance. The FES indicated that the mothers as a whole reported greater family cohesiveness ($p < 0.05$) than the normative mean, although all other scales were not significantly different from the normative mean. The PSI indicated that the parents' total reported stress was not significantly greater than the normative mean.

However, during the preoperative evaluation, family or patient psychiatric history was discovered in 20 (71%) of 28 patients screened preoperatively. The high level of psychiatric history in this sample may reflect referral patterns, in that physicians were able to identify those patients and families most at risk. This history included sessions with a school counselor, history of abuse, parental depression, incarceration or other legal difficulties of a parent or other close family member, and substance abuse of a family member. In some cases, parents were referred to local mental health practitioners for care prior to the patient's surgery.

Preoperative Preparation/Postoperative Support

The 56 patients who completed Ilizarov application were seen in the psychology department for an average of 3.1 preoperative sessions (range, 0 to 18) and an average of 8.9 (range, 1 to 28) postoperative sessions. The mean number of psychology sessions per patient was 12 (range, 1 to 33). Fifty-five percent received ten or fewer sessions, while 45% received 11 or more. Eighty-four percent of these patients received some type of intervention. A majority of patients (56%) received pain management training, with breathing exercises being the most common type of treatment. Biofeedback, relaxation training, distraction, and imagery/hypnosis were also used. Almost 40% of the patients required behavior modification and parent training to deal with problem behaviors. Coping skills training and counseling were used by 37.5% of patients, and 10.7% received assessment only. One patient's parent declined treatment for religious reasons.

Psychological and Behavioral Reactions During Reconstruction

Symptoms and reactions were classified according to severity (Table 1). Mild reactions remitted with little or no intervention. Moderate reactions eventually remitted, but required some type of formal intervention. Reactions were considered severe if they did not remit or if the eventual surgical outcome was affected.

Moderate to severe deteriorations in mental status were observed in almost half (48.2%) of the patients during Ilizarov application. The majority of these suffered from depression, ranging from adjustment disorders secondary to the procedure to major depression. Five patients expressed suicidal ideation, although there were no attempts. One patient did have to be transferred to a local psychiatric hospital for inpatient treatment as a result of suicidal and homicidal ideation and self-mutilation involving the pin sites. Other patients experienced anxiety, anger, and behavior problems. The majority of these remitted with psychological intervention. Six patients either did not remit or the psychological problems affected the outcome of the reconstruction.

Often deteriorations in mental status followed increases in pain. Almost half (48.2%) of the sample experienced moderate to severe pain at some point during the reconstruction process. The majority of these (85%) responded to ibuprofen, acetaminophen with codeine, or amitriptyline, in addition to psychological techniques of pain management. Other reactions included loss of sleep (26.7%), loss of appetite (8.9%), frustration caused by loss of normal activities (14.2%), concerns over body image (17.8%), concerns regarding peers (14.2%), and academic problems (14.2%).

Almost half (46.4%) of the sample experienced moderate to severe family stressors during, or just prior to, reconstruction. There were two divorces during reconstruction. Five parents suffered severe depression/anxiety. Three parents had serious drinking problems, possibly exacerbated by the stress of the patient's procedure, and one sibling was arrested for running away. One mother was diagnosed with breast cancer.

Table 1 Psychological/behavioral reactions of Ilizarov patients (n = 56)

Reaction	Mild	Moderate	Severe	None
Mental status problems	3	21	6	26
Pain	11	23	4	18
Family stressors	3	17	9	27
Sleep loss	8	10	5	33
Appetite loss	11	4	1	40
Frustration with loss of activity	4	6	2	44
Body image issues	5	8	2	41
Peer issues	9	6	2	39
Academic problems	5	5	3	43
Noncom*: exercise	2	11	7	36
Noncom*: pin care	0	9	1	46
Noncom*: bone distraction	1	1	0	54
Noncom*: psychology	12	0	0	44

*Noncom = Noncompliance. Noncompliance with psychological interventions was coded as either a "Yes" or "No" and shown as "mild"

Other significant issues occurring during reconstruction included those of noncompliance with exercise, pin care, and distraction. The most common problem was exercise, with 32% being in the moderate to severe category; noncompliance with pin care was observed in 17% of the sample. Only one patient experienced serious difficulties complying with distraction instructions. Most of the noncompliant patients responded to intervention, although there were eight patients whose outcome was affected, seven of these because of noncompliance with exercises. Over one fifth (21.4%) of the sample missed one or more psychology appointments or refused services.

Mental Status

The sample was divided into those patients who suffered moderate to severe mental status deteriorations and those who suffered no or only mild difficulties (Table 2). Patients suffering deterioration in mental status had significantly more psychology visits ($p = 0.0001$) than those who did not, although there were no differences between the two groups in total days spent in the hospital and total number of days in the fixator.

Compromised Versus Noncompromised Groups

The patients' physicians were asked which patients' outcomes were compromised due to psychological or behavioral factors. Eleven patients were identified as such and were placed in the compromised group. The other 45 patients became the noncompromised group (Table 3). Declines in mental status and noncompliance with exercise were most associated with treatment

Table 2 Factors in Ilizarov patients with good versus poor mental status

Factors	Good Mental Status (n = 29)		Poor Mental Status (n = 27)		Fisher Exact p value
	n	%	n	%	
Pain	10	34.5	17	63.0	0.031
Sleep	3	10.3	12	44.4	0.004
Appetite	0	0.0	5	18.5	0.021
Frustration with activity loss	0	0.0	8	29.6	0.002
Body image issues	2	6.9	8	29.6	0.029
Family stressors	6	20.7	20	74.1	0.001
Noncompliance: exercise	6	20.7	12	44.4	0.053
Noncompliance: pin care	2	6.9	8	29.6	0.029

failure in our sample. The compromised group was significantly more likely to suffer from sleep difficulties and loss of appetite than the noncompromised group. These symptoms are common neurovegetative signs in depression, and it could be argued that this group was more likely to suffer from a depressive disorder. In the compromised group, the families experienced significantly more family stressors just before or during reconstruction. There was a suggestive, but not conclusive, trend for the compromised group to have a positive family psychiatric history than the noncompromised group. However, there were no differences between the two groups in patient premorbid psychiatric diagnosis. There were no significant differences between the two groups in total number of days in the fixator or total days in the hospital. There were also no differences between the two groups in number of Ilizarov applications. The compromised group did receive significantly more psychology visits ($p = 0.046$) than did the other group because of their more significant problems.

Multiple Fixator Applications

Forty-six patients were seen for their first Ilizarov application, and ten patients were seen for their second or third application. Three patients were seen during the first Ilizarov and a later one. The first-time patients were then compared with the second- or third-time patients on the psychological and behavioral variables (Table 4). The three patients seen for both first and subsequent applications were placed in the latter category. Data indicated that patients experiencing multiple applications tend to be more compliant with exercise with later applications. There were no other differences on any of the other psychological or behavioral variables between the two groups. These data indicate that patients undergoing multiple stage applications do no worse from a mental status standpoint than patients undergoing only one procedure. In fact, they appear to do better in one area, compliance with exercise.

Table 3 Psychological/behavioral reactions in compromised versus non-compromised groups

Reactions	Noncompromised (n = 45)		Compromised (n = 11)		Fisher Exact p value
	n	%	n	%	
Sleep	9	20.0	6	54.5	0.030
Appetite	2	4.4	3	27.3	0.047
Family stressors	18	40.0	8	72.7	0.053
Mental status decline	18	40.0	9	81.8	0.015
Family psychiatry history	19	37.8	8	72.7	0.069
Noncompliance: exercise	9	20.0	9	81.8	0.001
Noncompliance: pin care	4	8.8	6	54.5	0.002

Table 4 Psychological/behavioral reactions in first fixator versus second or third fixator

Factor	First Fixator (n = 46)		Second or Third Fixator (n = 10)		Fisher Exact p value
	n	%	n	%	
Pain	21	45.7	5	50.0	0.726
Sleep loss	12	26.1	3	30.0	0.748
Appetite loss	5	10.9	0	0.00	0.359
Mental status decline	22	47.8	4	40.0	0.787
Frustration with loss of activity	6	13.0	3	30.0	0.192
Body image issues	8	17.4	0	0.00	0.184
Peer issues	5	10.9	3	30.0	0.143
Family stressors	21	45.7	5	50.0	0.726
Academic problems	6	13.0	1	10.0	0.769
Noncompliance: exercise	16	34.8	0	0.00	0.024
Noncompliance: pin care	9	19.6	0	0.00	0.145
Noncompliance: psychology	11	23.9	1	10.0	0.309
Presence of psychiatric disorder	11	23.9	3	30.0	0.105
Family psychiatry history	23	50.0	4	40.0	0.413

Discussion

The psychological cost of reconstruction with an external fixator, in this case, the Ilizarov, can be considerable, to both patients and their families, as others[3] have also reported. Moderate to severe deterioration in mental status and pain during the procedure were the most common psychological side effects reported in almost one-half the sample, which is less than that reported by others.[3] Because the data indicate that the average patient was functioning in the normal range psychologically prior to surgery, it may be assumed that the reconstructive procedure contributed to these mental status problems. However, it should also be noted that the sample consisted only of those patients referred to the Psychology Department and may represent an at-risk group, as the high level of premorbid psychiatric history would indicate. Noncompliance with exercise occurred in approximately one third, and loss of sleep in more than one fourth of the sample. During reconstruction, significant family stressors, which probably exacerbated the patients' psychological and behavioral problems, occurred in almost half the patients. In contrast with other reports,[2] length of hospitalization was not found to contribute to decline in mental/behavioral status.

Approximately one fifth of the patients in the sample of 56 experienced compromised medical outcome because of a psychological or behavioral factor. Factors most associated with this were noncompliance with exercise and mental status decline. Loss of sleep/appetite, family stressors during or immediately preceding the procedure, and, possibly, presence of premorbid family psychiatric history also appear to contribute to treatment failure.

Many patients need to have multiple stages of reconstruction with an external fixator. Data indicate that these patients are at no greater risk for psychological or behavioral problems than patients needing only one application. In fact, patients may even do better in the area of compliance with exercise on their second or third application than patients undergoing an initial application. This may be a result of increased maturity in children and adolescents by the second or third application, or of inoculation to the stressors of the procedure by undergoing it previously, or both. In addition, families may be more supportive of exercise regimens at a later application as they learn more about the procedure and the possible outcomes and consequences of noncompliance.

It is possible that the availability of psychological services to patients and families ameliorated the problems to some degree. Data suggest that the majority of the problems were transitory and remitted with appropriate treatment, which is consistent with Ghoneem and associates'[5] findings that the Ilizarov did not cause long-term psychological maladjustment.

Aggressive treatment of pain, sleep, and appetite problems should be a part of any protocol for reconstruction with an external fixator. Early identification of patients prone to noncompliance with exercise and/or pin care is important so that treatment strategies can be initiated. In addition, psychological screening can be helpful in identifying the presence of family stressors and psychiatric history so that appropriate decisions may be made regarding the reconstruction. For example, the presence of these factors may be sufficient to consider alternative treatments or postponement of the procedure. Data indicate that, in many cases, support for the family as well as the patient is critical for a successful outcome.

Because this review includes only those patients referred by physicians to the Psychology Department, the sample may have higher proportions of psychopathology than the overall population. Therefore, prospective studies are needed to determine conclusively factors for success or failure in limb reconstruction. Studies also are needed to compare psychological and social outcomes with those of alternative treatments, such as amputation.

Acknowledgments

The author gratefully acknowledges the assistance of Karl Koch, BS, in data collection, Richard Brown, PhD, in data analysis, Freddie Fain in manuscript preparation, and John Birch, MD, for guidance and support.

References

1. Herring J, Barnhill B, Gaffney C: Syme amputation: An examination of the physical and psychological function in young patients. *J Bone Joint Surg* 1986;68A:573–578.

2. Lavigne JV, Faier-Routman J: Psychological adjustment to pediatric physical disorders: A meta-analytic review. *J Pediatr Psychol* 1992;17:133–157.

3. Hrutkay JM, Eilert RE: Operative lengthening of the lower extremity and associated psychological aspects: The Children's Hospital experience. *J Pediatr Orthop* 1990;10:373–377.

4. Paley D: Problems, obstacles, and complications of limb lengthening by the Ilizarov technique. *Clin Orthop* 1990;250:81–104.

5. Ghoneem HF, Wright JG, Cole WG, Rang M: The Ilizarov method for correction of complex deformities: Psychological and functional outcomes. *J Bone Joint Surg* 1996;78A:1480–1485.

6. Dahl MT, Gulli B, Berg T: Complications of limb lengthening. *Clin Orthop* 1994;301:10–18.

7. Young N, Bell DF, Anthony A: Pediatric pain patterns during Ilizarov treatment of limb length discrepancy and angular deformity. *J Pediatr Orthop* 1994;14:352–357.

8. Friedman R, Sobel D, Myers P, Caudill M, Benson H: Behavioral medicine, clinical health psychology, and cost offset. *Health Psychol* 1995;14:509–518.

9. Butcher JN, Williams CL, et al: *MMPI-A: Manual for Administration, Scoring, and Interpretation.* Minneapolis, MN, University of Minnesota Press, 1992.

10. Hathaway SR, McKinley JC (eds): *MMPI-2: Manual for Administration and Scoring.* Minneapolis, MN, University of Minnesota Press, 1989.

11. Kovacs M (ed): *Children's Depression Inventory.* North Tonawanda, NY, Multi-Health System, 1992.

12. Reynolds CR, Richmond BO (eds): *Revised Children's Manifest Anxiety Scale (RCMAS).* Los Angeles, CA, Western Psychological Services, 1985.

13. Piers EV (ed): *The Piers-Harris Children's Self-Concept Scale: Revised Manual.* Los Angeles, CA, Western Psychological Services, 1984.

14. Moos RH, Moos BS (eds): *Family Environment Scale Manual,* ed 2. Palo Alto, CA, Consulting Psychologists Press, 1986.

15. Achenbach TM (ed): *Manual for the Child Behavior Checklist/4-18 and 1991 Profile.* Burlington, VT, University of Vermont Department of Psychiatry, 1991.

16. Abidin RR (ed): *Parenting Stress Index.* Charlottesville, VA, Pediatric Psychology Press, 1990.

Consensus

The Indications for Limb Lengthening in Fibular Deficiency

Affected children and their parents should be well-educated as to the advantages and disadvantages of each treatment modality. An ideal means to accomplish this is through contact with other families who have had similar treatment.

Specialized limb-deficiency clinics offer significant advantages in the management of these children, especially when multiple special areas of expertise are represented. These clinics also facilitate contact between families and children for educational purposes.

Family, cultural, and social factors must be taken into consideration in planning treatment and follow-up care. There is general agreement that epiphysiodesis or limb-lengthening with or without epiphysiodesis is appropriate for patients with (1) a foot with four rays or more; (2) a predicted discrepancy of the limb of 8 cm or less; (3) a stable, mobile ankle; (4) a plantigrade foot; and (5) a capable, multidisciplinary team to carry out treatment and follow-up care.

There is general agreement that amputation is appropriate for patients with a predicted limb-length discrepancy > 25 cm at maturity and a poor foot and ankle. Boyd modifications may improve function; however, further research is needed in this area. Although lengthening in this group is performed at some centers, long-term follow-up is not currently available.

The decisions about treatment are difficult in patients with intermediate deficiencies. The number of lengthenings and degree of difficulty should be considered. Consultation with surgeons versed in both lengthening and amputation approaches along with contact with experienced children and families should be available.

Cost analyses may be misleading, and managed care organizations should not determine treatment based solely on economic considerations. Well-conceived outcome studies that examine function and quality of life are needed before firm recommendations can be made. All investigators face a dilemma in that there is no long-term follow-up of current limb lengthening technology, because the techniques are evolving rapidly.

Section 4
Tibial Deficiency

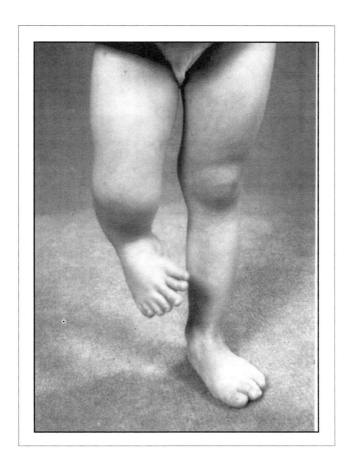

Chapter 18
Tibial Deficiency

Perry L. Schoenecker, MD

Congenital longitudinal deficiency of the tibia is a rare anomaly characterized by total absence or deficiency in the tibia and a relatively intact fibula.
The knee joint, as such, is grossly abnormal, and the extremity is markedly
shortened distally, with the foot in a pronounced equinovarus position.
Associated terminal longitudinal deformities of the foot include both duplication and deficiencies (Fig. 1). Longitudinal deficiencies of the tibia are
easily distinguishable from longitudinal deficiencies of the fibula. In the longitudinal tibial deficiencies, the unstable equinovarus foot is present at the
end of a very short, relatively functionless leg. In longitudinal fibular deficiencies, the foot typically is in an equinovalgus attitude articulating on the
lateral aspect of the variably shortened, often anteriorly bowed leg. For
patients with longitudinal deficiencies of the tibia, knee joint disarticulation
is the typical treatment of choice, and patients generally function well as
above-the-knee joint amputees. For patients with longitudinal deficiency of
the fibula, definitive treatment often is a more distal (foot) amputation, and
resulting function is predictably excellent.

Classification

Congenital anomalies of the tibia have been described as longitudinal deficiencies, either complete or incomplete, meromelia tibia, and intercalary
paraxial tibial hemimelia, either complete or incomplete. Patients with this
rare longitudinal deficiency of the lower limb have unique clinical findings
that vary in severity. Originally, Jones and associates[1] and, subsequently,
Schoenecker and associates[2] found it feasible to classify longitudinal deficiencies of the tibia into four radiographic types that are very useful in planning definitive surgical and prosthetic care (Fig. 2). A relatively intact fibula that often is proximally migrated is characteristic of all four types. The
normal fibular articulations, proximally with the tibia and distally at the
ankle, appear very distorted.

In type 1, the tibia is totally absent on initial radiographs. Clinically, the
deformity is pronounced, with a severely deficient leg, gross knee and
ankle joint instability, and equinovarus foot deformity. There is essentially no semblance of a knee or ankle joint and no potential for their development. Type 1 is the most commonly occurring deficiency and the most

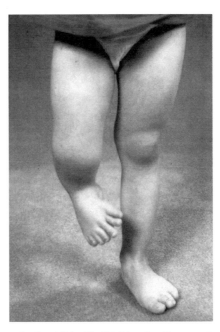

Fig. 1 *Clinical photograph of a child with tibial hemimelia; note the severely shortened limb, the equinovarus position, and the commonly associated partial duplication of the foot.*

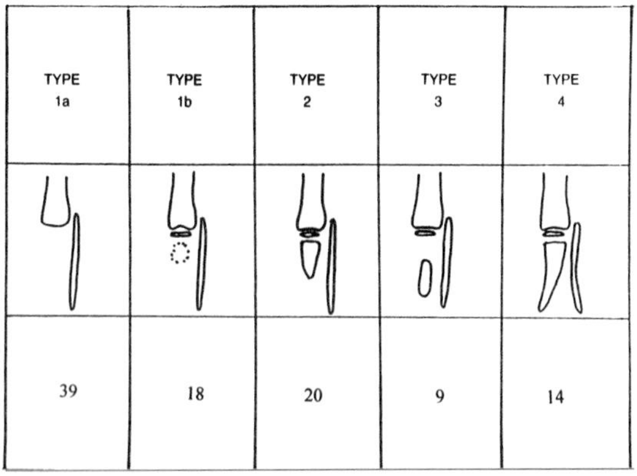

TYPE 1a	TYPE 1b	TYPE 2	TYPE 3	TYPE 4
39	18	20	9	14

Fig. 2 *Diagrammatic representation of radiographic types and total number of limbs with each type in the combined studies of Jones and associates[1] and Schoenecker and associates.[2] The majority of patients have the most significant deficiency, type 1. (Adapted with permission from Jones D, Barnes J, Lloyd-Roberts GC: Congenital aplasia and dysplasia of the tibia with intact fibula: Classification and management. J Bone Joint Surg 1978;60B:31–39.)*

likely to be bilateral. With growth and development, type 1 can be subdivided into types 1a and 1b. In type 1a, the tibia is completely absent and the distal end of the femur is relatively hypoplastic. In type 1b, a rudimentary tibia (nonossified in the infant) articulates with the distal end of a relatively abnormal distal femur. In type 2, the proximal end of the tibia is visible radiographically at birth and articulates with a near normal appearing distal femur. Approximately two thirds of the distal tibia is absent and never develops. Type 3, the rarest form, is characterized by an amorphous segment of bone, which appears to represent a foreshortened broadened segment of tibial diaphysis. Rudimentary articulations representative of knee and ankle joints eventually develop. Weightbearing potentiates severe proximal migration of the usually bowed fibula. In type 4, the proximal end of the tibia is well developed; the distal end is relatively shortened. The distal tibia and fibula do not form a component mortice, but rather are widely separated giving the appearance of a congenital diastasis.[3] The limb length inequality in type 4 deformity is subtle in the newborn. The clinically striking severe equinovarus position of the foot may be mistaken for a clubfoot, and the tibial dysplasia may be appreciated only after failure of "clubfoot" treatment.

Etiology

The clinical deformity that is seen with congenital longitudinal deficiency of the tibia varies according to the degree of deficiency. In the most severe deficiencies (type 1a), the tibia is totally absent or is represented only by a rudimentary development of the proximal end. As a consequence, true knee and ankle joints are nonexistent and the articulations that are present are unstable and cannot be reconstructed. The involved limb is extremely shortened, with the nonfunctional foot in a pronounced equinovarus position. In the deficiencies that occur less commonly (types 1b, 2, 3, and 4), at least partial development of the tibia eventually occurs, and a relatively functional knee joint will be present. Combining the two large clinical studies provides 100 deformities for review.[1,2] The types that occur most frequently (types 1a and 1b, 57 extremities) are characterized by the greatest degree of tibial deficiency, and bilateral involvement is more common (16 of 57 type 1 patients) (Fig. 3). There were 20 patients with type 2 deficiency in the combined studies, nine patients with the very rare and vaguely defined type 3 deficiency, and 14 with type 4 deformity (the only type amenable to reconstruction of an ankle joint). Only two of the 14 patients who had the less severe type 4 deficiency had bilateral involvement.

Patients with longitudinal deficiencies of the tibia frequently have a wide range of other congenital abnormalities. In a retrospective review of the experiences of three limb deficiency clinics over 22 years (1961–1983), Schoenecker and associates[2] noted associated congenital anomalies in 34 patients. Anomalies of the hip, hand, or spine occurred alone or in various combinations. Of 12 patients who had a deformity of the spine, six had a hypoplastic vertebra or a hemivertebra. A congenital anomaly of the hip

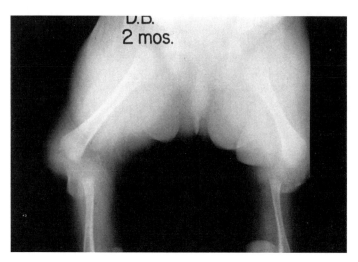

Fig. 3 *Radiograph of an infant with bilateral type 1a deficiencies; bilateral tibial hemimelia occurred more often in patients who had the more severe type 1 deficiency. (Reproduced with permission from Schoenecker PL, Capelli AM, Millar EA, et al: Congenital longitudinal deficiency of the tibia.* J Bone Joint Surg *1989;71A:278–287.)*

joint was documented in 22 patients: ten had congenital dislocation of the hip, five had congenital femoral deficiency, and seven had coxa valga. Seventeen hands had a deformity: five had syndactyly, three had absent or hypoplastic digits, six (five patients) had cleft hand deformity, one had radial dysplasia, and two had triphalagism of the thumb. There was no relationship between the type of tibial dysplasia and the incidence of associated congenital anomalies. Terminal foot deformities were documented in 17 of the involved extremities. In 11 feet, preaxial polydactyly of varying degree was noted; no total duplication of the foot was seen. In six extremities, there was a longitudinal deficiency of the foot.

The noted pattern of associated anomalies of the hip, hand, and spine may arise sporadically or in families in which tibial deficiency is inherited. At least two autosomal dominant syndromes that are associated with tibial deficiency have been described.[4,5] Two of our patients appeared to fit the first of these, in which tibial dysplasia is associated with triphalangeal thumbs and prehallucal polydactyly.[2] There is greater variability of associated anomalies in the second autosomal dominant syndrome, in which tibial deficiency is associated with split-hand deformities and femoral bifurcation or ulnar defects. Five of our patients had a cleft hand deformity.[2] In addition to dominant inheritance of tibial meromelia, several reports have suggested autosomal recessive inheritance.[6,7]

The etiology of longitudinal deficiency of the tibia for the most part remains obscure. Jones and associates[1] noted exposure to thalidomide in two cases and Schoenecker and associates[2] noted a positive family history of congenital anomalies in 20 of 57 patients. Schoenecker and associates[2] have reported a greater than 50% incidence of associated congenital anomalies, including the upper extremity and the spine. It is, therefore, not surprising that they also noted the frequent occurrence of congenital anomalies of the upper extremities in close relatives of their 57 patients. A relatively increased incidence of congenital anomalies of the spine may have been found in family members had radiographs been taken of them. The occurrence of longitudinal deficiency of the tibia in family members of affected patients is of great interest. Schoenecker and associates[2] noted three patients and Jones and associates[1] noted one who had a close relative with tibial deficiency. Otherwise, there has been only rare documentation of the occurrence of tibial deficiency in the same family.[8] Familial occurrence of longitudinal pre- and/or postaxial limb deficiencies of the upper and lower extremities has been reported far more frequently for the relatively rare tibial deficiency than for the much more common fibular or radial deficiencies. Moreover, other musculoskeletal anomalies occur frequently both in patients with longitudinal deficiency of the tibia and in their relatives.

Treatment

Treatment guidelines are based on the classification schema described earlier (Fig. 2). Definitive surgical treatment of longitudinal deficiency of the tibia in most cases (types 1 to 3) includes ablative surgery, either a knee disarticulation or a Symes or Chopart's amputation. Only patients with the uncommon type 4 deficiency are truly candidates for attempted reconstruction of an ankle joint. Patients who have a unilateral or bilateral type 1a deformity are best managed by a disarticulation of the knee joint. Amputation is optimally performed at about 12 months of age, although it is often deferred until the parents are convinced the extremity is and will be nonfunctional. A knee disarticulation is performed using a long curved transverse incision with the anterior flap larger than the posterior. The remnant of the quadriceps mechanism is reattached medially and laterally to identifiable hamstrings. The dressing, with or without a plaster shell, must be secured with suspension about the pelvis.

Definitive prosthetic fitting is appropriate when the patient is securely pulling to stand. Prosthetic design of choice consists of an endbearing knee disarticulation type. Pelvic suspension is often necessary, especially for bilateral deformity. Although eventual function for a patient with type 1a deformity is generally very good, lack of an anatomic knee joint lessens the functional potential in comparison to patients with types 1b to 4 deficiencies or those with longitudinal deficiency of the fibula. In attempting to anatomically reconstruct a functional knee joint, Brown[9] proposed transposing the proximal fibula into the distal femoral groove. In the retrospective review of the collective experiences of three major limb deficiency clinics at the Greenville, Chicago, and St. Louis Shriners Hospitals, generally unsatisfactory results were reported either secondary to instability or deformity (typi-

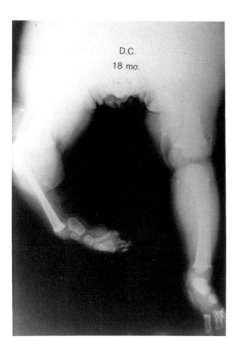
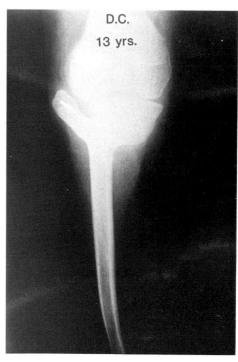

Fig. 4 *Radiographs of a patient with type 1b deficiency on the right.* **Left,** *Patient at 18 months. Note shortened limb, equinovarus foot; well-developed distal femur suggests the presence of an as yet unossified proximal tibial anlage.* **Right,** *Same patient at 13 years of age, 10 years after Syme amputation and 8 years after synostosis of proximal fibula to proximal tibial anlage; a functional knee joint allows use of a below-knee prosthesis. (Reproduced with permission from Schoenecker PL, Capelli AM, Millar EA, et al: Congenital longitudinal deficiency of the tibia. J Bone Joint Surg 1989;71A:278–287.)*

cally a flexion contracture) and poor function in ten of 14 limbs so treated; a knee disarticulation was subsequently done in six and a knee fusion in four.[2] For most surgeons,[2,10–12] the Brown procedure has not consistently proved to be a satisfactory means of salvaging a knee joint in a limb with a type 1a deficiency. As such, fibular centralization is not recommended in an attempt to preserve a knee joint in type 1a deficiency.

Satisfactory results can be obtained in some extremities with type 1b deficiency after synostosis of the fibula to the remnant of the proximal end of the tibia, distal to the intact functional knee joint (Fig. 4). It is possible to differentiate type 1b from type 1a deficiencies by arthrography, by direct surgical exploration of the knee joint, and most recently, by computed tomography, magnetic resonance imaging, or ultrasonography. If a cartilaginous remnant of the proximal end of the tibia is identified (type 1b), disarticulation of the knee joint should be deferred, the foot should be ablated, and a conventional below-knee prosthesis fitted. Because there is potential for the development of a relatively functional articulation between the distal

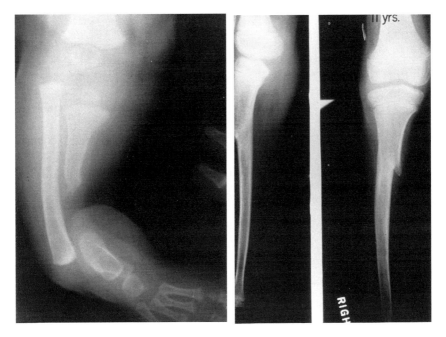

Fig. 5 *Radiographs of a patient with type 2 deficiency.* **Left,** *Patient at 10 months. Absence of distal tibia is apparent; note the relatively unusual associated longitudinal deficiency of the foot as opposed to the more commonly associated diplopodia.* **Right,** *At 11 years of age a stable, well-developed knee joint is present, allowing efficient use of a below-knee prosthesis; a tibiofibular synostosis was performed at 3 years of age and a Syme amputation at 4 years. (Reproduced with permission from Schoenecker PL, Capelli AM, Millar EA, et al: Congenital longitudinal deficiency of the tibia. J Bone Joint Surg 1989;71A:278–287.)*

end of the femur and the proximal tibial remnant, it may later be possible to perform tibiofibular synostosis, and a functional knee joint may then be preserved.

Type 2 deformity can be recognized early by the presence of ossification of a remnant of the proximal end of the tibia. The tibia is represented by a more fully formed proximal tibia with potential for development of a relatively functional articulation with the distal femur (Fig. 5). Patients who have a type 2 deformity are optimally treated with preservation of the knee joint and amputation of the foot; a subsequent tibiofibular synostosis is performed, usually before the child is 2 years of age. Using internal fixation as a supplement to cast immobilization makes it possible to obtain a synostosis in optimal alignment. Resection of the proximal protruding fibula should be considered when joining the fibula to the tibia. Left intact, the protruding proximal fibula potentially can adversely affect prosthetic fit and function. Once a stable synostosis is achieved, patients with a type 2 deformity usually function very well as below-knee amputees. However,

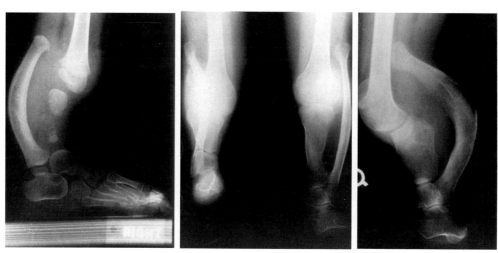

Fig. 6 *Radiographs of a patient with bilateral type 3 tibial hemimelia.* **Left,** *Lateral of leg at 3 years of age shows characteristic amorphous tibial segment and posteriorly bowed, proximally migrated fibula; note associated polydactyly. Bilateral Chopart amputations were done. Anteroposterior* **(center)** *and lateral* **(right)** *view at 21 years of age shows persistence of fibular bowing and proximal migration limiting knee flexion; the patient wore bilateral below-knee prostheses and was employed as a nurse. (Reproduced with permission from Schoenecker PL, Capelli AM, Millar EA, et al: Congenital longitudinal deficiency of the tibia.* J Bone Joint Surg *1989;71A:278–287.)*

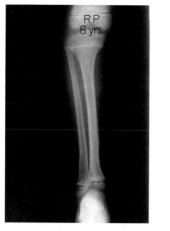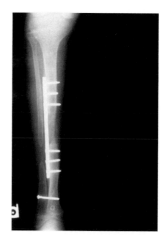

Fig. 7 *Radiographs of a patient with a relatively mild type 4 tibial deficiency.* **Left,** *At age 8 years there is dysplasia of the distal tibia with anticipated limb length inequality of 6 cm.* **Right,** *At completion of 5-cm lengthening by the Wagner method. (Reproduced with permission from Schoenecker PL, Capelli AM, Millar EA, et al: Congenital longitudinal deficiency of the tibia.* J Bone Joint Surg *1989;71A:278–287.)*

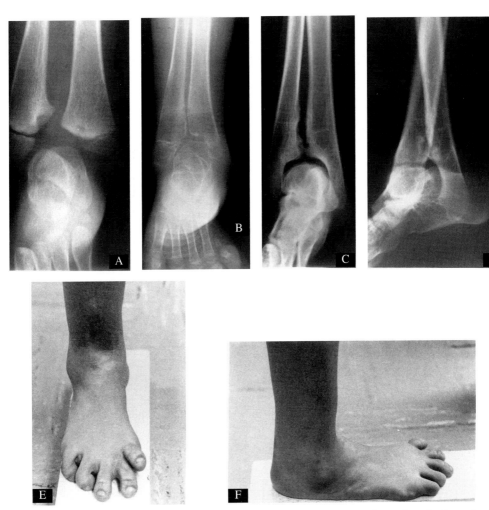

Fig. 8 Radiographs of a patient with type 4 tibial hemimelia. *A,* At 4 years of age, there is diastasis of the ankle and absence of the first ray; clinically the patient was noted to have moderate equinovarus. *B,* Four months after open reduction of the diastasis. *C* and *D,* At skeletal maturity the ankle was pain free and stable with dorsiflexion to neutral and 25° plantarflexion. *E* and *F,* Clinical photographs at skeletal maturity show a plantigrade foot; the length discrepancy had been treated with epiphysiodesis. *(Reproduced with permission FROM Sedgwick WG, Schoenecker PL: Congenital diastasis of the ankle joint: Case report of a patient treated and followed to maturity.* J Bone Joint Surg *1982;64A:450–453.)*

lack of normal ligamentous knee joint stability and muscle control of the proximal tibia sometimes necessitates the use of proximal thigh suspension to assure a functional stable prosthetic fit.

In patients with the very rare type 3 deformity, a unique amorphous osseus structure develops, representative of the shaft of the tibia. Eventually, a representative though rudimentary knee-ankle articulation develops. The scant information available reveals that patients who have a type 3 deficiency have functioned relatively well as below-the-knee amputees following Syme or Chopart amputation (Fig. 6).

In patients who have a type 4 deficiency, a functional articulation of the foot at the ankle is possible. However, following a successful reconstruction of the congenital diastasis of the ankle, significant limb length inequality (in some patients anticipated to be greater than 8 cm) remains a problem. Leg lengthening may be considered and performed successfully (Fig. 7). However, parental concerns with both the noted leg-length inequality and the magnitude of the lengthening procedure necessary frequently have resulted in amputation of the foot, either primarily, or after surgical treatment of the ankle deformity. Six of the nine patients with type IV deformity who had a leg-length inequality eventually treated with a Syme amputation had previously had successful reconstruction of the ankle joint, while three retained their foot (Fig. 8). I advise treatment of type 4 deficiencies on an individual basis, offering either reconstruction and eventual lengthening or primary amputation and conversion to a below-the-knee prosthesis.

References

1. Jones D, Barnes J, Lloyd-Roberts GC: Congenital aplasia and dysplasia of the tibia with intact fibula: Classification and management. *J Bone Joint Surg* 1978;60B:31–39.

2. Schoenecker PL, Capelli AM, Millar EA, et al: Congenital longitudinal deficiency of the tibia. *J Bone Joint Surg* 1989;71A:278–287.

3. Sedgwick WG, Schoenecker PL: Congenital diastasis of the ankle joint: Case report of a patient treated and followed to maturity. *J Bone Joint Surg* 1982;64A:450–453.

4. Clark MW: Autosomal dominant inheritance of tibial meromelia: Report of a kindred. *J Bone Joint Surg* 1975;57A:262–264.

5. Lenz W: Genetics and limb deficiencies. *Clin Orthop* 1980;148:9–17.

6. McKay M, Clarren SK, Zorn R: Isolated tibial hemimelia in sibs: An autosomal recessive disorder? *Am J Med Genet* 1984;17:603–607.

7. Mahloudji M, Farpour H: An unusual deformity in an inbred community. *Birth Defects* 1974;10:75–80.

8. Agarwal RP, Jain D, Ramesh Babu CS, Garg RK: A hereditable combination of congenital anomalies. *J Bone Joint Surg* 1996;78B:492–494.

9. Brown FW: Construction of a knee joint in congenital total absence of the tibia (paraxial hemimelia tibia): A preliminary report. *J Bone Joint Surg* 1965;47A:695–704.

10. Jayakumar SS, Eilert RE: Fibular transfer for congenital absence of the tibia. *Clin Orthop* 1979;139:97–101.

11. Loder RT, Herring JA: Fibular transfer for congenital absence of the tibia: A reassessment. *J Pediatr Orthop* 1987;7:8–13.

12. Kalamchi A, Dawe RV: Congenital deficiency of the tibia. *J Bone Joint Surg* 1985;67B:581–584.

Chapter 19

Brown's Fibula-Femur Transfer for Congenital Absence of the Tibia

John E. Hall, MD

It is generally agreed upon that when dealing with deficiencies in children's limbs, whether congenital or acquired, all useful length should be saved and all functional joints should be spared. Applying the principle to congenital absence of the tibia, Fred Brown[1] devised his procedure in an attempt to produce a limb with a useful knee and below-knee segment.

The advantages of this approach are self-evident (a proprioceptive knee joint with active flexion and extension) if it can be made to work. Here the controversy arises. Most authors have felt that the results of this operation have not been good enough to justify its use.

In 1965, I invited Fred Brown to come and operate on a child with bilateral complete absence of the tibias. Unfortunately, this person has been lost to follow-up, but at 5 years, function was judged to be superior to bilateral knee disarticulations. Since that time, I have used this procedure routinely in children with active quadriceps function. The results in five patients operated on between 1976 and 1988 were published in 1996.[2] At that time, all seven affected limbs were functioning satisfactorily, but one limb in a patient with bilateral tibial deficiencies has been converted to a knee disarticulation, which is, of course, the alternative if the Brown procedure fails. Knee disarticulation leaves the child with the same level of amputation as if it had been done primarily.

Another controversy concerning the Brown procedure is whether or not an attempt should be made to preserve the foot. Because a stable ankle is an unlikely result, bracing would have to be used permanently unless an eventual ankle arthrodesis was performed. The function of a braced ankle and a Syme's amputation is similar, and the end-bearing amputation residual limb makes control of leg length much simpler.

Materials and Methods

The patients on whom my experience has been based are those described in the article by Simmons and associates[2] plus one additional subsequent patient with both legs affected.

Surgical Technique

Technique was as described in the article by Simmons and associates.[2] Points to be emphasized include the shortening procedure (usually of the femur if necessary), the remodeling of the upper fibula, and the necessity to leave extremely long flaps for the Syme's type of amputation to avoid closure under tension.

The operation begins with a longitudinal incision along the lateral border of the quadriceps. The incision is carried down to the area where the patellar tendon blends with the anterior fascia of the leg. Through this opening the surgeon can ascertain whether or not there is an anlage of the upper tibia. If there is no upper tibial remnant, the surgeon can proceed with the fibular transfer. If an upper tibial component is present, the best course of action is to delay a transfer until the tibial segment is ossified. The fibular epiphysis must be dissected free enough to transpose it, but at least half of the area should be left with soft-tissue attachments to preserve blood supply. The proximal tip is cut with a knife to fit the condylar notch area of the femur.

Results

At follow-up in 1993, all seven limbs had been preserved. However, it recently was learned that one child with a bilateral transfer developed a severe knee flexion contracture of one knee. He had a knee disarticulation rather than an attempt to correct the contracture.

All "knee" joints were unstable in a medial and lateral direction, but this was controlled by a thigh cuff and knee hinges. All patients had knee flexion contractures of approximately 20°, which were accommodated easily in a modified patellar tendon-bearing type of socket. The average limit of flexion was to 70°, leaving an active range of 50° of movement. This is a limited but functional range, which allows most activities short of kneeling, sitting on the haunches, or squats.

Surgical complications were few but included one wound breakdown in the Syme's type incision when the flaps were closed under some tension. There were no wound infections or neurovascular problems. Further surgical procedures were necessary in four of the seven limbs; one to reposition the heel pad, two tendon transfers of hamstring to quadriceps to improve knee extension, and one subsequent revision to a knee disarticulation. Each patient had a planned operation to remove the internal fixation used to position the knee and to stabilize the shortening procedure if it was necessary.

Discussion

Most parents, given the choice, tend to opt for any procedure that preserves as much of a child's limb as possible. If a surgeon does not believe that this operation is worthwhile, it is very easy to transfer this belief to the patient, making it the surgeon's rather than the patient's choice.

How many of these limbs will survive into adult life, I do not know. Advances in prosthetic design with newer methods of swing and stance phase control and even improved proprioception will probably lessen the advantage of the Brown procedure. At the moment, I still consider it advantageous, particularly for the child with bilateral problems.

Summary

The primary indication for the Brown procedure, in my opinion, is a patient who has a well-developed lower end of the femur, preferably a patella, certainly a functioning quadriceps mechanism, and does not have an upper end of the tibia by current imaging techniques.

If a proximal tibial anlage is present, a tibiofibular synostosis procedure is indicated when the tibial component is ossified.

References

1. Brown FW: Construction of a knee joint in congenital total absence of the tibia (paraxial hemimelia tibia). *J Bone Joint Surg* 1965;47A:695–704.
2. Simmons ED Jr, Ginsburg GM, Hall JE: Brown's procedure for congenital absence of the tibia revisited. *J Pediatr Orthop* 1996;16:85–89.

Chapter 20

Fibular Transfer for Congenital Absence of the Tibia (Brown Procedure)

Randall T. Loder, MD

Introduction

Congenital absence of the tibia has a wide spectrum of abnormality. In some cases it is associated with a femoral deficiency, and in these cases the femoral deficiency takes precedence in selecting treatment. In other circumstances it is an isolated lesion, either unilateral or bilateral; this chapter addresses only isolated congenital absence of the tibia.

There are two major types of congenital tibial anomalies.[1] In most cases, the tibia is short with associated aplasia or dysplasia of the fibula; the lateral ray(s) of the foot typically are reduced as well. Less commonly, the tibia is absent or dysplastic and the fibula is relatively normal; the foot may be augmented in this type. This last type, an absent or dysplastic tibia with a relatively normal fibula, has been classified by Jones and associates[1] into four types based on radiographic appearance (Fig. 1). This classification scheme is of utmost importance in selecting appropriate surgical management. Type 1 is radiographic absence of the proximal tibia; type 2 is radiographic presence of the proximal tibia; type 3 is radiographic presence of only the distal tibia; and type 4 is a short tibia with distal tibiofibular diastasis. Type 1 is subdivided into type 1a with a hypoplastic lower femoral epiphysis and type 1b with a normal lower femoral epiphysis. This distinction is crucial. The presence of a normal lower femoral epiphysis (type 1b) implies the presence of a proximal tibia (analogous to a normal acetabulum implying the presence of a proximal femur prior to the appearance of any epiphyseal ossification).

Surgical Options

The goal of treatment is to obtain knee function that will allow as normal a gait as possible. The first step is to address the fixed foot deformity, typically an equinovarus position. Amputation and prosthetic fitting is usually the best treatment for the foot deformity, because reconstructive attempts universally fail, with recurrence of a deformed, rigid nonplantigrade foot, and because the associated limb-length discrepancy at maturity can be problematic.

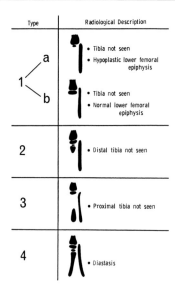

Type		Radiological Description
1	a	• Tibia not seen • Hypoplastic lower femoral epiphysis
	b	• Tibia not seen • Normal lower femoral epiphysis
2		• Distal tibia not seen
3		• Proximal tibia not seen
4		• Diastasis

Fig. 1 *The four radiographic types of congenital aplasia of the tibia. (Reproduced with permission from Jones D, Barnes J, Lloyd-Roberts GC: Congenital aplasia and dysplasia of the tibia with intact fibula: Classification and management.* J Bone Joint Surg *1978;60B:31–39.)*

The next and most important management decision concerns the knee. It is here that the Jones classification becomes extremely important. If a proximal tibial remnant is present (type 2), then the preferred management is a tibiofibular synostosis. The fibula is medially transposed and synostosed into the tibial remnant, creating a one-bone leg. Although there is some residual lateral knee instability, the prosthesis used to address the foot ablation can provide knee stability. The quadriceps and hamstring muscles have normal insertions because the proximal tibia and fibula exist; therefore, knee function with regards to active flexion and extension is quite good.

When no proximal tibial remnant is seen radiographically (type 1), the distinction between a type 1a and 1b anomaly becomes very important. The presence of a normal lower femoral epiphysis (type 1b) implies the presence of a proximal tibia (albeit cartilaginous), and the treatment should be a tibiofibular synostosis when adequate ossification of the proximal tibia has occurred. This treatment should result in excellent function. For the type 1a anomaly, there are two major treatment options: knee disarticulation with prosthetic fitting or reconstruction of a tibia by transposing the fibula into the intercondylar notch (Brown procedure). The hope is that the fibula will hypertrophy and develop into a tibia-like structure with satisfactory knee function.

History of the Brown Procedure

The description of fibular transfer for complete congenital absence of the tibia has been credited to Brown.[2] However, the first actual description of this transposition in the English literature was by Myers,[3] who, in 1904, performed a fibular transplantation under the femoral condyles in a 2-year-old boy. Follow-up 11 months later was encouraging. Sulamaa and Ryöppy[4] described the same procedure one year before Brown. Nevertheless, fibular transfer for congenital absence of the tibia typically is called the Brown procedure.

Brown[2] first reported on three cases with very encouraging results. A 15-year follow-up study of 40 cases further defined the indications and surgical technique.[5] If the indications, surgical procedure, and postoperative management were followed, Brown and Pohnert[5] believed that the child would have an extremity with proprioception and a functional knee joint adaptable for a below-knee prosthesis. However, this 15-year follow-up study was published only in abstract form and does not allow the reader to closely examine the cases and results. Although Brown has reported good results with fibular transposition,[2,5] most other authors report very poor results and no longer recommend the procedure.

Poor outcome results primarily from inadequate quadriceps power, which causes a progressive knee flexion contracture and poor function. Many authors have stated that a strong quadriceps is an absolute prerequisite for a successful Brown procedure. To further understand the successes and failures of treatment for type 1 congenital absence of the tibia, I have undertaken an analysis of all cases published in the English-speaking literature with adequate information.[6–11] Unfortunately, the information provided in the Brown and Pohnert study[5] is inadequate for inclusion in this compiled analysis.

Compiled Results for the Brown Procedure

Eighty-seven cases of type 1 tibial deficiency were described in the literature. Detailed information was gathered for each case; parameters covered are listed in Table 1. If a Brown procedure had been performed, it was also determined if a knee disarticulation was later recommended or performed. The results of treatment for the Brown procedure were graded using the criteria of Jayakumar and Eilert,[12] who are strong proponents of the procedure provided a strong quadriceps is present. Their criteria for a good result are the minimal requirements for an acceptable gait: active knee motion from 10° to 80°, varus or valgus instability < 5°, and no flexion contracture. If active knee motion was < 10° to 80°, a varus or valgus instability of > 5° existed, or there was a flexion contracture > 10°, then the result was considered poor. The recommendation or performance of a knee disarticulation or fusion was also considered a poor result. The reason for the poor result was also determined (instability, flexion contracture, or other [eg, leg-length discrepancy]).

There were 43 unilateral cases and 44 bilateral cases; 56 involved the right and 28 the left lower extremity (laterality not known in three). The first surgical procedure for the knee was a knee disarticulation in 18 cases, a Brown procedure in 62 cases, a knee arthrodesis in two cases, a soft-tissue release in one case, and a tibiofibular synostosis in two cases (unknown in two cases). The time of follow-up was known for 80 cases and averaged 12.3 years (range, 2.2 to 29.7 years). The median quadriceps power was grade 2 (range, 1 to 5); the average age at the first surgery was 1.5 ± 2.5 years (range, 0.25 to 15.0 years).

Type 1a Versus Type 1b

There were 75 type 1a and 12 type 1b tibial deficiencies. The differences between the type 1a and 1b cases are shown in Table 1. There were statistically significant differences between the 1a and 1b groups for both quadriceps power ($1a = 1.8 \pm 1$, $1b = 4.8 \pm 0.4$, $p = 0.0002$) and results ($1a = 98\%$ poor results, $1b = 55\%$ poor results, $p = 0.001$). There were no other statistically significant differences between the groups.

The Brown Procedure for Type 1a or Type 1b Tibial Deficiency

The 62 cases of the Brown procedure were extracted and analyzed separately; there were 56 type 1a and six type 1b cases (Table 2). Here again there was a highly significant difference in quadriceps power between these groups. There was no difference between the groups in overall results (results known in 61 cases). However, when the poor results were selected and the reason for the poor results analyzed, only one of six type 1b cases had a flexion contracture; the other five had only valgus/varus knee instability. This was reversed in the 1a group, where 53 cases had flexion contractures, one had valgus/varus instability, and one a major limb-length discrepancy. This difference was highly significant ($p = 0.000001$). Thus, 53 of 55 cases in which the Brown procedure was used for type 1a congenital absence of the tibia developed flexion contractures that led to poor results. The poor results in the 1b cases were due to valgus/varus knee instability. This valgus/varus instability is easily controlled by the prosthesis for the foot amputation, whereas persistent and recurrent knee flexion contractures are not permanently correctable. These flexion contractures eventually lead to knee disarticulation or arthrodesis.

It is clear from this literature review that the Brown procedure uniformly fails in the treatment of Jones type 1a tibial deficiency. I believe it should not be attempted in the "hopes that it might work," because it will always end in failure at long-term follow-up. The psychological trauma of a child undergoing multiple surgeries with eventual amputation must be kept in mind. Compared to a knee disarticulation within the first year of life, which the child will not remember, the financial costs of unsuccessful, multiple surgeries in this era of medical-care cost containment must also be considered.

Table 1 Comparison between 87 combined cases of type 1a and 1b tibial deficiency

Parameter	Total	Type 1a	Type 1b	p value
Number of cases	87	75	12	-
Gender (M/F)	21/8	18/6	3/2	0.60
Unilateral/bilateral	43/44	33/41	9/3	0.07
Quadriceps power*	2.4 ± 1.6	1.8 ± 1.0	4.8 ± 0.4	0.0002
First surgery (Kd/Br/Kf/St/Tfs)†	18/62/2/1/2	16/56/2/1/0	2/6/0/0/2	0.05
Age at first surgery	1.5 ± 2.5	1.5 ± 2.5	1.6 ± 1.8	0.79
Eventual knee disarticulation (Y/N)	41/45	39/35	2/10	0.028
Results (good/poor)	5/62	1/57	4/5	0.001
Cause of poor result (Fc/Ins)§	55/6	55/1	0/5	0.00001
Final follow-up	12.3 ± 7.0	12.5 ± 7.0	11.2 ± 7.1	0.54

* 1 = no active extension, 2 = a flicker of extension, 3 = active extension with gravity eliminated, 4 = active extension against gravity, and 5 = full strength of active extension against resistance
† Kd = knee disarticulation, Br = Brown procedure, Kf = knee arthrodesis, St = soft-tissue release, and Tfs = tibiofibular synostosis
§ Fc = flexion contracture, Ins = instability

Table 2 Comparison between 62 cases of the Brown procedure for types 1a and 1b tibial deficiency

Parameter	Type 1a	Type 1b	p value
Number of cases*	55	6	-
Quadriceps power	1.9 ± 1.1	4.8 ± 0.4	0.0003
Age at Brown procedure	1.0 ± 0.7	0.6 ± 0.2	0.07
Results (good/poor)	1/54	1/5	0.19
Cause of poor result (Fc/Ins)†	53/1	0/5	0.000001
Final follow-up	12.6 ± 7.2	14.2 ± 7.0	0.59

* Results were known in 55 of 56 type 1a cases

† Fc = flexion contracture, Ins = instability

Functional Results of Knee Disarticulation

The results of knee disarticulation are remarkably good. To my knowledge there is only one series[13] in which the functional results of pediatric knee disarticulations are analyzed. In this series of six children studied by gait analysis, the child's gait velocity averaged 81% of normal and the time for a single gait cycle averaged 131% of normal. The energy expenditure as measured by the physiologic cost index ([heart rate walking – heart rate at rest]/gait velocity) was within the normal range. Most importantly, the prosthetic knee showed good flexion during swing phase and absence of flexion during stance, allowing for a stable, extended knee with weightbearing. There were no residual limb problems. Although none of the six children were in organized sports, one child was able to ski recreationally with modified equipment. Nevertheless, as anticipated, their running was markedly decreased, with the time for the 50-yard dash below the fifth percentile for age.

Conclusion

The literature is uniformly in favor of knee disarticulation for Jones type 1a tibial deficiency, whereas tibiofibular synostosis is recommended for Jones type 1b tibial deficiency. If this distinction cannot easily be made radiographically, ultrasonography[14] should be used to determine the presence or absence of a proximal tibial cartilaginous anlage. With this information, early and appropriate counseling to the parents can be made regarding the recommended method of treatment and functional expectation.[15,16]

References

1. Jones D, Barnes J, Lloyd-Roberts GC: Congenital aplasia and dysplasia of the tibia with intact fibula: Classification and management. *J Bone Joint Surg* 1978;60B:31–39.

2. Brown FW: Construction of a knee joint in congenital total absence of the tibia (paraxial hemimelia tibia): A preliminary report. *J Bone Joint Surg* 1965;47A: 695–704.

3. Myers TH: Congenital absence of the tibia: Transplantation of head of fibula. Arthrodesis at the ankle-joint. *Am J Orthop Surg* 1905;3:72–85.

4. Sulamaa M, Ryöppy S: Congenital absence of the tibia. *Acta Orthop Scand* 1963;33:262–270.

5. Brown FW, Pohnert WH: Abstract: Construction of a knee joint in meromelia tibia (congenital absence of the tibia): A fifteen-year follow-up study. *J Bone Joint Surg* 1972;54A:1333.

6. Christini D, Levy EJ, Facanha FA, Kumar SJ: Fibular transfer for congenital absence of the tibia. *J Pediatr Orthop* 1993;13:378–381.

7. Epps CH Jr, Tooms RE, Edholm CD, Kruger LM, Bryant DD III: Failure of centralization of the fibula for congenital longitudinal deficiency of the tibia. *J Bone Joint Surg* 1991;73A:858–867.

8. Loder RT, Herring JA: Fibular transfer for congenital absence of the tibia: A reassessment. *J Pediatr Orthop* 1987;7:8–13.

9. Schoenecker PL, Capelli AM, Millar EA, et al: Congenital longitudinal deficiency of the tibia. *J Bone Joint Surg* 1989;71A:278–287.

10. Simmons ED Jr, Ginsburg GM, Hall JE: Brown's procedure for congenital absence of the tibia revisited. *J Pediatr Orthop* 1996;16:85–89.

11. Wehbé MA, Weinstein SL, Ponseti IV: Tibial agenesis. *J Pediatr Orthop* 1981;1:395–399.

12. Jayakumar SS, Eilert RE: Fibular transfer for congenital absence of the tibia. *Clin Orthop* 1979;139:97–101.

13. Loder RT, Herring JA: Disarticulation of the knee in children: A functional assessment. *J Bone Joint Surg* 1987;69A:1155–1160.

14. Grissom LE, Harcke HT, Kumar SJ: Sonography in the management of tibial hemimelia. *Clin Orthop* 1990;251:266–270.

15. Epps CH Jr, Schneider PL: Treatment of hemimelias of the lower extremity: Long-term results. *J Bone Joint Surg* 1989;71A:273–277.

16. Pattinson RC, Fixsen JA: Management and outcome in tibial dysplasia. *J Bone Joint Surg* 1992;74B:893–896.

Consensus

The Indications for the Brown Procedure in Tibial Deficiency

The Brown procedure for complete absence of the tibia usually fails. When there is a well-developed distal femur and the quadriceps and patella are present, there are some successful cases, but longer-term follow-up is needed.

The proximal tibia may be present but not ossified in the infant and if it is present, will allow a synostosis procedure when the tibial fragment ossifies. Early evaluation with palpation, ultrasound, and arthrography may delineate this type of tibia.

Section 5
Acquired Amputations

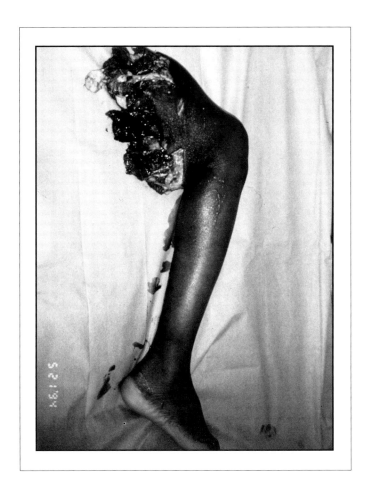

Chapter 21

Epidemiology and Prevention of Traumatic Amputations in Children

Merv Letts, MD, FRCSC
Darin Davidson

Epidemiology of Childhood Trauma

Trauma is the major cause of morbidity and mortality among children. Since the mid 1930s, trauma has been the leading cause of death in persons from 1 to 44 years of age, far exceeding death from infections (Fig. 1). In those younger than 35 years, morbidity and mortality resulting from injury far exceeds that from cancer and heart disease (Fig. 2). In the United States alone, in 1988, approximately 16,614,000 children were injured as a result of trauma.[1] In 1993, it was estimated that between 20 and 25 thousand children died as a result of unintentional trauma, with four times that number suffering permanent disability.[2]

Thus, injuries to children constitute the major public health problem in North America. Although injuries have grown in importance as a cause of incapacitation of youth as a result of better control of infection and disease, injury prevention largely has been ignored by politicians, the press, funding agencies, and, to a lesser extent, by pediatric orthopaedic surgeons. There is a widespread belief that injuries to children are the inevitable consequence of immaturity and as such are not preventable. In fact, these injuries are greatly affected by demographic factors, many of which can be modified to reduce morbidity and mortality. Over 70% of catastrophic injuries resulting in major morbidity or death are preventable.

Analysis of mortality rates in Canada and the United States (mortality statistics are meticulously recorded by public health authorities) indicates that 45% of all deaths in those 1 to 4 years of age, 46% in those 5 to 14 years of age, and 78% in those 15 to 24 years of age are from injuries. Before the 1940s injuries in children, although common, were overshadowed by the overwhelming virulence of infectious diseases. However, by 1980, death rates from these diseases had declined by 99%; whereas deaths from injuries had declined by only about 30%.[3] This premature loss of life is a tragic loss of productivity and an immeasurable cost to society. A recent estimate[4] of total lifetime costs of all injuries that occurred during the year 1985 in the United States was 158 billion dollars. This was four times the loss for cancer and more than six times the loss for cardiovascular disease. Thus, the morbidity and mortality of childhood injuries is a major economic disaster that is continuing to occur at an unacceptable rate in both Canada and the United States.

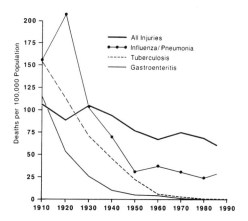

Fig. 1 *Death rates from injuries and infectious diseases by year.*

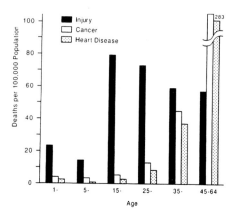

Fig. 2 *Death rates by cause and age.*

The most common causes of unintentional injury deaths in children are motor vehicle accidents, drowning, and house fires.[3] Car pedestrian deaths in childhood peak at age 6 years and then decline, whereas deaths from gunshot injuries increase in the teens. Death rates for most unintentional injuries are highest in the more rural areas. For example, farm machinery death rates are high among young children, although only 2% of children live on farms. The most common cause of farm machinery death among young children is being run over by tractors, farm wagons, combines, or fork lifts. Augers and power takeoffs are also major causes of death and injury in young children.[5] The farm injury death rate per hundred thousand population was 0.25 in

1930 and 0.27 in 1986, an increase of 8%, while the death rate from drowning has decreased by 61% over the same period.

Unintentional injury is obviously a major public health problem in the pediatric age group and basically is the last "human plague" waiting for adequate scientific investigation and understanding.

Epidemiology of Traumatic Amputations in Children

Although meticulous statistics on childhood mortality are kept by most developed countries, the documentation of limb loss in children is unfortunately lacking. There are sporadic excellent reports from some districts and hospitals concerning amputations in children, but overall there is a woeful lack of consistency in this documentation. Traumatic amputation is a devastating injury in a child and almost always is preventable. Great advances have been made in the prevention of childhood accidents over the past decade. However, the initiation and maintenance of an adequate data base on injuries, such as amputations, that cause severe disability will provide the understanding needed to improve trauma-prevention techniques. As trauma registries are set up at trauma centers throughout North America, the computerized data base must include the ICD-9 CM codes 885 to 887 and 895 to 897 for amputation injuries. Data collected are important not only in the prevention of such injuries, but also in the analysis of success in limb salvage and revascularization techniques.

A recent review on pediatric amputation injuries[6] can serve as a model of how a national, comprehensive profile of childhood amputations should be compiled. In this study of 74 children who sustained amputations, 53% were unsupervised at the time of the injury. Power lawnmowers accounted for 42% of all amputations to children under 10 years of age. Motor vehicle accidents accounted for 16% of amputations; farm injuries, 13%; and gunshot wounds, 8%. In this study, 61% of injuries to the upper extremity and 15% to the lower extremity resulted in limb salvage through replantation or revascularization. Most of these were digits amputated by a sharp mechanism.

The Association of Children's Prosthetic/Orthotic Clinics (ACPOC) have conducted periodic reviews of their amputee populations in Canada and the United States. In the most recent ACPOC review,[7] acquired amputations were outnumbered 2:1 by congenital limb deficiencies. Among 1,366 children with acquired amputations, the most common amputation was below knee, 354; followed by above knee, 259; below elbow, 128; and ankle disarticulation, 126. Although some of these amputations resulted from reconstruction of congenital malformations, these figures indicate how many acquired amputations are being dealt with by juvenile amputee clinics.

The gender distribution of traumatic amputations is consistent in most studies as having a 2:1 male to female predominance. Denmark has a very efficient amputations register, which provides dependable data for population-based studies concerning the epidemiology of amputation. This register, established in 1972 to collect data on major upper and lower extremity amputations in Denmark, would seem to be a model for such registries. The most recent report from this registry[8] indicated that the percentage of traumatic amputations in Denmark has remained unchanged during the last decade despite the improvements in replantation, plastic, vascular, and orthopaedic surgery; a considerable decrease in the number of road traffic collisions; and improvements in industrial safety. Seventeen percent of all traumatic lower limb amputations occurred in the childhood age group.

Causes of Traumatic Amputations in Childhood

Lawnmower Amputations

Epidemiology

The power lawnmower is the most frequent cause of traumatic amputation in children according to most current reviews of acquired limb loss. The majority of these amputations involve the lower limbs of children, who usually are younger than 14 years of age. Most of these injuries involve children riding on a power mower with a parent rather than playing in the vicinity of a power push mower. These injuries are devastating because the limb confronts a blade rotating at 3,000 revolutions per minute, creating tremendous kinetic energy and resulting in severe injury to the extremity despite minimal contact with the blade. Such amputations are very contaminated and the part is traumatized from several contacts with the blade, making reimplantation impossible. The most common type of amputation is amputation of a portion of the foot. There is almost a 3:1 male to female incidence of these amputations, and most children are injured playing near the lawnmower or falling off a riding lawnmower and being run over by the blades.[9–11]

Prevention

These amputations are preventable. Children should not be allowed to play in the vicinity of a lawnmower and should never be taken on rides on a power lawnmower. Because the lawnmower is such a ubiquitous piece of machinery, the family often loses respect for its potential hazards. A program of continuous safety instruction should be made available to schools to educate families and, in particular, children about the hazards of lawnmowers in an attempt to maintain the child's respect for this powerful piece of machinery that resides in the family garage. Most lawnmowers are now equipped with safety features to allow the operator to shut the machine down quickly, and lawnmowers without these safety features should not be purchased. The use of grass catchers eliminates the dangers of missile injury from stones and metal. Teenagers using lawnmowers must be mature, responsible, and aware of the dangers of the lawnmower before being allowed to operate the machine.

Farm Machinery Amputations

Epidemiology

Farm machinery accidents are one of the most common causes of traumatic limb loss in childhood and in many areas are second only to amputations from lawnmowers. In North America, farm machinery accidents account for 50% of all deaths from machinery accidents although farmers account for less than 7% of the population. The auger, in particular, is a major cause of childhood limb loss.[12] Archimedes designed the first auger to deliver water up a hill by encasing a screw device within a cylinder. The principles of today's augers are the same except that the power has increased from that of single ox to that of a modern tractor. Portable grain augers, the most common form used by farmers in rural America, have diameters of up to 120 cm and a speed of 500 to 600 revolutions per minute. They are powered by an electric motor, a gas engine, or a tractor power takeoff. The intake of the auger must of necessity be accessible to the grain. The grain may be fed to it from a hopper, or the lower end may simply be buried within a pile of grain, thus being hidden, so that a child investigating a moving pile of grain may not comprehend the potential hazard. Augers are not easily stalled, even when a limb becomes caught in the device. Although a tremendous labor-saving device for the farmer, the auger is one of the most hazardous pieces of farm equipment. In the few reviews available on trauma caused by farm machinery, the tractor has been mentioned as the main cause of agricultural accidents and the auger is the second most common.[13–15]

Boys are injured much more frequently than girls, comprising as high as 80% of cases in some series. The age at injury is usually under 7 years, indicating that most children are not injured helping out at harvest but rather playing in the vicinity of the machinery. In this type of injury, the level of amputation is usually very high; because of the tremendous power of the machinery, the limb literally becomes screwed into the machine within seconds with disastrous consequences to the limb (Fig. 3). Limb reattachment is almost always not possible because of the severe trauma that the entire limb has sustained, and subsequent prosthetic fitting may be difficult because of the high level of amputation and the considerable scarring that often results. Of 23 children with auger injuries at the Winnipeg Children's Hospital, ten had high above knee or above elbow amputations.[12]

Prevention

Amputations suffered by children as a result of farm machinery accidents can be prevented. In most industrial situations, great strides have been made in eliminating or reducing occupational hazards, largely through regulations that are enforced by employers, unions, and government agencies. Such regulatory mechanisms, however, are not operative in the case of the farmer, whose safety precautions are self imposed and who is free to operate with or without them as he chooses, usually with meager instruction. Safety shielding for power takeoff shafts, cutting blades, and augers are still optional

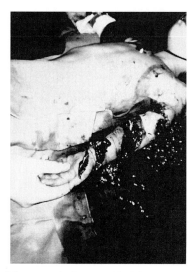

Fig. 3 *Appearance of the arm of a 7-year-old child that became entangled in an auger as he was poking it with a stick.*

accessories in some countries and, because of their cost and their real or imagined decrease in efficiency, usually are not obtained by farmers.13 More research is needed in safety, engineering, and design for farm equipment. Currently available protective devices are inadequate for preventing a child's limb from becoming entangled (Fig. 4). Orthopaedic surgeons can encourage farm groups and government to: (1) determine the true incidence of childhood trauma and amputations caused by farm equipment accidents; (2) provide better safety education for not only the farmer but also the entire family, because the average farm is a family operation; (3) encourage farm equipment manufacturers to improve machine safety; (4) develop good rural emergency and first aid programs to deal with catastrophic farm injuries; and (5) develop realistic rehabilitation programs for the injured farm member so that the farm operation may continue.

Individually, surgeons can do little but try to save life and limb, but collectively, we may be able to influence farm groups, manufacturers, and perhaps even governments, to attempt to reduce the incidence and severity of farm injuries to children.

Motor Vehicle Trauma Amputations

Epidemiology

Accidents involving motorized vehicles, including cars, recreational vehicles, and trains, are usually the second or third commonest cause of childhood amputations. The resulting injuries are usually crush injuries of the

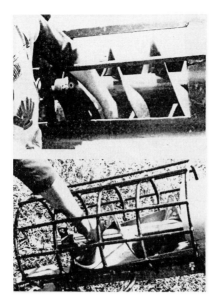

Fig. 4 *Protective devices for augers currently do not prevent a child's limb from contacting the auger.*

extremity and often are associated with a mangled extremity with degloving of skin.[16] The most common type of amputation caused by this type of injury is below knee or knee disarticulation. Children frequently are exposed to motorized vehicles, such as snowmobiles,[17] all-terrain vehicles,[18] motorcycles,[19] and, as pedestrians, the ubiquitous cars, trucks,[20] and trains.[21] In most instances, the child's limb is run over and crushed by the wheels of the vehicle, resulting in major soft-tissue trauma, vascular insufficiency, and an unsalvageable extremity. In younger children, the extremity may become entangled in the spokes of a wheel while riding double on a motorcycle or motor bike,[22] or the foot may become entangled in the treads of a snowmobile,[17] resulting in amputation of the toes and feet. Although most motor vehicle accidents result in a single limb amputation, train accidents often result in bilateral lower extremity amputations (Table 1). A common pattern of a transfemoral amputation on one side with a transtibial amputation on the other occurs as the child falls beneath the wheels of a boxcar[23,24] (Fig. 5).

Vehicle-pedestrian accidents often result in the so-called mangled extremity, and amputation may follow a prolonged attempt to salvage the limb. Often, the limb is severely traumatized from the crush injury as well as severe soft-tissue trauma from degloving of the surrounding skin and open Gustillo type III C fractures. Avulsions of nerves and blood vessels frequently render such limbs unsalvageable. Care must be taken in applying the mangled extremity score[25-27] to children, because a lower extremity that is completely denervated with a tenuous blood supply and major skin

Table 1 Type of traumatic amputation caused by trains*

Type of Amputation	Number of Amputations
Below-knee	18
Below-knee plus contralateral foot	7
Above-knee	6
Above-elbow	4
Below-elbow	1
Hand	1

* An amalgamation of data from five recent reports of childhood amputations secondary to train accidents

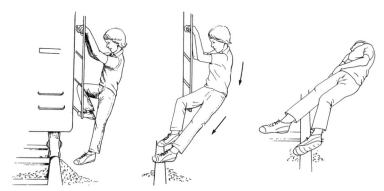

Fig. 5 *Child attempting to board the ladder of a boxcar, slipping off the high step, and slipping obliquely across the rails, often incurring an amputation of the foot and a below-knee amputation of the opposite limb. (Reproduced with permission from Thompson GH, Balourdas GM, Marcus RE: Railyard amputations in children.* J Pediatr Orthop *1983;3:443–448.)*

loss will be much less functional in weightbearing than a prosthesis. Limbs run over by tires are particularly prone to degloving injuries, which are caused by sudden, severe shearing strain that results in complete disruption of all attachments between the skin and underlying fascia. The loss of the vasculature to the degloved skin is the major reason for the inevitable skin necrosis. The degloving injury superimposed on an already crushed limb often renders the limb incapable of being salvaged, and amputation is the inevitable result.[16]

Prevention

The prevention of motor vehicle injuries can be greatly facilitated by vehicle safety education, including bicycle safety because many children sustain their injuries while riding bicycles. Legislation is necessary to prevent children from operating high-powered vehicles, such as all-terrain vehicles, snowmobiles, and motorized dirt bikes, because their motor skills are not well enough developed to allow safe operation of these types of vehicles. Because it is difficult to enforce existing legislation in remote areas, families must be educated regarding the dangers of children operating such high-powered machinery.[28] The ubiquitous motor vehicle places children constantly at risk, and they need to be "street proofed" with recurrent safety instruction from both the family and the schools. In addition, improved child restraints in motor vehicles are needed to help decrease the small number of amputations that occur as a result of motor vehicle accidents. Providing safe playgrounds that include safe areas for bicycling will help reduce motor vehicle-child pedestrian trauma in cities.

The most obvious way to prevent train accidents is to separate children from railroad yards and to educate them on the dangers of climbing on freight trains. Development of safety devices that preclude access for children to the rear ladder of train cars would greatly reduce the frequency of childhood train accidents, and this area needs to be addressed.[29]

Commercial Machinery Amputations

Epidemiology

Unfortunately, in their homes and communities, children frequently come into contact with powerful machines, such as snowblowers, commercial washing machines, power tools, chainsaws, meat grinders, and paper cutters, that can produce traumatic amputations. Most frequently these are amputations of the upper extremity, primarily fingers and hands. A major male predominance is characteristic of all commercial machine accidents. Many of the children involved in commercial machine accidents were operating the machine, either helping their parents or working at a commercial establishment.[30] Amputations from snowblowers usually occur when a teenager uses a hand to unclog a snowclog shoot and subsequently becomes entangled in the blade.[31] Chainsaw amputations usually occur when the saw strikes a solid object, such as a knot in the wood or a piece of metal, and kicks backwards, hitting the child's arm or hand.[32] Table saws and jointers are the most dangerous types of home power tools and are currently responsible for 78% of traumatic hand amputations in the workplace, with many instances of injury to inexperienced teenage operators.[33]

Prevention

Carelessness and inexperience in the use of a dangerous piece of equipment is the commonest cause of amputation in children. A lack of attention while working and a lack of experience with poor respect for the piece of equipment they are working with predispose many children to accidents. A lack of effective safety devices no doubt contributes to many amputations in children because most safety devices are designed for an adult operator. Failure to properly use installed safety devices and noncompliance with the guidelines and warnings have been reported to cause many injuries. Snowblower injuries could be prevented by design changes to decrease the frequency of clogging of the chute and the development of safety devices to more effectively prevent the operator from using a hand to unclog the machine. Many safety devices, such as protective clothing, face shields, body pads, proper gloves, and footwear are available, but often the accident occurs because the child does not use them. The enforcement of compliance with child labor laws that preclude children from being exposed to dangerous machinery would help decrease the incidence of amputations in the workplace.

Amputations Secondary to Burns in Children

Epidemiology

Severe burns from fire, electricity, or frostbite, although uncommon as a cause of major amputation, often result in loss of portions of the fingers or toes in children.[34] Thermal burns are less common in developed countries, but are a major cause of morbidity in areas where wood and coal still are used as fuel. In a Northwestern University review of 800 traumatic amputations in children, thermal burns were a cause of 47 amputations (6%).[35] The average age of the child who suffered a thermal burn resulting in an amputation was 5 years. Again, a significant male predominance was observed, with the most common cause of the thermal burn being an open flame (Fig. 6).

In colder climates, frostbite is a cause of fingertip amputations and, in more severe cases, amputations of portions of the feet and hands. Electric burns are more severe than thermal burns, and amputation (usually of an upper extremity) is a more likely outcome. In a large review of electric burns in Western Scotland, it was found that children sustained 47% of the burns.[36] Children who suffer amputations as a result of electric burns average 13 years of age, and 80% are male. Many severe electric burns result from the child coming into direct contact with a high-voltage current, usually from mischievous activities, ignorance, and insufficient safeguards to prevent children from climbing electric poles or breaking into transformer stations.

Prevention

Although the predominant prevention of all burns is probably common sense and good judgment, fire safety education is especially useful in areas where wood-burning fires are a necessity. Parental supervision of younger children around fires is mandatory. Education of children at an early age regarding the hazards and safe use of electric current is essential. Effective warning signs around high-voltage areas, increased security, and the use of safety devices around power lines and electric outlets help to decrease access to children.

Amputations Caused by Vascular Catheterizations in Neonates

Epidemiology

Specific vascular problems predispose to amputation in children. One of the most devastating is vascular insufficiency of a limb in a newborn infant. This

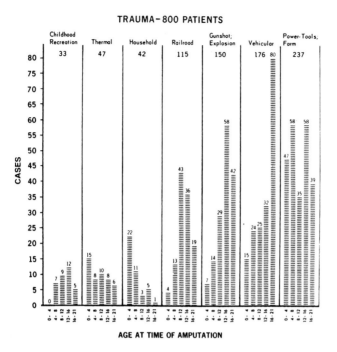

Fig. 6 *Etiology of acquired amputations secondary to trauma. (Courtesy of Northwestern University Medical School Prosthetic-Orthotic Program.)*

condition, which has been called neonatal gangrene, occurs in children who have certain predisposing factors to vascular occlusion. These factors include prematurity, polycythemia, umbilical artery catheterization, or other invasive procedures required in the intensive-care treatment for life-threatening illnesses in newborn infants.[37] The lower extremity is affected most commonly, and the condition often results in amputation of portions of the foot or below-knee amputations. In very young children and infants, care should always be taken not to amputate prematurely and to await definitive demarcation of the gangrenous portion. Amputation in children should also always be designed to preserve growth plates wherever possible to ensure an adequate residual limb for prosthetic fitting in the older child.

Other acquired conditions may cause vascular insufficiency. For example, meningococcemia can result in a devastating coagulopathy, which necessitates multiple amputations and often results in growth plate arrests secondary to vascular insufficiency of the physis. Vascular insufficiency resulting from fractures, so-called Volkmann's ischemia, if unrecognized may be so severe that the extremity ultimately may require amputation, if only to remove a useless appendage.

All vascular insufficiencies are major emergencies that require aggressive management to reestablish vascularity. In a recent 15-year review of neonatal gangrene at the Children's Hospital of Eastern Ontario, ten infants required amputation for vascular insufficiency out of a total of 5,550 neonates who had been treated in the neonatal nursery for an incidence of 0.2%. These children must deal with the amputation for the rest of their lives, and the vascular insult is a threat to life as well as limb at this young age.

Prevention

Prevention of vascular insufficiency requires extreme vigilance in monitoring of the extremity in the face of circumstances that predispose to vascular occlusion, especially arterial catheterizations. A risk scale for neonatal vascular insufficiency has been proposed (Table 2) that should increase the awareness of infants at risk for vascular occlusion. The best management is early recognition and aggressive treatment with good hydration, attempts to promote fibrinolysis of clots, and occasionally surgical removal of vascular obstruction. All children with meningococcemia should be watched carefully for any signs of vascular insufficiency although treatment is extremely difficult in these very ill children.

Vascular insufficiency after fractures of the upper and lower extremity should always be kept in mind and the limb monitored accordingly. Careful observation of the pulse, warmth, color, movement, and sensation of the extremity following a fracture and closed reduction is mandatory. Immediate pain relative to the fracture should suggest the diagnosis of a compartment syndrome. Early treatment includes removal of all tight bandages and casts. Compartment measurements may confirm the diagnosis and early fasciotomy may avert disastrous compartment necrosis.

Landmine Amputations

Epidemiology

Landmine explosions in countries previously devastated by war are a major cause of limb loss in children. Although the exact incidence is unknown, it is now realized that in such countries as Cambodia, Afghanistan, Vietnam, Mozambique, and Bosnia, death and limb loss from landmines and unexploded ordnance are a major public health problem.[38–41] After conflict in which there has been extensive use of landmines, landmine-related casualties are almost exclusively civilian and a significant proportion of those maimed are children. Mine contamination of a country leaves a deadly legacy that not only results in hundreds of childhood amputations but also makes it difficult to farm the lands, to adequately carry out vaccination campaigns in rural areas, and to provide humanitarian aids. In such countries, children are often required to perform tasks, critical to the very survival of the family, such as herding animals, fetching water or firewood, or scavenging for food. The impact of a landmine explosion on a child is much greater than on an adult. Because of the small body frame of the often underdeveloped child, the mine results in much higher amputations than in the soldier it is designed to maim. In these underdeveloped countries, prosthetic management is often

Table 2 Risk scale for neonatal vascular insufficiency

Risk	Point
Prematurity	3
Umbilical artery catheter	3
Polycythemia > 20 g Hb	3
Diabetic mother	2
Twin	2
Septicemia	2

inadequate, and the child can no longer contribute to the family. Thus, the result of the landmine blast is much greater than simply a loss of limb to the child.

A review of 1,177 nomad families in Afghanistan representing 8,793 individuals indicate that 63% of the families had lost animals to landmines, and 214 members of the family, 17% of whom were younger than 15 years of age, had been injured by landmines.[41] In Cambodia in 1994, it was estimated that the number of mine amputees was 36,000 out of a population of 8.5 million. Approximately one in every 236 Cambodians had lost one or more limbs from landmine injuries.[38]

Prevention

Landmines continue to be a major public health hazard in many countries trying to recover from the ravages of war. Most mine injuries involve civilians, often women and children. Survivors of mine blasts often require lengthy hospital stays, multiple operations, and prolonged prosthetic management. Orthopaedic surgeons can contribute to the care of landmine victims and assist with their rehabilitation through volunteer work with Orthopaedics Overseas or similar organizations. Clearing of landmines is of utmost urgency. Continued and active lobbying of politicians to support a ban on the use of mines by modern armies is essential. Although a ban on exports from major countries including the United States and Canada has been implemented, the United Nations General Assembly resolution calling for a permanent worldwide moratorium on the exports of antipersonnel landmines needs to be instituted.[40] There currently are as many as 110 million buried landmines in 60 countries. These will continue to maim or kill 26,000 people a year, and most of the survivors will have an amputation of one or more extremities. Intensified efforts to demine affected countries is urgently needed.

Amputations Resulting From Gunshot Wounds and Blast Injuries

Epidemiology

Approximately 1,200 children die and 8,000 are injured annually in the United States from accidental gunshot wounds and explosive blasts. There has been a tremendous increase in the incidence of gunshot wounds in children over the past decade.[42] Although gunshot amputations most commonly involve the toes and digits of the hand, high-velocity bullets have also resulted in amputations of the foot and hand. Gunshot wounds and explosive injuries accounted for 150 of 800 amputations in children or 19% of all traumatic amputations in the Northwestern University review.[35] Explosive blasts from fireworks or homemade bombs most commonly result in amputations of the fingers or hands because they usually explode while being carried in the child's hands.[43] Higher amputations occur as well.

Prevention

The escalation of gunshot wounds to children is a major public health problem in many areas of the United States. The increased availability of weapons, especially hand guns, has precipitated most of these gunshot wounds. Increased gun control legislation is needed. The unsafe storage of unused fireworks also has been a major factor preceding many blast injuries. Gang wars in some cities have also contributed to an increase in amputations from gunshot wounds and the use of explosive devices. An increased crackdown on gangs, violent crime, and terrorism, and increased regulation of hand guns would significantly abate this problem.

Prevention of Psychosocial Effects of Traumatic Amputations in Children

Children between 1 and 3 years of age think of their bodies as separate from the rest of the world; the so-called body image. Surgeons must help these children heal the psychic as well as the body damage. Doll playing is an excellent method to accomplish this. The portion of the body to be operated on is explained together with any defect that will be left, the casting, and in cases of amputation, the artificial limb. Acceptance in home and school is also dealt with.

The changes caused by surgery in these young children disturb concepts of body image that are often fundamental to their sense of self-esteem. The child or parents do not say "you've hurt my child's self-esteem by removing a foot or toe" but it may be reflected in an apprehensive, anxious, depressed, or confused child.[44]

Quiet discussions in which children act out with doll play and ventilate their anxieties about their bodies often relieve them of unrealistic and unwarranted anger at the surgeon or the circumstances of the accident. Children, although they are physically recovering well, may be left emotionally distressed and perhaps even furious because they feel their bodies were wantonly invaded and injured. The medical team may be perceived as adversaries, especially the surgeon. Doll play and puppetry provide an opportunity to work out these feelings for children younger than 6 or 7 years of age.

Older children benefit from contact with other child amputees through the Juvenile Amputee Clinic. Participation in sports programs also helps to improve and maintain self esteem.

Summary and Overview

Traumatic amputations in children, aside from being a devastating traumatic event for the child, also impose an ongoing burden on the family and limitations on the child for future employment opportunities. At the present time, the ability to gather national statistics on childhood amputations is limited. Such data would assist in future preventive measures, because almost every traumatic amputation in a child is preventable. Much needs to be done to prevent serious trauma and amputations in children. It is ironic that childhood amputations are actually increasing in incidence and severity in some parts of the world, primarily because of the improved technology and ease of planting landmines. All orthopaedic surgeons must act as catalysts to bring their experience with limb loss in children to the attention of the media, public health officials, and governments to reduce the incidence of amputations in the childhood age group.

References

1. Scheidt PC, Harel Y, Trumble AC, Jones DH, Overpeck MD: The epidemiology of nonfatal injuries among US children and youth. *Am J Public Health* 1995;85: 932–938.

2. Allshouse MJ, Rouse T, Eichelberger MR: Childhood Injury: A current perspective. *Pediatr Emerg Care* 1993;9:159–164.

3. Baker SP, O'Neill B, Ginsburg MJ, Li G (eds): *The Injury Fact Book*, ed 2. New York, NY, Oxford University Press, 1992.

4. Rice DP, Mackenzie EJ (eds): *Cost of Injury in the United States: A Report to Congress, 1989.* San Francisco, CA, Institute for Health and Aging, University of California, 1989.

5. Rivara FP: Fatal and non-fatal farm injuries to children and adolescents in the United States. *Pediatrics* 1985;76:567–573.

6. Trautwein LC, Smith DG, Rivara FP: Pediatric amputation injuries: Etiology, cost, and outcome. *J Trauma* 1996;41:831–838.

7. Krebs DE, Fishman S: Characteristics of the child amputee population. *J Pediatr Orthop* 1984;4:89–95.

8. Ebskov LB: Trauma-related major lower limb amputations: An epidemiologic study. *J Trauma* 1994;36:778–783.

9. Dormans JP, Azzoni M, Davidson RS, Drummond DS: Major lower extremity lawn mower injuries in children. *J Pediatr Orthop* 1995;15:78–82.

10. Anger DM, Ledbetter BR, Stasikelis PJ, Calhoun JH: Injuries of the foot related to the use of lawn mowers. *J Bone Joint Surg* 1995;77A:719–725.

11. Letts RM, Mardirosian A: Lawnmower injuries in children. *Can Med Assoc J* 1977;116:1151–1153.

12. Letts RM, Gammon WA: Auger injuries in children. *Can Med Assoc J* 1978;118:519–522.

13. Letts RM: Farm machinery accidents in children, in Dosman JA, Cockcroft DW (eds): *Principles of Health and Safety in Agriculture.* Boca Raton, FL, CRC Press, 1986, pp 357–361.

14. Stueland D, Layde P, Lee BC: Agricultural injuries in children in central Wisconsin. *J Trauma* 1991;31:1503–1509.

15. Cogbill H, Steenlage ES, Landercasper J, Strutt PS: Death and disability from agricultural injuries in Wisconsin: A 12 year experience with 739 patients. *J Trauma* 1991;31:1632–1637.

16. Letts RM: Degloving injuries in children. *J Pediatr Orthop* 1986;6:193–197.

17. Letts RM, Cleary J: The child and the snowmobile. *Can Med Assoc J* 1975;113:1061–1063.

18. Dolan MA, Knapp JF, Andres J: Three-wheel and four-wheel all-terrain vehicle injuries in children. *Pediatrics* 1989;84:694–698.

19. Yong-Hing K, Howlett E, Owen JS: Child-operated motorcycle accidents: The pattern, severity, and sequelae of injuries, in Dosman JA, Cockcroft DW (eds): *Principles of Health and Safety in Agriculture*. Boca Raton, FL, CRC Press, 1989, pp 362–364.

20. Paulson JA: The epidemiology of injuries in adolescents. *Pediatr Ann* 1988; 17:84–86,89–96.

21. Shapiro MJ, Luchtefeld WB, Durham RM, Mazuski JE: Traumatic train injuries. *Am J Emerg Med* 1994;12:92–93.

22. Perks AG, Penny M, Mutimer KL: Finger injuries to children involving exercise bicycles. *Med J Aust* 1991;155:368–370.

23. Thompson GH, Balourdas GM, Marcus RE: Railyard amputations in children. *J Pediatr Orthop* 1983;3:443–448.

24. Moore TJ, Wilson JR, Hartman M: Train versus pedestrian accidents. *South Med J* 1991;84:1097–1098.

25. Helfet DL, Howey T, Sanders R, Johansen K: Limb salvage versus amputation: Preliminary results of the Mangled Extremity Severity Score. *Clin Orthop* 1990;256:80–86.

26. Slauterbeck JR, Britton C, Moneim MS, Clevenger FW: Mangled Extremity Severity Score: An accurate guide to treatment of the severely injured upper extremity. *J Orthop Trauma* 1994;8:282–285.

27. Bonanni F, Rhodes M, Lucke JF: The futility of predictive scoring of mangled lower extremities. *J Trauma* 1993;34:99–104.

28. Pyper JA, Black GB: Orthopaedic injuries in children associated with the use of off–road vehicles. *J Bone Joint Surg* 1988;70A:275–284.

29. Nixon J, Corcoran A, Fielding L, Eastgate J: Fatal and nonfatal accidents on the railways: A study of injuries to individuals, with particular reference to children and to nonfatal trauma. *Accid Anal Prev* 1985;17:217–222.

30. Cooper SP, Rothstein MA: Health hazards among working children in Texas. *South Med J* 1995;88:550–554.

31. Millea TP, Hansen RH: Snowblower injuries to the hand. *J Trauma* 1989;29:229–233.

32. Haynes CD, Webb WA, Fenno CR: Chain saw injuries: Review of 330 cases. *J Trauma* 1980;20:772–776.

33. Justis EJ, Moore SV, LaVelle DG: Woodworking injuries: An epidemiologic survey of injuries sustained using woodworking machinery and hand tools. *J Hand Surg* 1987;12A:890–895.

34. Burke JF, Quinby WC Jr, Bondoc C, McLaughlin E, Trelstad RL: Patterns of high tension electrical injury in children and adolescents and their management. *Am J Surg* 1977;133:492–497.

35. Tooms RE: The amputee, in Morrissy RT (ed): *Lovell and Winter's Pediatric Orthopaedics*, ed 3. Philadelphia, PA, JB Lippincott, 1990, vol 2, pp 1023–1070.

36. Gordon MW, Reid WH, Awwaad AM: Electrical burns: Incidence and prognosis in Western Scotland. *Burns Ind Therm Inj* 1986;2:254–259.

37. Blank JE, Dormans JP, Davidson RS: Perinatal limb ischemia: Orthopaedic implications. *J Pediatr Orthop* 1996;16:90–96.

38. Stover E, Keller AS, Cobey J, Sopheap S: The medical and social consequences of land mines in Cambodia. *JAMA* 1994;272:331–336.

39. Coupland RM, Krover A: Injuries from antipersonnel mines: The experience of the International Committee of the Red Cross. *Br Med J* 1991;303:1509–1512.

40. Geiger HJ, Cook-Deegan RM: The role of physicians in conflicts and humanitarian crises: Case studies from the field missions of Physicians for Human Rights, 1988 to 1993. *JAMA* 1993;270:616–620.

41. Abramson B: Children's rights in the age of landmines, in *The Impact of Landmines on Children.* UNICEF Office for Europe, 1994.

42. Stucky W, Loder RT: Extremity gunshot wounds in children. *J Pediatr Orthop* 1991;11:64–71.

43. Kon M: Firework injuries to the hand. *Ann Chir Main Memb Super* 1991;10:443–447.

44. Letts M, Stevens L, Coleman J, Kettner R: Puppetry and doll play as an adjunct to pediatric orthopaedics. *J Pediatr Orthop* 1983;3:605–609.

Chapter 22

Management of Pediatric Mutilating Extremity Injuries and Traumatic Amputations

John P. Dormans, MD

Introduction

Trauma is the leading cause of amputation in children.[1-3] Traumatic injuries resulting in amputation most commonly are caused by power tools and machinery (such as lawn mowers), followed by vehicular accidents, gunshot wounds, explosions and railroad injuries, household accidents, and thermal or electrical injuries.[3,4] Malignant tumors result in more amputations in children than any other single disease process and are exceeded only by trauma as a cause of acquired amputations. Better public education is needed to lessen the frequency of these injuries. The Pediatric Orthopaedic Society of North America recently initiated an effort in this regard.

Children Are Not Small Adults

Children requiring amputation for trauma deserve specialized attention in their evaluation, stabilization, surgical treatment, postoperative management, and rehabilitation. The basic differences between the child and adult that affect the evaluation and management of a child with a severely injured extremity are (1) the child's potential for future growth (ie, the physis), (2) the potential problem of residual limb overgrowth, (3) the better healing potential of children, and (4) the emotional and psychological issues that affect rehabilitation.

Children, as opposed to adults, have the potential for further growth. As a result of this potential, discrepancies in limb length may become amplified with time. A thigh segment (residual limb) that is 80% of the length of the opposite thigh segment after above-knee amputation in an infant can become a thigh segment (residual limb) that is only 20% of the length of the opposite thigh segment with time and growth because of the loss of the distal femoral physis. The cardinal rule, therefore, is to attempt to conserve all the limb length, including the chondroepiphysis and growth plate when possible and appropriate, consistent with the appropriate treatment for the injury necessitating the amputation.[3] In addition, the potential for further growth may be associated with the potential for angular deformity if there is partial injury to an open growth plate of the residual limb.

Children also have the potential problem of residual limb overgrowth[5] (Chapter 23). As a result of this, whenever possible, it is best to perform a disarticulation rather than a supraepiphyseal or transdiaphyseal amputation in a growing child.[6,7] This procedure preserves the longitudinal growth of the remaining skeleton (ie, ultimately, a longer limb segment by leaving the growth center), lessens the likelihood of limb overgrowth, and provides a sturdy end-bearing stump to enhance prosthetic use.

The remarkable healing potential in children makes it possible to attempt more aggressive limb-salvage surgery for trauma. Injuries that may result in amputation in an adult may at times have a better chance of healing in the child. It is important, however, not to subject a child to repeated attempts at limb salvage when amputation is clearly the best option. Unlike adults, skin grafts may be used successfully for soft-tissue coverage in children to conserve limb length without compromising wound healing or incurring subsequent prosthetic use problems.[6] In contrast to adults, scarring of the residual limb from trauma or skin grafting is well tolerated by most children, with the necessity of prosthetic modification to dispense weightbearing forces and diminish shear at the stump-socket interface.[8] Some patients with insufficient soft-tissue coverage on below-knee amputation stumps have been successfully treated with free-tissue transfer surgery to preserve a functional below-knee prosthetic level.[9] Further lengthening of short amputation residual limbs is becoming more of a reality (Chapter 24).

Finally, other differences that may enhance or detract from the effectiveness of the surgical and prosthetic care of the child amputee are the child's psychological and emotional immaturity, the child's dependence on others for basic needs, and the variability of the quality of care given by parents or guardians. Rapid growth and the child's high demand on the prosthetic device necessitate frequent maintenance and replacement.[10] Frequent clinic visits are needed initially for optimal adjustment to prosthetic use; the child amputee is often best managed in a specialized multidisciplinary setting.[7,11]

General Evaluation

The patient's general condition (as reflected in the "ABC approach" to trauma management) is the most important factor in initial assessment, and in some cases it will determine and influence ultimate treatment of the extremity injury.[12] A potential danger in dealing with serious extremity injuries is to be sidetracked by a striking extremity injury and not evaluate other potential life-threatening injuries. Often, considerable blood loss has occurred with these injuries and early aggressive volume resuscitation is required. Further details on stabilization of the child with multiple trauma are available elsewhere.[12]

Care of an Amputated Part in the Field

The handling of an amputated part in the field may determine whether successful limb or digit replantation can be carried out. The current recommendations are that the amputated part be wrapped in a slightly moistened (sterile saline) sponge and placed in a sterile container (usually a plastic zip-lock type of bag). The container is placed on ice and is transported, as soon as possible, with the patient to the trauma center.[13]

With incomplete injuries, the injured area is dressed with a bulky sterile dressing. If there is excessive bleeding, a pressure dressing should be used. Avoid clamping or tying a vessel and avoid using a tourniquet in the field.

Emergency Room Care

Children with multiple injuries are best treated under the guidance of a pediatric trauma team. The details of the injury, especially such factors as mechanism of injury, warm ischemic time, tetanus status, initial early outside treatment, and handling of amputated parts, are especially important in the management of children with extensive extremity injuries or traumatic amputations.

When an extremity has suffered a major injury, initial evaluation in the emergency room is important for assessment of circulation, sensation, and function. Most children require formal surgical intervention in the operating room. Radiographs are obtained in the emergency room or in the operating room, when this is more appropriate. The emergency room evaluation is beneficial in preparing the operating room personnel and also planning for the procedure. For most replantation cases, blood transfusion is necessary, so typing and cross matching for blood should be done early after arrival at the hospital.[14]

Most authors recommend the use of prophylactic antibiotics for open mutilating lower extremity injuries or traumatic amputations to reduce the bacterial load, which is believed to be the most important determinant of postoperative infections.[15]

Operating Room Care

Initial Surgical Decision Making

Once the child has been properly anesthetized, the bandages are removed and the extremity inspected. The extent of injury is evaluated, including the posture of extremity, the extent of devascularization, and damage to soft tissues. Consultation with other surgical specialists (plastic, hand, vascular, and general surgery) may be helpful at this point if special expertise of these specialists could be useful in addressing specific surgical issues. Photographs at this point are often very useful in documenting the extent of injury for both medical and medicolegal reasons. If replantation of a traumatic amputation is considered, two teams of surgeons are ideal, with each debriding, irrigating, and identifying corresponding neurovascular structures.

The first decision faced by the team treating a child with a mangled extremity is that of reconstruction versus early amputation. Inappropriate attempts at limb salvage surgery may lead to multiple operations, prolonged hospitalization, and prolonged suffering by the patient and family. An early independent review by the surgical teams, with the aim of establishing an accurate prognosis for salvaging a useful limb, may help prevent such problems.[16] This review must take into account many factors, including the presence of neurovascular injury, warm ischemic time, wound contamination, and the extent of damage to the skin, bone, growth plates, articular cartilage, and muscle.[16,17]

Objective criteria can be used to predict the necessity of amputation after lower extremity trauma in adults. In children, however, such specific criteria have not yet been established. Because of the presence of the growth plate and the potential for healing and remodeling, attempts at limb salvage or replantation can be considered in children that may not be considered appropriate in an adult. With severe injuries for which reconstruction is not possible, however, early amputation is not a failure but an appropriate first step in the rehabilitation.

Considerable discussion has taken place regarding criteria used to predict successful limb salvage in adults.[18] Predictive indices have been described in the literature to identify limbs for which attempted salvage will be successful. These include criteria for primary amputation after open tibial fractures with vascular injury,[19] the mangled extremity syndrome index (MESI),[20] the predictive salvage index system (PSI),[21] the mangled extremity severity score (MESS),[22] the limb salvage index (LSI),[23] and the NISSSA Scoring System.[24] Further details have been provided by Dirschl and Dahners.[18]

The MESS system is the most thoroughly validated of the mangled scoring systems and is also the simplest to apply.[18] This system was based on four clinical criteria, including skeletal and soft-tissue injury, limb ischemia, shock, and age (Table 1). Although originally based on retrospective review of 26 mangled lower extremities, this system was further evaluated in a prospective trial of 26 patients treated at a separate trauma center. In both trials, a MESS of less than seven predicted salvage with 100% accuracy,[22,25] and a MESS of greater than or equal to seven predicted amputation with 100% accuracy.[25] Although this evaluation system has some subjective aspects, in most cases all of the information necessary for scoring is available at the time of the initial evaluation.

In a retrospective review of 152 patients with lower extremity requiring vascular soft-tissue reconstruction, Robertson[26] found that all patients with an MESS of 7 or more eventually required amputation, whereas all 43 patients who ultimately had limb salvage had a score of less than seven. However, only 16 of the 65 patients who underwent delayed amputation had a MESS of seven or more at the time of initial evaluation. The authors concluded that the MESS system had a 100% specificity but lacked sensitivity.

Table 1 Mangled Extremity Severity Scoring System*

Factor	Score
Skeletal/soft-tissue injury	
Low energy (stab, fracture, civilian gunshot wound)	1
Medium energy (open or multiple fracture)	2
High energy (shotgun or military gunshot wound, crush)	3
Very high energy (above plus gross contamination)	4
Limb ischemia	
Pulse reduced or absent but perfusion normal	1*
Pulseless, diminished capillary refill	2*
Patient is cool, paralyzed, insensate, numb	3*
Shock	
Systolic blood pressure always > 90 mm	0
Systolic blood pressure transiently < 90 mm	1
Systolic blood pressure persistently < 90 mm	2
Age, years	
< 30	0
30 to 50	1
> 50	2

*Double value if duration of ischemia exceeds 6 hours
(Adapted with permission from Johansen K, Daines M, Howey T, Helfet D, Hansen ST Jr: Objective criteria accurately predict amputation following lower extremity trauma. *J Trauma* 1990;30:568–573.)

McNamara and associates[24] retrospectively applied the MESS system to 33 patients with grade III open tibia fractures and found that a MESS value of four was 100% sensitive, a value of seven was 100% specific, and a value of seven or more was 100% predictive of amputation. Slauterbeck and associates[27] applied the MESS system in a retrospective review of 43 patients with mangled upper extremities. They found that all nine patients with a MESS of seven or more had undergone amputation while 34 patients with a MESS of less than seven had undergone successful salvage procedures. These authors concluded that the MESS system was an accurate predictor of amputation of a severely injured upper extremity and advocated its use as an objective aid to augment the surgeon's clinical experience for these patients.[27]

In 1991, Russell and associates[23] proposed the LSI based on a retrospective review of 70 lower extremity injuries. It related the likelihood of salvage to the duration of ischemia in the presence and severity of injury to six types of tissue: artery, bone, muscle, skin, nerve, and vein (Table 2). All 51 patients whose limbs were salvaged had an LSI of less than six, while all 19 who had amputation had an LSI of six or greater. Ninety five percent of amputated limbs were associated with complete disruption of the sciatic, tibial, or peroneal nerves.

Bonnani and associates[28] applied the LSI retrospectively and concluded that it had a sensitivity of 61% and a specificity of 43%. These authors found that extensive surgical evaluation was required for accurate application and that for accurate scoring in the skin category, definitive treatment in this outcome must be known. They concluded that the LSI could not be reliably used in the decision-making process.

Table 2 Limb Salvage Index System

Factor	Score
Arterial injury	
Contusion, intimal tear, partial laceration	0
Occlusion of two or more shank vessels, no pedal pulses	1
Occlusion of femoral, popliteal, or three shank vessels	2
Nerve injury	
Contusion, stretch, minimal clean laceration	0
Partial transection or avulsion of sciatic nerve	1
Complete transection or avulsion of sciatic nerve	2
Bone injury	
Closed fracture or open fracture with minimal comminution	0
Open fracture with comminution or large displacement	1
Bone loss > 3 cm; type IIIB or IIIC fracture	2
Skin injury	
Clean laceration, primary repair, first-degree burn	0
Contamination, avulsion requiring split-thickness skin graft or flap	1
Muscle injury	
Laceration involving single compartment or tendon	0
Laceration or avulsion of two or more tendons	1
Deep vein injury	
Contusion, partial laceration, or avulsion	0
Complete laceration, avulsion, or thrombosi	1
Warm ischemia time, hours	
< 6	0
6 to 9	1
9 to 12	2
12 to 15	3
> 15	4

(Adapted with permission from Russell WL, Sailors DM, Whittle TB, Fisher DF Jr, Burns RP: Limb salvage versus traumatic amputation: A decision based on a seven-part predictive index. *Ann Surg* 1991;213:473–481.)

There are several problems with those classification systems as they apply to children. First and foremost, they have been developed based on retrospective series of adults with mangled extremities. Second, with the exception of the small prospective series in which the MESS system was not validated, all of these systems have been assessed retrospectively, applying retrospective criteria to patients with known outcomes. Third, the current classifications all have shortcomings. None have been validated in studies using large numbers of patients in a prospective multi-institutional evaluation. Finally, there are problems with definitions. Salvage in these studies has been defined as preservation of a viable lower extremity without regard to limb function. Only a few investigators have compared functional outcome and cost of early amputation versus that of limb salvage surgery.[18,19] Russell and associates[23] defined functional failures on the basis of there being a nonweightbearing extremity without sensory or motor function. Bonanni and associates[28] defined functional failure as an inability to walk a minimum of 150 feet independently, climb 12 stairs, or independently transfer from bed to chair. The strict definition of failure used in these series is likely responsible for the low specificity and sensitivity of the scoring systems reported by Bonnani and associates.[28]

In the case of a mangled lower extremity, there are significant differences between injuries above and below the knee. Functional outcomes differ widely. The functional outcome and prosthetic function after an above-the-knee amputation is poorer than that after a below-the-knee amputation. Outcome after nerve repair above the knee is often poorer, whereas reconstruction of vascular injuries is frequently easier above the knee than below. Reconstruction of both bone and soft tissue appear easier above the knee, with the thick soft-tissue envelope. As a result, more consideration for limb salvage should be given for an above-the-knee injury than for a similar injury in the leg unless the sciatic nerve is disrupted.

Functional results of salvage of the upper extremity are better than those of the lower extremity, and functional prognosis after amputation of the upper extremity is poor. Therefore, criteria for salvage of the upper extremity are often necessarily different from those of the lower extremity.

Attempts at classifying severity of extremity injury and correlating these findings with functional outcome is a worthy goal. At present, however, there is no predictive scale that can be used with confidence to decide on limb salvage versus amputation in children. The surgeon is left with clinical judgment and experience. For certain severe injuries, initial early amputation is the best option for the patient. The belief that an amputation of a mangled extremity represents a treatment failure can lead to costly, demoralizing, complicated, and sometimes lethal attempts at reconstruction of functionless extremities.[29]

Surgical Principles in Children

Define the extent of the injury. This is done with the history and the physical examination in both the emergency department and the operating room. Radiographs are taken not only of the injured extremity, but also looking for other associated injuries. Occasionally other diagnostic evaluations, such as arteriography, arthrograms, and magnetic resonance imaging, will be helpful.

Debride and irrigate all open wounds properly. As with adults, proper wound debridement and irrigation are key in lessening the chances of early wound infection. For traumatic amputations, debridement usually is done under tourniquet control. All nonviable and contaminated tissues are excised except for vital structures such as vessels and nerves. Revitalized or avulsed muscle is excised. Debridement, irrigation, and curettage of bone ends is done. Structurally relevant bone fragments may be retained for maintenance of structural integrity. Divided nerve ends are excised to healthy appearing fascicles, and contused nerves are cleansed of contaminants. Major vessel ends are excised to healthy intima in preparation for repair. Smaller branches are ligated. Skin and subcutaneous tissue are sharply debrided to healthy skin. After initial debridement, and further inspection for bleeding or nonviable tissue, the tourniquet is released. The wound is thoroughly irrigated with sterile normal saline or Ringer's lactate solution. Culture swabs are taken at completion of debridement and irrigation. The role of qualitative cultures is not clear at this stage.[30]

The idea of what constitutes proper wound debridement varies among authors. Some authors have recommended preservation of viable tissue on the basis that such tissues will "declare themselves" in a few days. This concept of conservative debridement may, however, predispose to latent infection. Delayed debridement leaves the wounds exposed to hospital pathogens without overlying skin protection. Godina[31] has shown that early aggressive wound excision and flap coverage within 72 hours is associated with a postoperative infection rate of 1.5% compared to 17.5% for delayed reconstruction in which the average delay was 90 days. Some other authors suggest that the term "debridement" should be replaced by "wound excision." [14]

Whenever possible, the surgeon should preserve length. For both the upper and lower extremity, the preservation of length will allow for a more functional extremity, if satisfactory closure and coverage can be achieved without undue risk.

If possible, the surgeon should maintain the cartilaginous surface (epiphysis and articular surface) at the end of the residual skeletal segment to avoid potential problems of stump overgrowth. This preservation of the epiphyseal (and physeal) portion of the residual limb segment also allows for continued growth of the extremity. The distal femoral epiphysis, for example, provides 80% of the growth of the femur and an above-the-knee amputation done at an early age leads to significant limb-length discrepancy. At the ankle, the medial and lateral malleoli are not usually prominent and should be removed only in patients who are approaching skeletal maturity.[32,33]

In addition, it is important to use early and appropriate wound coverage. Patients with severe open fractures should return to the operating room early for formal repeat debridement and irrigation. Delayed primary closure should be done only when satisfactory tissue for coverage is available and closure can be achieved without excessive tension. Early coverage with a free flap is technically easier than secondary free flap reconstruction, which is more difficult as a result of edema obscuring tissue planes and difficulty in the handling of vessels.[9]

Principles of skeletal stabilization for open and associated closed fractures are paramount in allowing for restoration of anatomy and early return to function. Principles of skeletal stabilization in the child are well outlined in standard pediatric orthopaedic fracture texts.[34]

Replantation

Sharp, clean traumatic amputations have a much better chance of success with replantation than do injuries with crush or stretching components. Moreover, longer ischemic times are related to a poor prognosis after replantation.[13] Warm ischemic time is defined as that period of time from injury to initial cooling of the amputated part. Poor prognosis for replantation is expected with warm ischemic time of over 10 hours for a digit and 4 hours for a limb. For partial amputations, with poor or no perfusion of the partially amputated part, there is often a prolonged warm ischemic time and, thus, a poor prognosis. Cold ischemic time is defined as the period of time from initial cooling to revascularization. Poor prognosis is again expected with cool ischemic times of over 48 hours for digits and over 10 hours for limbs. Total ischemic time, therefore, is the total time from injury to revascularization. Shorter total ischemic times are related to improved function.

Successful replantation requires a team approach. The sequence of repair for replantation after traumatic amputation depends on the individual circumstances and type of injury, but in general is as follows: bony stabilization, followed by arterial repair (venous repair can be done first if there would be a high anticipated blood loss from a large arterial repair), nerve repair, and musculotendinous repairs. Nerve grafting or muscle transfers may be useful options for difficult situations.

Approximately 50% of failures occur within the first 72 hours after replantation. During this time, sympathetic nervous system stimulation causing vasoconstriction is avoided. Adequate pain control and avoidance of nausea and vomiting and hypothermia are needed. Thorazine may be used to cause sympathetic vasodilatation.

Finally, replantation requires a motivated patient because of the often lengthy rehabilitation process. Protective sensation is key for satisfactory function. The more proximal the injury, the less likely the nerve function will be adequate (Fig. 1).

Postoperative Treatment After Amputation

There is controversy regarding immediate postsurgical prosthetic fitting (IPSF) in children.[2,10] Some authors believe that IPSF may be hazardous to young children in that it may result in wound dehiscence if the child resumes full weightbearing in the early period.[2] At the Children's Hospital of Philadelphia, postoperative treatment of the child amputee usually involves the use of a soft dressing or cast for the first 5 to 7 days. This is replaced by a new rigid dressing, which incorporates a pylon and prosthetic foot as a temporary prosthesis. Gait training under supervision may begin and be increased gradually over 6 to 8 weeks postoperatively, at which time the fitting for a definitive prosthesis can be performed. Early ambulation, resumption of normal activities, and the diminution of the psychological impact of limb loss are desirable goals of early management that are made possible with the technique of immediate or early postsurgical prosthetic fitting.[7,10,35] Because of their remarkable rehabilitation potential, children with amputation are able to function in a comparable fashion to their peers regardless of increased energy consumption and altered gait patterns.[36]

Delayed Amputation

If after revascularization and skeletal stabilization, the extremity is nonviable or remains insensate, delayed amputation can be done under elective conditions. Once attempts at salvage have been made, however, it may become increasingly difficult for the patient (and surgeon) to accept the prospect of amputation.[34] A subjective assessment of long-term functional outcome in above- and below-the-knee amputations implied that there was little difference between early and delayed amputations; however, the delayed group

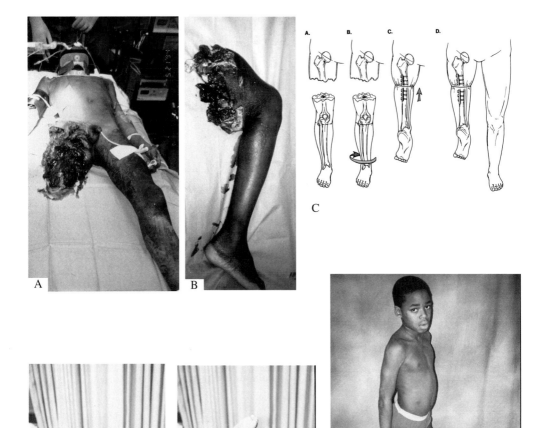

Fig. 1 A and **B,** *A 12-year-old boy was brought to our institution with a traumatic amputation of the right lower extremity 1 hour after being run over by a train. Irrigation, debridement, and eventual closure would have left the child with a very short above-the-knee residual limb level, and he would likely have rejected a prosthesis. Because of the intercalary crush injury to the extremity, primary replantation could not be accomplished without significant shortening of the extremity.* **C,** *A rotationplasty shortening replantation with microvascular anastomosis of the leg allowed for above knee function as compared to the function of a high above-the-knee amputation for this child.* **D, E,** and **F,** *At 3-year follow-up, the patient has active "knee" plantar and dorsiflexion with protective sensation and proprioception; he has no pain and ambulates independently with a modified rotationplasty type prosthesis, without the aid of crutches.*

was more satisfied with the end result.[37] Furthermore, lengthening of short residual limbs is becoming more successful as additional experience is gained in this area[38] (Chapter 24).

Lawn Mower Injuries

Lawn mower injuries are a common cause of morbidity for children, with an estimated annual occurrence of 75,000 in the United States.[39] These injuries often are complicated by extreme contamination with dirt and grass. Further, severe damage to bone and soft tissue is encountered. Although most injuries involve the distal ends of the extremities (hands and feet), injuries are at times segmental, with severe damage to bone and soft tissue in an intercalary fashion. In severe injuries of this type where amputation is indicated, tissue from the distal segment may be used as a flap.

In a series of 16 children with 18 extremity lawn mower injuries, injuries were classified into two main types: shredding, and pauci laceration. The most common type of lawn mower injury was the shredding type, which was either intercalary or distal. The distal shredding injury resulted in amputation in 14 children, all of whom eventually had satisfactory results. Two attempted salvages in children with intercalary shredding were considered to have poor results, and two-limb salvage attempts in the pauci laceration category were considered to have good results. Limb salvage was associated with prolonged hospitalizations, a higher incidence of surgical problems, a longer treatment course, and more complications than early ablative procedures.[39]

Summary

The child with a traumatic amputation or major extremity injury is managed differently than an adult with a similar injury. The potential for future growth, the often better healing potential, and the psychological and emotional differences are factors that make these injuries different. Recent efforts toward prevention of these injuries should be encouraged and promoted. Although rating scales to predict the need for early amputation have been useful in adult patients, none of these scales take into account the unique differences of children with these injuries. An early, thorough evaluation and aggressive support with appropriate management of the extremity injury will help lessen the impact and improve the outcomes of these children.

References

1. McIntire MS (ed): *Injury Control For Children and Youth*. Elk Grove Village, IL, American Academy of Pediatrics, 1987.

2. Herring JA, Cummings DR: The limb-deficient child, in Morrissy RT, Weinstein SL (eds): *Lovell and Winter's Pediatric Orthopaedics*, ed 4. Philadelphia, PA, Lippincott-Raven, 1996, vol 2, pp 1137–1180.

3. Tooms RE: The amputee, in Morrissy RT (ed): *Lovell and Winter's Pediatric Orthopaedics*, ed 3. Philadelphia, PA, JB Lippincott, 1990, vol 2, pp 1023–1070.

4. Tooms RE: Acquired amputations in children, in Bowker JH, Michael JW (eds): American Academy of Orthopaedic Surgeons *Atlas of Limb Prosthetics: Surgical, Prosthetic, and Rehabilitation Principles*, ed 2. St. Louis, MO, Mosby-Year Book, 1992, pp 735–741.

5. Abraham E, Pellicore RJ, Hamilton RC, Hallman BW, Ghosh L: Stump overgrowth in juvenile amputees. *J Pediatr Orthop* 1986;6:66–71.

6. Aitken GT: Surgical amputation in children. *J Bone Joint Surg* 1963;45A:1735–1741.

7. Aitken GT: The child amputee: An overview. *Orthop Clin North Am* 1972;3:447–472.

8. Aitken GT: Prosthetic fitting following amputation for bone tumors. *ICIB* 1964;3:1.

9. Gallico GG III, Ehrlichman RJ, Jupiter J, May JW Jr: Free flaps to preserve below-knee amputation stumps: Long-term evaluation. *Plast Reconstr Surg* 1987;79:871–878.

10. Burgess EM, Romano RJ: Immediate postsurgical prosthetic fitting of children and adolescents following lower extremity amputations. *ICIB* 1967;7:1.

11. Brooks MB, Mazet R Jr: Prosthetics in child amputees. *Clin Orthop* 1957;9:190–204.

12. Alexander RH, Proctor HJ (eds): *Advanced Trauma Life Support Program for Physicians: ATLS Student Manual*, ed 5. Chicago, IL, American College of Surgeons, 1993, pp 261–281.

13. Buncke HJ (ed): *Microsurgery: Transplantation-Replantation: An Atlas-Text*. Philadelphia, PA, Lea & Febiger, 1991, pp 587–683.

14. Gupta A, Wolff TW: Management of the mangled hand and forearm. *J Am Acad Orthop Surg* 1995;3:226–236.

15. Breidenbach WC III: Emergency free tissue transfer for reconstruction of acute upper extremity wounds. *Clin Plast Surg* 1989;16:505–514.

16. Pozo JL, Powell B, Andrews BG, Hutton PA, Clarke J: The timing of amputation for lower limb trauma. *J Bone Joint Surg* 1990;72B:288–292.

17. Poole GV, Agnew SG, Griswold JA, Rhodes RS: The mangled lower extremity: Can salvage be predicted? *Am Surg* 1994;60:50–55.

18. Dirschl DR, Dahners LE: The mangled extremity: When should it be amputated? *J Am Acad Orthop Surg* 1996;4:182–190.

19. Lange RH, Bach AW, Hansen ST Jr, Johansen KH: Open tibial fractures with associated vascular injuries: Prognosis for limb salvage. *J Trauma* 1985;25:203–208.

20. Gregory RT, Gould RJ, Peclet M, et al: The mangled extremity syndrome (M.E.S.): A severity grading system for multisystem injury of the extremity. *J Trauma* 1985;25:1147–1150.

21. Howe HR Jr, Poole GV Jr, Hansen KJ, et al: Salvage of lower extremities following combined orthopedic and vascular trauma: A predictive salvage index. *Am Surg* 1987;53:205–208.

22. Johansen K, Daines M, Howey T, Helfet D, Hansen ST Jr: Objective criteria accurately predict amputation following lower extremity trauma. *J Trauma* 1990;30:568–573.

23. Russell WL, Sailors DM, Whittle TB, Fisher DF Jr, Burns RP: Limb salvage versus traumatic amputation: A decision based on a seven-part predictive index. *Ann Surg* 1991;213:473–481.

24. McNamara MG, Heckman JD, Corley FG: Severe open fractures of the lower extremity: A retrospective evaluation of the Mangled Extremity Severity Score (MESS). *J Orthop Trauma* 1994;8:81–87.

25. Helfet DL, Howey T, Sanders R, Johansen K: Limb salvage versus amputation: Preliminary results of the Mangled Extremity Severity Score. *Clin Orthop* 1990;256:80–86.

26. Robertson PA: Prediction of amputation after severe lower limb trauma. *J Bone Joint Surg* 1991;73B:816–818.

27. Slauterbeck JR, Britton C, Moneim MS, Clevenger FW: Mangled extremity severity score: An accurate guide to treatment of the severely injured upper extremity. *J Orthop Trauma* 1994;8:282–285.

28. Bonanni F, Rhodes M, Lucke JF: The futility of predictive scoring of mangled lower extremities. *J Trauma* 1993;34:99–104.

29. Hansen ST Jr: Editorial: The type-IIIC tibial fracture: Salvage or amputation. *J Bone Joint Surg* 1987;69A:799–800.

30. Marshall KA, Edgerton MT, Rodeheaver GT, Magee CM, Edlich RF: Quantitative microbiology: Its application to hand injuries. *Am J Surg* 1976;131:730–733.

31. Godina M: Early microsurgical reconstruction of complex trauma of the extremities. *Plast Reconstr Surg* 1986;78:285–292.

32. Herring JA, Barnhill B, Gaffney C: Syme amputation: An evaluation of the physical and psychological function in young patients. *J Bone Joint Surg* 1986;68A:573–578.

33. Tachdjian MO (ed): *Pediatric Orthopedics*, ed 2. Philadelphia, PA,WB Saunders, 1990.

34. Hensinger RN: Complications of fractures in children, in Green NE, Swiontkowski (eds): *Skeletal Trauma in Children*. Philadelphia, PA, WB Saunders, 1993.

35. Tooms RE: General principles of amputations, in Crenshaw AH (ed): *Campbell's Operative Orthopaedics*, ed 7. St. Louis, MO, CV Mosby, 1987.

36. Waters RL, Perry J, Antonelli D, Hislop H: Energy cost of walking of amputees: The influence of level of amputation. *J Bone Joint Surg* 1976;58A:42–46.

37. Walker CR, Ingram RR, Hullin MG, McCreath SW: Lower limb amputation following injury: A survey of long-term functional outcome. *Injury* 1994;25:387–392.

38. Younge D, Dafniotis O: A composite bone flap to lengthen a below-knee amputation stump. *J Bone Joint Surg* 1993;75B:330–331.

39. Dormans JP, Azzoni M, Davidson RS, Drummond DS: Major lower extremity lawn mower injuries in children. *J Pediatr Orthop* 1995;15:78–82.

Consensus

The Prevention of Traumatic Amputations

We would strongly encourage the gathering of meaningful data to document the incidence of and factors related to traumatic amputations in children. Prevention of these amputations should be a high priority for our various professional organizations. Special efforts toward public education need to be ongoing and should emphasize changing risk-taking behavior. We should stress the concept that these "accidental injuries" usually are preventable. The importance of such activities as awareness days, pressure on manufacturers, political lobbying, and other measures cannot be overstressed.

Land mines represent an enormous, world-wide plague in which children are the primary victims. Public awareness and political activism must be brought to bear for removal of existing mines and to BAN the manufacture and use of mines.

We encourage the use and teaching of techniques to improve the residual limb, such as saving or transplanting cartilage surfaces, using defatted skin flaps, delaying amputation until viability is certain.

Surgeons managing traumatized extremities in children should whenever possible save any viable and potentially functional portion of that extremity. Consideration should be given to covering bone ends with residual cartilagenous fragments and to defatting of degloved skin.

Chapter 23

Terminal Bony Overgrowth of the Residual Limb: Current Management Strategies

Jon R. Davids, MD

Problems associated with the residual limb in the juvenile amputee may be primarily related to the skin, the soft-tissue envelope, or the bone. Examples of primary skin problems include contact dermatitis, folliculitis, dermal inclusion cysts, and ulcers over a split thickness skin graft. A deficient soft-tissue envelope is often seen following acquired amputations associated with significant burns, high-energy trauma, and systemic illnesses such as purpura fulminans. Skeletal problems seen in physiologically immature individuals include overgrowth occurring at the tip of the residual limb, and progressive angular deformity relating to a partial physeal arrest. Each type of problem may occur in isolation or in combination. Appropriate prosthetic and surgical management begins with an appreciation of all of the component problems present. The remainder of this chapter will deal with terminal bony overgrowth of the residual limb, the problem most unique to children with limb deficiencies.

Definition/Epidemiology

Terminal bony overgrowth of the residual limb in juvenile amputees is characterized by swelling, warmth, and tenderness at the distal aspect of the residual limb, and in many cases, by formation of a bursa over the tip of a bony spike that is contiguous with the end of the underlying bone (Fig. 1). In extreme cases, the tip of the spike may perforate the soft-tissue envelope of the residual limb, causing pain and creating an avenue for infection. The diagnosis is confirmed radiographically by the presence of terminal overgrowth of bone with cortical radiodensity. The overgrowth involves the whole diameter of the bone, with distal tapering to a narrow tip, the so-called licked candy sign (Fig. 2). At surgery, the skin and subcutaneous tissues are generally normal, except at the tip of the bony spike, where progressive attenuation and ulceration are found. When present, the bursa is well delineated by a thick fibrous shell that is contiguous with the base of the bony spike. The bursa may contain clear fluid, occasionally with multiple rice bodies, and is lined by villous appearing tissue (Fig. 3). Histologic analysis of the bony spike has revealed mature lamellar bone peripherally

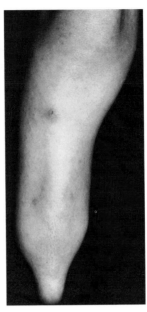

Fig. 1 *Photograph of the residual limb of an 8-year-old girl who had sustained a traumatic below-the-knee amputation on the right side when she was 5 years old. The distal tip of the limb was erythematous, warm, and tender to touch. A small bursa and a spike of bone were palpable. (Reproduced with permission from Davids JR, Meyer LC, Blackhurst DW: Operative treatment of bone overgrowth in children who have an acquired or congenital amputation.* J Bone Joint Surg *1995;77A:1490–1497.)*

and immature woven bone centrally.[1,2] Analysis of the soft tissues has shown reactive connective tissue stratification, and the bursa has been found to be lined with synovial and mucin-producing cells.[3,4]

Overgrowth is thought to be the most common problem of the residual limb seen in the child with a limb deficiency, and its prevalence has been reported at 4% to 35%.[3–10] This lesion is seen following diaphyseal and metaphyseal amputations and affects, in order, the tibia/fibula, humerus, and occasionally, the femur.[1,9–11] Overgrowth of the radius or ulna has not been reported. This condition most commonly occurs prior to the age of 12 years and has not been reported in an individual older than 15 years of age.[1,9] It may be seen following both acquired and congenital amputations.[1,3,11] The earlier controversy surrounding the occurrence of overgrowth in congenital amputations can be resolved when this group is further divided into deficiencies caused by early amnion rupture sequence (also known as amniotic band syndrome, congenital constriction bands, or Streeter's dysplasia) and those caused by a failure of normal, genetically-controlled embryologic development. The former condition, while resulting in a limb deficiency that is present at birth (hence the term "congenital") is actually a traumatic amputation in utero of a genetically normal limb, and like postnatally acquired amputations is at risk for overgrowth. In congenital limb deficiencies caused by failure of normal embryologic development, the

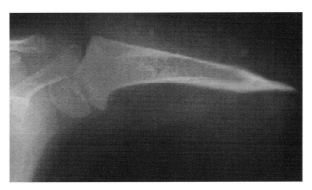

Fig. 2 *Anteroposterior radiograph of a 3-year-old boy with congenital transverse deficiency of the humerus, proximal, of the left arm. The end of the bone tapered distally to a narrow, sharp tip that was painful and threatening to pierce through the soft-tissue envelope. (Reproduced with permission from Davids JR, Meyer LC, Blackhurst DW: Operative treatment of bone overgrowth in children who have an acquired or congenital amputation.* J Bone Joint Surg *1995;77A:1490–1497.)*

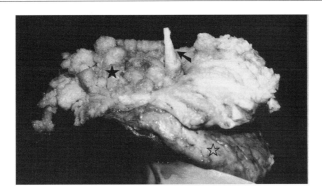

Fig. 3 *Intraoperative photograph taken at the time of resection revision in a 6-year-old boy who had sustained a traumatic above-the-elbow amputation on the right in a lawn mower accident 2 years earlier. The bone spike from the humerus (arrow), the villous tissue lining the bursa surrounding the spike (solid star), and the normal subcutaneous tissue (open star) are seen. (Reproduced with permission from Davids JR, Meyer LC, Blackhurst DW: Operative treatment of bone overgrowth in children who have an acquired or congenital amputation.* J Bone Joint Surg *1995;77A:1490–1497.)*

subsequent development all of the tissue types of the extremity is presumably affected and the phenomenon of overgrowth is not seen.

Etiology/Pathophysiology

The etiology of residual limb overgrowth has long been a source of debate and controversy. The earliest investigators felt that overgrowth was due to contracture of the soft-tissue envelope in association with the disuse atrophy that is invariably seen following acquired amputations.[5,7,10,12] Surgical management was focused on leaving an ample soft-tissue flap at the time of amputation or revision. Recognizing the association between overgrowth and skeletal immaturity, subsequent investigators believed that the overgrowth was a consequence of disproportionate growth between the skin and soft tissues and growth of the bone.[7,12,13] In this scenario the proximal physis, by contributing to longitudinal growth of the bone, was a significant factor. This hypothesis was supported by the observation that the most commonly affected bones (eg, the tibia/fibula and humerus) were those in which the majority of longitudinal bone growth came from the preserved proximal physis. This observation led several investigators to recommend proximal epiphyseodesis as a management strategy for bony overgrowth; however, none have reported the results of this procedure to confirm its efficacy.[3,12,13] Although most subsequent investigators have considered proximal epiphyseodesis to be ineffective, none offer objective clinical evidence to support their clinical impressions.

Little is known about the function of the proximal physis following amputation. Christie and associates[14] compared actual growth to "expected" growth of the proximal tibia in 18 children with below-the-knee (BK) amputation and found that only 50% of expected physeal growth occurred. Diminished physeal function in a congenital amputation may be a consequence of the underlying limb bud insult. In an acquired amputation, altered loading may affect physeal function, as described by the Heuter-Volkmann law. A related observation that proximal physeal growth was responsible for the different longitudinal growth rates between the tibia and fibula, allowing one bone to grow longer than the other following amputation, led other investigators to recommend distal synostosis in BK amputations.[15,16] Although this procedure might address the problem of differential longitudinal growth between the tibia and fibula, it does not directly address the problem of distal overgrowth and introduces the possibility of progressive angular deformity with subsequent growth. Documentation of outcome following distal synostosis is poor, and this procedure has not subsequently been used as a management strategy for bony overgrowth.

Aitken[4] was the first to show that overgrowth was primarily the consequence of a local (occurring at the end of the bone) biologic phenomenon. He placed metallic markers at the end of the tibia and fibula at the time of amputation or revision and showed radiographically that subsequent overgrowth occurred distal to the markers. His work led other investigators to examine what occurs at the bony end of the residual limb following amputation in a variety of animal models. Vascular perfusion studies and histologic analysis of specimens revealed a wound-healing sequence identical to that seen during healing of a fracture. In the skeletally immature animals, biologic sealing of the medullary canal at the site of amputation occurred consistently, presumably in an attempt to normalize the vascular dynamics of the marrow cavity.[16–18] Subsequent overgrowth developed from the biologic seal, and histologic studies have variably implicated the periosteum, endosteum, enchondral ossification of hematoma, and direct metaplasia of fibrous tissue as principal contributors to the overgrowth phenomenon.[19–23] Elegant studies by Speer[2] have determined that the normal wound contracture mechanism may pull the periosteum into the medullary canal, placing it in contact with the endosteum. Subsequent collagen fibers are oriented longitudinally about the end of the bone, with new bone deposition occurring at the periosteal, endosteal, and apical margins. Speer's wound contracture model would seem to explain many of the clinical observations of overgrowth. Further work has shown that if the medullary canal is occluded or plugged with muscle or bone, the local sealing mechanism of the canal is disrupted and the subsequent development of overgrowth does not occur.[22,23]

When all of this information is considered within the context of current knowledge of the biology of bone healing, further observations concerning the pathophysiology of overgrowth are possible. This phenomenon occurs only in the skeletally immature, and the only phase of normal bone healing that is unique to children is the ultimate modeling phase, characterized by the resorption and formation of mature lamellar bone, which alters the micro- and macroscopic contours of the bone[24] (Fig. 4). This process is driven by local mediator mechanisms collectively known as a regional acceleratory phenomenon (RAP).[24,25] The RAP accelerates the modeling response to local mechanical strains, such as shear and compression, that result from muscle loading, body weight, and externally applied loads. Most bone healing problems (usually inadequate healing) are the result of malfunction of the local mediator mechanisms leading to inadequate RAP. In overgrowth, the altered mechanical milieu surrounding the end of the bone leads to excessive RAP, resulting in excessive modeling with development of the characteristic bony spike that grows faster than the surrounding soft tissues.

Occlusion of the medullary canal prevents the development of overgrowth. In the last decade, it has been clearly established that the bone marrow contains multiple osteoinductive agents as well as undifferentiated, pluripotential cells that have the capacity to become bone-forming cells when activated by the appropriate biologic signals.[26,27] These cells contribute to fracture healing, reactive bone formation around infections and neoplasms, and ingrowth to prostheses. Exposure of the marrow cavity elements to extramedullary stimuli, be they chemical, electrical, or mechanical, is necessary for the development of overgrowth. These observations further support the hypothesis that overgrowth is a consequence of the malfunction of established mechanisms of wound healing and normal bone growth.

Management Strategies

Prosthetic management of the child with established bony overgrowth, or at risk for its development, is focused on the prevention of circumstances that increase the mechanical loading of the end of the residual limb. The two most common problems leading to excessive loading of the residual limb are end

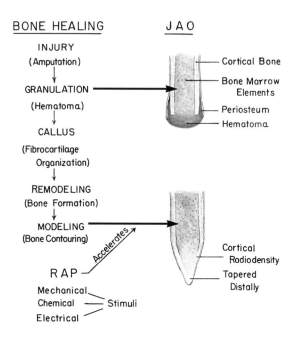

Fig. 4 *Residual limb overgrowth (JAO) may be the consequence of the malfunction of established mechanisms of normal fracture healing and bone growth. In this hypothesis, excessive regional acceleratory phenomenon (RAP), generated primarily by local mechanical stimuli, leads to excessive modeling activity and subsequent development of the characteristic bony spike.*

bearing and hammocking. As the child grows, the length of the residual limb consistently increases, while the girth of the limb may either increase or decrease. If the limb girth decreases, as the child grows out of the socket and loses the proximal fit and control, the tip of the limb will come into excessive contact with the base of the socket, leading to end bearing when the limb is loaded. If the limb girth increases, the soft-tissue envelope is subjected to proximally based traction as the limb is forced into the socket, resulting in a hammocking effect, which increases the pressure on the skin at the end of the residual limb. Optimal prosthetic management of the growing child, therefore, requires frequent prosthetic examinations and the resources to modify or replace the prosthesis as frequently as every 6 months during growth spurts.

The variety of surgical management strategies used over the years is a reflection of the incomplete understanding of the pathophysiology of overgrowth. The clinical experience with proximal epiphyseodesis and distal synostosis for the management of overgrowth has been poorly documented, and both procedures have been largely abandoned. Other management strategies described in the literature include dynamic skin traction and denervation of the residual limb.[28,29]

The historic standard for the surgical management of bony overgrowth has been resection revision.[3,5–8,10] This procedure involves exposure of the bony spike, excision of all bursal and scar tissue, resection of the spike proximally through the normal diaphysis or metaphysis, and 1 to 3 cm more proximal resection of the periosteum. Closure of the soft-tissue envelope is in layers, with a myodesis performed when possible. Resection revision is quick and technically simple, but sacrifices length of the residual limb and often is followed by recurrence of the overgrowth within several years, as would be expected given the current view that overgrowth is a consequence of the malfunction of normal bone healing mechanisms. Recognition that plugging the bony medullary canal prevented the development of overgrowth in animal models led some investigators to attempt distal capping with a variety of synthetic and biologic materials. Synthetic implants used to plug the medullary canal in children include metallic, silastic, and high density polyethylene caps.[11,30,31] These devices generally have performed poorly, with short and long-term complications related to inadequate soft-tissue coverage, failure of fixation at the implant-bone interface, fracture of the implant, infection, and local inflammation.

Marquardt and associates are generally credited as being the first to propose placement of a biologic cap to treat overgrowth.[32-35] Recognizing that overgrowth did not occur in children following disarticulation, they developed a technique for the transfer of an autologous cartilage-bone graft consisting of the distal tibial physis complex (metaphysis-physis-epiphysis-articular cartilage) or calcaneal apophysis at the time of primary amputation in the child at risk for developing overgrowth. For the management of established overgrowth, they recommended using the proximal fibular physis complex or iliac apophysis as a biologic cap. They initially believed that the growth potential of the transferred physis was preserved, and that the overlying articular cartilage was viable. Subsequent investigations have shown that the growth potential is poor following partial or complete nonvascularized free physeal transfer.[36,37] Recognizing the value of plugging the medullary canal, Davids and associates[11] modified the procedure by substituting a tricortical iliac crest graft. Following exposure and appropriate resection of bursal and scar tissue, the apex of the overgrowth segment is resected, and an osteotome is used to split the remaining bone longitudinally for several centimeters, creating two pillars in the coronal plane (Fig. 5). The bone graft from the iliac crest is then wedged into the apex between the pillars (Fig. 6). Fixation is often adequate as is because children's bones are able to deform in an elastic fashion. When necessary, fixation can be augmented with Kirschner wires or the placement of a nonabsorbable suture through a transverse drill hole.

The results of resection revision, synthetic capping with a high density polyethylene implant, and biologic capping with an autologous iliac crest bone graft have been directly compared.[11] Survival analysis revealed that subsequent surgical procedures for recurrent overgrowth were necessary in 84% of the cases managed by resection revision, 78% of those receiving synthetic capping, and only 31% of those managed with a biologic cap. Mean survival time (ie, time to a subsequent surgery for overgrowth) was

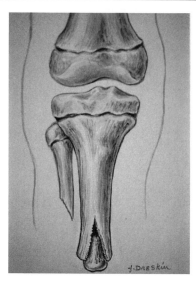

Fig. 5 *Diagram of the modified Marquardt technique for application of a biologic cap (usually an autologous tricortical iliac crest bone graft) to the distal tibia. (Reproduced with permission from Davids JR, Meyer LC, Blackhurst DW: Operative treatment of bone overgrowth in children who have an acquired or congenital amputation.* J Bone Joint Surg *1995;77A:1490–1497.)*

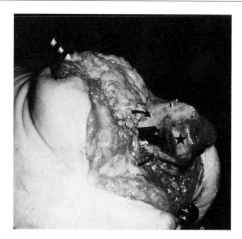

Fig. 6 *Intraoperative photograph showing placement of a biologic cap into the tibia of a 9-year-old boy with a right lower extremity transverse deficiency due to early amnion rupture sequence. The tibial pillars (arrows) and the position of the iliac crest bone graft (star) are evident. The graft in this case was stabilized with two Kirschner wires. (Reproduced with permission from Davids JR, Meyer LC, Blackhurst DW: Operative treatment of bone overgrowth in children who have an acquired or congenital amputation.* J Bone Joint Surg *1995;77A:1490–1497.)*

42 months for the resection revision group, 46 months for the synthetic capping group, and 60 months for the biologic capping group. The investigators concluded that biologic capping with autogenous iliac crest bone graft was the most efficacious technique and, therefore, the treatment of choice for established bony overgrowth.

Current Recommendations/Investigations

Several investigators have recommended a proactive, prophylactic strategy for the management of children who are at risk for developing overgrowth following an acquired amputation.[11,32,33,38] At the time of the initial amputation, biologic capping with an autologous bone graft is performed on the tibia/fibula and humerus. For BK amputations, the ipsilateral fibular head, the dome or head of the talus, and the base of the great toe metatarsal have all been described as potential bone graft donor sites. This approach is justified in all children younger than 12 years of age in whom a transdiaphyseal or transmetaphyseal amputation is being performed.

Biologic capping is the current treatment of choice for children younger than 12 years of age. When the bony spike has penetrated the soft-tissue envelope, leading to contamination of the bursa or subcutaneous tissues, or when obvious infection is present at the tip of the residual limb, the procedure should be performed in a staged manner. The first stage should consist of a resection revision with appropriate debridement of necrotic, infected tissues and perioperative antibiotic therapy. One to 2 months later, once all of the soft tissues have healed and the infection has resolved, the biologic cap can be placed.

Application of a synthetic cap remains a theoretically attractive alternative. The ideal material should be biologically friendly, or at least inert, and the implant design should be appropriately durable and allow for adequate fixation to the bone at the end of the residual limb. Such a material has yet to be identified. Clinical trials at my institution are underway, examining the use of polytetrafluoroethylene (PTFE, also known as Teflon) felt (Meadox Medicals, Oakland, NJ). This fabric has been used extensively by cardiovascular surgeons for the repair of vascular wall defects and is extremely durable and biologically inert. PTFE felt comes in a sheet, and an appropriately sized cruciform implant is fashioned intraoperatively with scissors. A pursestring stitch of nonabsorbable suture is placed around the margin of the implant and is used to anchor it to the end of the bone through two transverse drill holes. This effectively caps the medullary canal, preventing communication between external mediator mechanisms and the bone marrow elements. Although our early experience (approximately 3 years) is encouraging, longer follow-up is required before this procedure can be recommended.

Finally, inspired by reports of the Ertl procedure in young adults, I have reconsidered the use of distal tibiofibular synostosis. The Ertl osteoplasty was designed to facilitate end bearing through a transdiaphyseal amputation by increasing the distal bony surface area by creation of a wide, broad

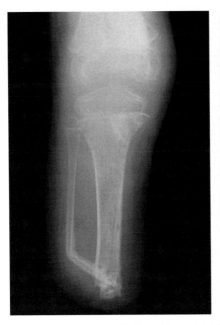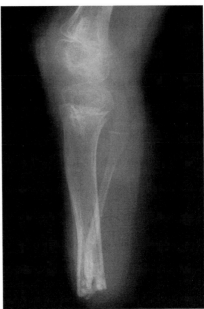

Fig. 7 *Anteroposterior (**left**) and lateral (**right**) radiographs of the left lower extremity in a 4-year-old girl with bilateral below-the-knee amputations due to purpura fulminans. Overgrowth of the tibia and fibula was treated by distal tibiofibular synostosis. Morcellized fragments of the resected bone are packed around the distal fibula to fill the space between the tibial pillars.*

distal synostosis (derived from a tibial periosteal tube that is attached to the distal fibula).[39,40] The synostosis procedure currently utilized at my institution involves shortening the tibia to a level 1 to 2 cm proximal to the distal tip of the fibula and then performing a longitudinal osteotomy of the tibia, creating two pillars in the sagittal plane. A greenstick fracture of the fibula (apex lateral) 1 cm proximal to the end of the tibia is created, and the distal fibula is displaced medially into the space between the tibial pillars (Fig. 7). When necessary, a nonabsorbable suture is used to stabilize the fibula to the tibia. This creates a biologic cap for the tibia and a wide, broad synostosis between the two bones. Although early experience with this procedure is encouraging, longer follow-up is required before it can be recommended.

References

1. O'Neal ML, Bahner R, Ganey TM, Ogden JA: Osseous overgrowth after amputation in adolescents and children. *J Pediatr Orthop* 1996;16:78–84.
2. Speer DP: The pathogenesis of amputation stump overgrowth. *Clin Orthop* 1981;159:294–307.
3. Abraham E, Pellicore RJ, Hamilton RC, Hallman BW, Ghosh L: Stump overgrowth in juvenile amputees. *J Pediatr Orthop* 1986;6:66–71.

4. Aitken GT: Overgrowth of the amputation stump. *Inter Clin Info Bull* 1962;1:1–8.
5. Frantz CH, Aitken GT: Management of the juvenile amputee. *Clin Orthop* 1959;14:30–49.
6. Jorring K: Amputation in children: A follow-up of 74 children whose lower extremities were amputated. *Acta Orthop Scand* 1971;42:178–186.
7. Kurtz AD, Hand RC: Bone growth following amputation in childhood. *Am J Surg* 1939;43:773–775.
8. Lambert CN: Amputation surgery in the child. *Orthop Clin North Am* 1972;3:473–482.
9. Pellicore RJ, Sciora J, Lambert CN, Hamilton RC: Incidence of bone overgrowth in the juvenile amputee population. *Inter Clin Info Bull* 1974;8:1–8.
10. Romano RL, Burgess EM: Extremity growth and overgrowth following amputations in children. *Inter Clin Info Bull* 1966;5:11–12.
11. Davids JR, Meyer LC, Blackhurst DW: Operative treatment of bone overgrowth in children who have an acquired or congenital amputation. *J Bone Joint Surg* 1995;77A:1490–1497.
12. Beekman F: Amputations during childhood. *Surg Clin North Am* 1938;18: 425–431.
13. Vom Saal F: Epiphysiodesis combined with amputation. *J Bone Joint Surg* 1939;21:442–443.
14. Christie J, Lamb DW, McDonald JM, Britten S: A study of stump growth in children with below-knee amputations. *J Bone Joint Surg* 1979;61B:464–465.
15. Barber CG: Amputation of the lower leg with induced synostosis of the distal ends of the tibia and fibula. *J Bone Joint Surg* 1944;26:356–362.
16. Mercer W: Reflections on the amputation stump. *J R Coll Surg Edinb* 1962; 8:52–69.
17. Hellstadius A: An investigation, by experiments on animals, of the role played by the epiphysial cartilage in longitudinal growth. *Acta Chir Scand* 1947;95:156–166.
18. Hulth A, Olerud S: Studies on amputation stumps in rabbits. *J Bone Joint Surg* 1962;44B:431–435.
19. Erikson U, Olerud S: Healing of amputation stumps, with special reference to vascularity and bone. *Acta Orthop Scand* 1966;37:20–28.
20. Hansen-Leth C, Reimann I: Amputations with and without myoplasty on rabbits with special reference to the vascularization. *Acta Orthop Scand* 1972;43:68–77.
21. Hansen-Leth C, Reimann I: Knee disarticulation: An experimental study. *Acta Orthop Scand* 1973;44:75–86.
22. Hansen-Leth C: Muscle blood flow after amputation with special reference to the influence of osseous plugging of the medullary cavity: Assessed by 133 xenon and histamine. An animal experiment. *Acta Orthop Scand* 1976;47:613–618.
23. Hansen-Leth C: Bone vascularization and bone healing in the amputation stump: An experimental study. *Acta Orthop Scand* 1979;50:39–47.
24. Frost HM: The biology of fracture healing: An overview for clinicians. Part II. *Clin Orthop* 1989;248:294–309.
25. Bogoch E, Gschwend N, Rahn B, Moran E, Perren S: Healing of cancellous bone osteotomy in rabbits: Part I. Regulation of bone volume and the regional acceleratory phenomenon in normal bone. *J Orthop Res* 1993;11:285–291.
26. Diduch DR, Coe MR, Joyner C, Owens ME, Balian G: Two cell lines from bone marrow that differ in terms of collagen synthesis, osteogenic characteristics, and matrix mineralization. *J Bone Joint Surg* 1993;75A:92–105.
27. Wolff D, Goldberg VM, Stevenson S: Histomorphometric analysis of the repair of a segmental diaphyseal defect with ceramic and titanium fibermetal implants: Effects of bone marrow. *J Orthop Res* 1994;12:439–446.
28. Friedman LW, Friedman L: The conservative treatment of the bony overgrowth problem in the juvenile amputee. *Inter Clin Info Bull* 1985;20:17–23.
29. Bunch WH, Deck JD, Romer J: The effect of denervation on bony overgrowth after below knee amputation in rats. *Clin Orthop* 1977;122:333–339.

30. Meyer LC, Sauer BW: The use of porous high density polyethylene caps in the prevention of appositional bone growth in the juvenile amputee: A preliminary report. *Inter Clin Info Bull* 1975;14:1–4.

31. Swanson AB: Silicone-rubber implants to control the overgrowth phenomenon in the juvenile amputee. *Inter Clin Info Bull* 1972;11:5–8.

32. Bernd L, Blasius K, Lukoschek M, Lucke R: The autologous stump plasty: Treatment for bony overgrowth in juvenile amputees. *J Bone Joint Surg* 1991;73B:203–206.

33. Marquardt E, Correll J: Amputations and prostheses for the lower limb. *Int Orthop* 1984;8:139–146.

34. Marquardt E: The multiple-limb-deficient child, in Bowker JH, Michael JW (eds): American Academy of Orthopaedic Surgeons *Atlas of Limb Prosthetics: Surgical, Prosthetic, and Rehabilitation Principles,* ed 2. St Louis, MO, Mosby-Year Book, 1992, pp 839–884.

35. Martini AK, Marquardt E: Stump plasty on congenital amputations. *Garyounis Med J* 1980;3(suppl):83–86.

36. Wang G-J, Baugher VM, Stamp WG: Epiphyseal transplant in amputations: Effects on overgrowth in a rabbit model. *Clin Orthop* 1978;130:285–288.

37. Zaleske DJ: Biology of epiphyseal transplantation, in Friedlaender GE, Goldberg VM (eds): *Bone and Cartilage Allografts: Biology and Clinical Applications.* Park Ridge, IL, American Academy of Orthopaedic Surgeons, 1991, pp 27–36.

38. Benevenia J, Makley JT, Leeson MC, Benevenia K: Primary epiphyseal transplants and bone overgrowth in childhood amputations. *J Pediatr Orthop* 1992;12:746–750.

39. Moll JH: More on the Ertl osteoplasty. *Amputee Clin* 1970;2:7–8.

40. von Ertl JW: The care of amputation stumps by osteo-myeloplastic according to v Ertl. *Z Plast Chir* 1981;5:184–189.

Chapter 24

Lengthening of Short Residual Limbs in Children

Hugh G. Watts, MD

Introduction

For children who have amputation residual limbs that are very short, the gain of even a small amount of length may provide an adequate lever to use a less extensive prosthesis. The potential advantages are decreased energy consumption, improved prosthetic control, decreased heat retention, increased comfort from the lighter prosthesis, and fewer components requiring repairs, as well as decreased cost.

Children with upper-extremity limb loss, especially if the loss is congenital, frequently will choose not to wear prostheses. However, longer limbs may allow for grasping objects in the midline between the residual limbs for "bimanual" activity without a prosthesis. Furthermore, the addition of a longer distal segment can allow objects to be grasped, for example, between a lenthened humeral residual limb and the chest, or between a lengthened forearm and the upper arm.

The goal of lengthening posttraumatic amputation residual limbs or short congenital residual limbs is not new.[1,2] The interest in Ilizarov's technique of callus lengthening has infused new enthusiasm for the idea. While Ilizarov is known to have lengthened a number of amputation residual limbs, the exact experience is not well documented[2–6] and none is in English with the exception of a comment by Ilizarov that "...the author's method can be employed to lengthen amputation stumps for improved prosthetic fitting."[7]

In the English literature there have been 12 case reports dealing mostly with adults.[8–14] At an ACPOC Workshop (1995), a request for presentations of current experience brought to light eight cases from seven surgeons (one previously reported) in addition to my own experience at that time of 23.

This chapter addresses the issues of lengthening short residual limbs in children using my personal experience as a guide. This chapter will not deal with lengthening of fingers, nor will it deal with techniques for getting longer residual limbs at the time of initial amputation.

Experience at Los Angeles Shriners Hospital

Patients

From 1990 to the present, 32 short residual limbs in 27 patients have been lengthened. Three patients underwent bilateral humeral lengthenings, one underwent bilateral tibial lengthenings, and two patients had bilateral femoral lengthenings. Bilateral lengthenings were done simultaneously.

Segments lengthened were: humerus, 11; ulna, two; femur, 12; tibia, four; feet, two; rib-to-scapula, one. There were 13 males and 14 females, ages 6 to 20 years. The etiology of amputation was: burn injury (including electrical), four; trauma, 12; tumor, three; and congenital, eight.

Six patients are still in treatment (femur, five; humerus, one). Although their functional results cannot be given, their increased length and complications are included here.

Technique

All patients were lengthened by gradual distraction using the biologic techniques described by Ilizarov, but employing a number of different distracting devices. All osteotomies were made by power saw rather than by an osteotome because the fragments were very small and required accurate cuts. Gradual distraction at 1 mm/day was started approximately 1 week following the osteotomy.

The apparatus used was determined by the anatomy of the very short segments: Ilizarov, two (one ulna; one foot); large Wagner, two (femurs); small Wagner, 11 (ten femurs, one ulna); large Hoffmann, four (tibias); small Hoffmann, 12 (11 humerus, one foot); none, one (one single-stage lengthening was performed where a vascularized rib segment was fused to the scapula into a skin bed previously stretched out with a tissue expander).

Results

Technical Results

The bone of the residual limb was lengthened an average of 8.7 cm (range, 3.4 cm in a cuneiform to 18.3 cm in a femur). Compared to the length of the original bone, this represented a mean lengthening of 110% (range, 45% to 220%).

The lengthening index (ie, the number of months the patient wore the external fixator per centimeter of length achieved) averaged 1.26 months/cm (range, 0.34 to 3.3 months). There was no difference in the lengthening index by anatomic site or age of the child. The total treatment time (ie, the length of time from the start of the lengthening to the fitting of the new prosthesis) averaged 15 months (range, 7 to 29 months).

Functional Results

All children who have completed lengthening of their femurs or tibias achieved sufficient length to be fitted with a prosthesis at one level more distal than before lengthening. Two children with partial foot deletions no longer require a partial foot prosthesis.

Children with upper extremity deficiencies are harder to assess because a longer residual limb can increase function even if a prosthesis is never worn. Three patients were lengthened with the anticipation that a prosthesis would *not* be used after lengthening. All are "users" in that they now grasp objects between the lengthened residual limb and trunk. Of the nine remaining patients who have completed their lengthenings, all but one wear their prostheses, but are not constant "users."[15] The one child who underwent the attempt to form a humeral residual limb by grafting the rib segment to the scapula wears a prosthesis and uses the residual limb to activate a control switch of a powered shoulder disarticulation prosthesis; however, this limb has been of limited functional benefit to her.

Complications

There were no deep wound infections, but pin tract infections and oozing were virtually universal. Pain was usually mild to moderate during lengthening; however, one child and her family became sufficiently distraught that she required hospitalization on two occasions for 3 days each to defuse the problem. One child undergoing lengthening of her femoral residual limb for a congenital lesion suffered a dislocation of the femoral head, which was managed successfully by closed reduction and the application of a spica cast for 6 weeks. She has retained full range of motion and went on to wear an above-knee prosthesis successfully. One boy with a very short ulnar segment suffered loss of motion of the elbow when the osteotomy was made too proximally (just at the level of the coronoid process) so that as the fragments separated, the proximal ulna was forced proximally, partly enlarging the joint. One patient who underwent lengthening of both short below-knee residual limbs required hamstring lengthening bilaterally as a result of knee flexion contractures that developed during the lengthening.

Assessment of Technical Results

Lengthening of Bone Versus Lengthening of Residual Limb

The evaluation of the amount of lengthening uses criteria that have been useful for assessing lengthening of intact limbs. However, in lengthening residual limbs, these criteria may not be appropriate. For example, children who have sustained very proximal amputations of the humerus usually have weak deltoid muscles with a resulting inferior subluxation of the humeral head. At the beginning of lengthening, the bone can be elongated as much as 3 cm before the upper end of the humerus abuts against the acromion. It is only at this point that further lengthening starts to change the effective length of the residual limb distally. In some femoral residual limb lengthenings, the bone can be lengthened a number of centimeters with loss of the flabby soft tissues at the end of the residual limb. In such a case, the residual limb may not have lengthened as much as the bone, yet this residual limb may be more easily fitted to a prosthesis and provide the child with better prosthetic control.

Percent Versus Absolute Lengthening

The use of "percent increase" in bone or residual limb length may not be a good measure of technical results because the starting residual limb lengths are often so very small. Is a 100% lengthening of a 3-cm tibial residual limb a worthwhile endeavor?

Assessment of Functional Results

Assessing Lower Extremity Function

Is energy consumption really decreased by residual limb lengthening? Waters and associates[16] indicate that for lower extremity amputees, each distal level of amputation increases the gait velocity by 20% and halves the O_2 consumption/meter. However, they studied a limited number of patients, and the lengths of the residual limbs were not given. There are no data to indicate whether an amputee with a femoral residual limb of, say 20 cm, would function significantly better with a residual limb of 30 cm.

Does the gait look better? A child with a short femoral residual limb usually has an abductor lurch. The longer the residual limb, the less the lurch. At what length of residual limb does the lurch significantly decrease? Gait laboratory analyses are needed to document the changes. Although a sample of children with different femoral residual limb lengths could be compared, there are enough differences due to age, size, and muscle strengths, that it would be preferable to study each child before and after lengthening. Yet even this procedure may result in misinterpretation because of the very long treatment time involved. Such studies would necessarily have to take place 2 to 3 years apart. Over that length of time, changes in the growth and development of the child could make significant differences unrelated to residual limb length. Consequently, for such studies, it would be preferable to evaluate patients who have reached skeletal maturity.

Assessing Functional Results in Children With Upper Extremity Deficiency

Children with congenital upper extremity limb deletions frequently choose not to use prostheses. Is it worthwhile, then, to lengthen upper extremity residual limbs? The answer is a qualified yes. As stated above, longer residual limbs may allow for grasping objects in the midline for bimanual activities without a prosthesis. Some functions, especially toileting, may be greatly enhanced by having longer residual limbs. For example, one child for whom I lengthened both humeral residual limbs became able to manipulate the zipper on the fly of his trousers so that he could use public toileting facilities without additional help. This is a function that he is very pleased to have gained.

Lengthening a humerus so that there is now space in the axilla between the humerus and the chest wall can allow objects to be grasped. A lengthened forearm allows grasping in the crook of the elbow between forearm and arm. These functions are useful in spite of the presence of water or dirt, which may damage a prosthesis.

Skin Coverage

A number of surgeons who have lengthened amputation residual limbs have had problems maintaining skin coverage, especially in those residual limbs resulting from burn injuries. Myocutaneous free flaps have been used. One potential problem with flaps is the limited sensation. If a residual limb has no, or limited sensation, an upper extremity prosthesis may not add function. In one girl who sustained a short below-elbow amputation due to a fire, the bone was lengthened under an abdominal flap. When length had been achieved, the flap was cut free. Subsequently the child did not use her prosthesis. She stated that the lack of sensation made her prosthesis "feel weird." Two years later, as a teenager, she became a full-time wearer and user. She now has some sensation, but the change in prosthetic wearing may merely be the result of the added desire for cosmesis driven by teenage emotions.

I have tried other strategies with less success. In one patient, I tried concomitant skin lengthening using stockinet stuck to the thigh with "super glue" but found that the glue did not hold successfully. I have not yet tried to do the same by attaching the stretcher to the skin by sutures.

Tissue expanders have not proved useful in our hands. In order for tissue expanders to be effective, they are placed superficial to the deep fascia. For an amputation residual limb the extra tissue provided is just skin and a little fat without the fascia and underlying muscle. The thin skin layer has not been able to withstand the abuses of prosthetic wear. If the expanders are placed deep to the fascia, only limited stretching is possible.

In one boy for whom the humerus was being lengthened, I attempted to bend the bone regenerate 180° and continued the lengthening (along the apex of the "U"-shaped residual limb where there was full-thickness soft tissue) with the plan to straighten out the "U" when length had been achieved. However, the regenerate began to coalesce across the "U," so the process was abandoned.

As experience with residual limb lengthening improves, orthopaedic surgeons may wish to change their strategy of acute amputation surgery. In limb reimplantations, it has been useful in some hands to shorten an extremity sufficiently to allow good healing and then to lengthen the limb to its original length.[17] The same principle could be used at the time of initial amputation. Good skin coverage could be achieved by shortening the bone in the anticipation of lengthening after healing is complete. This procedure would be especially useful if it allowed for the preservation of a knee joint (rather than proceeding immediately to do a through-knee amputation "because the tibial residual limb would have been too short to be useful anyway").

Prolonged Time to Complete the Treatment Process

A very long time is required from the start of lengthening to the fitting of the final prosthesis. Over a lifetime of prosthetic wear, the process seems to be a good investment of time. However, this prolonged treatment time can be very frustrating to all involved, no matter how this aspect is emphasized to patients and their parents prior to lengthening.

Our prosthetists have tried to obviate the problem of the long time the patient has to wait to get his or her prosthesis by fabricating a temporary leg that can be worn around the pins of the external fixators. They have tried this with success in three patients with femoral residual limb lengthenings. They had planned to do a similar set of prostheses for one boy undergoing bilateral below-knee lengthenings but consolidation occurred rapidly enough that they were not able to complete the temporary prosthesis before it was time to remove the fixators. They have not yet made temporary prostheses for a child with a humeral lengthening, but plan to do so.

Lengthening a residual limb over an intramedullary rod might allow for fitting as soon as sufficient length has been gained. Alternatively, after the length has been achieved, the external fixator could be replaced with an interlocked intramedullary rod. However, I have been reluctant to try these techniques for fear of creating a severe bone infection during a treatment that is still believed to be "experimental."

Role of Physical and Occupational Therapy

Does lengthening decrease the range of motion of the proximal joint? We have not found that to be a significant problem. While we encourage exercising the affected joint during lengthening, we have not insisted on a specific regimen.

A very short humeral residual limb that goes unused for a number of years after an amputation results in a very weak deltoid muscle and subluxation of the humeral head. This has been a problem, especially in those children who suffered traumatic amputations. It may be beneficial to strengthen the deltoid before lengthening. We wonder if there is a place for strengthening by electrical stimulation?

Age

At this point in our experience we remain uncertain as to the best age at which to consider lengthening. In a child with an open physis proximal to the level of amputation, there is a potential that subsequent growth itself might provide an adequate residual limb. We have waited to lengthen such a residual limb until we were able to document an absence of useful growth proximally.

What are the realistic limits of lengthening? Ilizarov lengthened a tibial stump until it reached the level of the opposite foot, then the stump was bent to 90° and lengthened further to provide a "foot" (ML Samchuhov, MD, Dallas, TX, personal communication, 1997). In a child it could be expected that the angled bone would straighten out by remodeling (as does a humerus after a Marquardt osteotomy in children). One has to doubt the capability of the skin under the "foot" to withstand pressure over the long term.

Surgical Problems Other Than Skin Coverage

Bone fixation has not proven to be a major problem. Prior to lengthening, most of the residual limb bones have been very porotic from disuse. However, the forces required to effect the lengthening appear to be less than those needed for lengthening intact bones. It has only been necessary to change pin locations in one child, who was undergoing lengthening of a congenital femoral deletion.

Is there an optimal external fixation apparatus? We do not feel that there is one apparatus that works best for all lengthenings. The apparatus we have used for a given bone has been predicated on our desire to select the smallest apparatus (for weight considerations) that will provide an adequate excursion. For femoral residual limbs we have settled on using the small Wagner lengthener, and for humeral residual limbs, the small Hoffmann.

Small lengtheners do not have long lengthening excursions. We have solved the problem when lengthening a humeral residual limb by using a small Hoffmann apparatus and selecting the pin clamps that have an extra post. When the full extent of lengthener has been reached, a jumper rod is fixed between the pin clamps (using these extra posts) to preserve the length already gained. The lengthener is then shortened back to the zero mark, and the jumper rod is removed. The lengthening is then continued. This can readily be done in the clinic.

It is essential when doing the lengthenings that the cuts in the bone are designed to allow the bone fragments to elongate without dragging the adjacent tendons with them. Such bone cuts may need to be oblique, stepped, or a complex shape. For example, in a short tibial residual limb, the cut in the bone needs to leave the patellar tendon and the hamstring tendons attached to the proximal segment, not to the distal one. Thus the cut is a half-barrel shaped one made from medial-to-lateral.

Research Needs

When we discuss the possibilities of lengthening a short amputation residual limb with a child and the parents, we stress that the process is still experimental. Many questions need answering. The following major areas of research could be beneficial.

We need reproducible, clinically meaningful, and simple means of defining the effective length of an amputation residual limb or congenital residual limb for each of the levels for which we provide prostheses. We need data that document the energy savings benefit to a patient of having a longer residual limb segment. We need gait analysis data that document the changes that result from the residual limb lengthenings. Upper extremity functional change is of importance to all aspects of the management of children with upper extremity limb deficiencies. It may be possible surgically to enhance the function in children who often prefer not to use prostheses. The development of instruments for the assessment of functional outcomes will be a great step forward.

Conclusion

Lengthening of short amputation residual limbs can be successful in children. The technique has potential for improving the function of amputees over a lifetime, but direct research is needed to prove the value of the surgery. The unification of assessment and reporting of results will enhance the analysis of residual limb lengthening surgery.

The lengthening of short residual limbs requires techniques different from those used for standard limb lengthenings. Many of these experiences with children should be applicable to adult amputees, except those with limbs lost to vascular disease, and they could alter the strategy for amputation surgery during the acute phase.

References

1. Marquardt E: The multiple limb-deficient child, in American Academy of Orthopaedic Surgeons *Atlas of Limb Prosthetics: Surgical and Prosthetic Principles*. St. Louis, MO, CV Mosby, 1981, pp 595–641.

2. Shatilov OE, Rozhkov AV: Lengthening of short stumps of the leg in children at the expense of rupture of the growth zone. *Ortop Travmatol Protez* 1972;33:58–60.

3. Ilizarov GA, Shevtsov VI, Kaliakina VI, Okulov GV: Methods of shaping and lengthening the foot. *Ortop Travmatol Protez* 1983;11:49–51.

4. Rozhkov AV, Iankovskii VM: A method for lengthening a very short stump of the leg and its prosthesis. *Ortop Travmatol Protez* 1988;10:61–63.

5. Rozhkov AV, Startseva TE, Batenkova GI, Lukashevich TA, Kudriavtsev VA: Method of reconstructing a short stump of the foot by the distraction method. *Ortop Travmatol Protez* 1983;5:48–50.

6. Voinova LE: Characteristics of surgical preparation of invalids for prosthesis after amputation of the upper limbs. *Ortop Travmatol Protez* 1984;11:10–14.

7. Ilizarov GA: Clinical application of the tension-stress effect for limb lengthening. *Clin Orthop* 1990;250:8–26.

8. Eldridge JC, Armstrong PF, Krajbich JI: Amputation stump lengthening with the Ilizarov technique: A case report. *Clin Orthop* 1990;256:76–79.

9. Fealy MJ, Most D, Struck S, Simms GE, Hui K: Femur lengthening with a vascularized tibia bone flap. *Ann Plast Surg* 1996;37:140–146.

10. Kour AK, Seo JS, Pho RW: Combined free flap, Ilizarov lengthening and prosthetic fitting in the reconstruction of a proximal forearm amputation: A case report. *Ann Acad Med Singapore* 1995;24(suppl 4):135–137.

11. Latimer HA, Dahners LE, Bynum DK: Lengthening of below-the-knee-amputation stumps using the Ilizarov technique. *J Orthop Trauma* 1990;4:411–414.

12. Moss AL, Waterhouse N, Townsend PL, Hannon MA: Lengthening of a short traumatic femoral stump. *Injury* 1985;16:350–353.

13. Persson BM, Broome A: Lengthening a short femoral amputation stump: A case of tissue expander and endoprosthesis. *Acta Orthop Scand* 1994;65:99–100.

14. Younge D, Dafniotis O: A composite bone flap to lengthen a below-knee amputation stump. *J Bone Joint Surg* 1993;75B:330–331.

15. Kruger LM, Fishman S: Myoelectric and body-powered prostheses. *J Pediatr Orthop* 1993;13:68–75.

16. Waters RL, Perry J, Antonelli D, Hislop H: Energy cost of walking of amputees: The influence of level of amputation. *J Bone Joint Surg* 1976;58A:42–46.

17. Betz AM, Stock W, Hierner R, Baumgart R: Primary shortening with secondary limb lengthening in severe injuries of the lower leg: A six year experience. *Microsurgery* 1993;14:446–453.

Chapter 25

Limb-Salvage Surgery Versus Amputation for Children With Extremity Sarcomas

John P. Dormans, MD

Introduction

Malignant tumors account for more than half the amputations done for disease processes in children.[1] Vascular malformations, neurogenic disorders, and a variety of miscellaneous disorders are responsible for the remainder of amputations for disease in children. Eight thousand cases of pediatric cancer are diagnosed in the United States each year. Bone and soft-tissue sarcomas make up 11% of this total (880 cases per year). Six hundred children die of cancer each year in the United States, making cancer the most common cause of death from disease in childhood and adolescence.[2]

Appropriate evaluation and management of children with malignant tumors is essential to optimizing survival and function and, necessarily, involves a multidisciplinary approach that includes the radiologist, pathologist, oncologist, prosthetist, social worker, and surgeon.[3]

Several significant advances have been made in the evaluation and treatment of malignant bone tumors in the last several years. Magnetic resonance imaging (MRI) has improved the surgeon's ability to visualize and assess these tumors preoperatively. Better chemotherapeutic regimens and refinement in radiotherapeutic and surgical techniques have resulted in significant improvements in long-term survival. In addition, molecular genetic findings have contributed greatly in the diagnosis of these tumors; the prognostic and treatment significance of these findings is still evolving.[4]

Epidemiology and Clinical Presentation

Osteogenic sarcoma (osteosarcoma) is the most common malignant bone tumor of childhood, and Ewing's sarcoma is the second most common.[5] Both osteosarcoma and Ewing's sarcoma usually affect children between the ages of 10 and 20 years, but they may occur at any age. Osteosarcoma usually affects the most rapidly growing metaphyseal end of long bones, with the most common sites being the distal femur, proximal tibia, and proximal humerus.[6] Unlike osteosarcoma, Ewing's sarcomas most often arise in the axial skeleton, particularly in the pelvis, but may arise in any bone. The humerus and femur are commonly affected, and when they occur in long bones, the lesions are often diaphyseal.[7] With both tumors, an accompanying soft-tissue mass is often seen.

Approximately 15% of patients with osteosarcoma present with clinically evident metastases, most commonly in the lungs, while 25% of patients with Ewing's sarcoma present with overt metastases, typically in the lungs, bone marrow, or bone. Metastasis at presentation is a poor prognostic sign for both of these malignant bone tumors.[5]

Patients with osteosarcoma usually present with pain. Pain and local swelling are the most common clinical findings in patients with Ewing's sarcoma. Constitutional symptoms, such as fever and malaise, may be seen in patients with Ewing's sarcoma, especially those with metastatic disease. The presence or absence of constitutional symptoms in patients with localized disease, however, is not predictive of outcome. These symptoms, along with common laboratory findings of high white cell counts and elevated sedimentation rates may suggest osteomyelitis as a differential diagnosis.

Rhabdomyosarcoma, a malignant tumor arising in muscle, is the most common soft-tissue sarcoma of childhood.[8] It accounts for around 5% of all childhood cancer. These lesions may present anywhere in the body, and typically present with either a painless mass or evidence of organ dysfunction caused by tumor growth. There are two major histologic subtypes of rhabdomyosarcoma, embryonal and alveolar. Embryonal tumors are typically found in the first decade of life, most often in the head and neck or the genitourinary tract, whereas alveolar rhabdomyosarcomas are more commonly seen in the second decade of life in the extremities and trunk. Alveolar tumors may spread to bone, but embryonal tumors rarely do so.[5]

Evaluation

The evaluation of a child with a suspected musculoskeletal sarcoma establishes the foundation for subsequent treatment. After a careful history and physical examination of the child, the first diagnostic test for a patient with a suspected malignant bone tumor is a plain radiograph.[9] Radiographs of osteosarcoma may show lytic or mixed lytic/destructive lesions, sometimes with calcification or evidence of new bone formation, most commonly in the metaphyseal region of long bones (Fig. 1). Extensive periosteal reaction (Codman's triangle) may be seen. Ewing's sarcomas demonstrate permeative, destructive bone changes, usually arising in the diaphyseal region of long bones or in flat bones of the axial skeleton. Reactive bone formation and onion skin or "hair-on-end" periosteal reaction may be seen.

MRI should include the entire involved portion of the extremity, including the joint above and below, to define the intra- and extraosseous extent of the tumor and to define the relationship of the tumor to adjacent neurovascular structures. A bone scan is obtained to look for bone metastasis or to diagnose skip lesions, and a computed tomography (CT) scan of the chest is done to look for lung metastases. Bone marrow sampling (aspirates

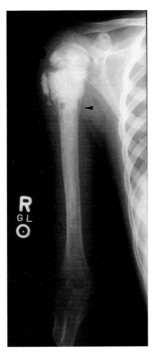

Fig. 1 *Plain radiograph of osteosarcoma of the proximal humerus showing a permeative lesion extending from the distal diaphysis (open arrow) into the epiphysis (closed arrow). Associated periosteal reaction (Codman's triangle, arrowhead) and calcification are shown. (Reproduced with permission from Himelstein BP, Dormans JP: Malignant bone tumors of childhood.* Pediatr Clin North Am *1996;43:967–984.)*

and biopsies from two sites) should be done at the time of the biopsy for Ewing's sarcomas and soft-tissue sarcomas. The prebiopsy clinical and radiographic evaluation of a child with a suspected musculoskeletal sarcoma is well described by Letson and associates.[3]

Staging

Careful "staging" of a suspected malignant tumor is required prior to biopsy. It is important to learn as much as possible about a lesion and its differential diagnosis prior to the biopsy so that mistakes that may alter the ultimate management of the child can be avoided.[10]

The staging system used most commonly by musculoskeletal tumor surgeons is that of Enneking.[10,11] With this classification, the histologic appearance is defined as low grade (G1) or high grade (G2), and the determination of the location of the lesion is defined as intracompartmental (T1), extracompartmental (T2), or metastatic (M).[11] Stage IA lesions are low grade, intracompartmental lesions, whereas stage IB lesions are low grade, extracompartmental. Stage IIA lesions are high grade, intracompartmental lesions, whereas IIB lesions are high grade, extracompartmental. Stage III lesions are associated with metastases. A compartment is an anatomic structure or space bounded by natural barriers to tumor extension. A whole bone, a joint, and a functional muscle group are each considered compartments.[11]

The Biopsy

It is estimated that approximately 50% of all malignant musculoskeletal neoplasms are initially treated inappropriately. Biopsy-related complications are five times more common in community hospital settings than in primary cancer referral centers. For these reasons, if the differential diagnosis for a child with an extremity lesion includes a malignant tumor, immediate referral to a tertiary care center is warranted. A survey of the Musculoskeletal Tumor Society in 1982 revealed the hazards involved in biopsy of patients with malignant skeletal and soft-tissue tumors.[12] Of 329 cases reviewed, 18.2% had major errors in diagnosis and had the optimum treatment plan altered as a result of problems related to the biopsy, 10.3% had nonrepresentative biopsies, and 4.5% received an unnecessary amputation because of problems with the biopsy. Because the biopsy-related problems occurred from three to five times more frequently when the biopsy was performed at a referring institution, the Society recommended that the biopsy be planned as carefully as the definitive surgery, with careful attention to asepsis, hemostasis, skin handling, and wound closure. The biopsy is probably the most important procedure, short of the operation, for definitive local tumor control in the management of children with bone and soft tissue sarcomas.[13,14] Needle aspiration may provide adequate tissue for a histologic diagnosis;[15] however, many oncologic surgeons prefer an incisional technique, which also provides additional tissue for newer molecular diagnostic studies and research. Incisional biopsy involves removing only a portion of the tumor without contaminating the surrounding soft-tissue structures, such as neurovascular structures, joints, muscles, or compartments not originally involved by the tumor.

Pathology

Osteogenic sarcoma is a malignant pleomorphic bone tumor in which the proliferating tumor cells produce new bone. Two pathologic findings are required for diagnosis of osteosarcoma, malignant sarcomatous cells and production of osteoid or new bone. Electron microscopy may occasionally be needed to confirm the presence of osteoid.

Ewing's sarcoma and the cytogenetically related primitive neuroectodermal tumor (PNET) are "small, round, blue-cell tumors" of childhood. Ewing's sarcomas are characterized by their lack of recognition by antibodies that are specific for other round-cell tumors, such as desmin in rhabdomyosarcoma. Immunostaining for vimentin, an intermediate filament, is typically positive, and most Ewing's sarcomas are found to have intracytoplasmic glycogen ultrastructurally. Recently, a new monoclonal antibody to the antigen determined by the *MIC2* gene, expressed in most Ewing's and PNET tumors, was developed and found to be very reliable in identifying these tumors immunohistochemically.[16]

Etiology and Molecular Genetics

While the exact cause of extremity sarcomas is unknown, cancer is now understood to be a genetic disease. The molecular biology, cytogenetics, and pathobiology of sarcomas is being better understood and will undoubtedly change the evaluation, treatment, and outcome of patients with musculoskeletal cancers.[4,17] Surgeons involved in the care of patients with these cancers should understand the advances made as part of the "genetic revolution." Sarcomas are being grouped by specific genetic alterations. These alterations may be prognostic and certainly have treatment implications. It is imperative that the biopsy of a suspected malignant extremity tumor be done in a center with immediate access to these newer tests because most currently require fresh tissue.

Treatment Principles

Musculoskeletal sarcomas are systemic diseases that also require local treatment of the primary tumor. Before the advent of systemic chemotherapy, most patients with localized osteosarcoma of the extremities were treated with amputation alone. Most of these patients succumbed to metastatic disease, with long-term survival of less than 25%.[18] These results suggested that such patients, without overt metastases at diagnosis, must have "micrometastatic disease," foci of tumor that are established but too small to see macroscopically or with CT scans of the lung. Without systemic chemotherapy to kill these tumor cell foci, they will grow. About 90% of patients with Ewing's tumors will also develop metastatic disease without systemic therapy, again supporting the notion that these are systemic tumors with local presentations.[19] Malignant bone tumors are therefore treated with a multimodal approach to achieve local control, to eradicate established micrometastases, and to prevent new systemic spread.

Treatment of Osteosarcoma and Ewing's Sarcoma

Several prospective randomized trials have demonstrated highly significant improvements in disease-free survival when systemic chemotherapy was added to surgical treatment for osteosarcoma, with current survival rates exceeding 60% for patients with localized primary tumors.[20] Multiagent chemotherapy is now given to most patients preoperatively (neoadjuvant) in order to decrease primary tumor viability and to treat micrometastatic disease present at diagnosis. This approach also permits more careful surgical planning. Protocols utilizing preoperative (neoadjuvant) chemotherapy use the extent of tumor necrosis at the time of definitive surgery as a measure of effectiveness and as a prognostic sign. In recent studies, the most significant prognostic factor for patients with osteosarcoma is the degree of chemotherapy-induced necrosis in the resection specimen.[21] Because osteosarcoma is unresponsive to radiation therapy, surgery is the mainstay of local control of the primary tumor.

Ewing's tumors are typically sensitive to both chemotherapy and radiotherapy. To improve local control and to reduce morbidity and associated functional impairments after radiation therapy, the use of neoadjuvant chemotherapy followed by delayed primary tumor control with surgical resection, when possible, is now the standard of care for Ewing's sarcoma. For nonmetastatic Ewing's sarcoma of bone, surgical resection is the mainstay of local control. For osteosarcoma, surgical resection involves removal of the tumor with wide margins. For large pelvic tumors, outcome may be improved with wide surgical resection, suggesting that aggressive surgery may be indicated in selected cases.[22] For metastatic Ewing's tumors, the prognosis is still poor.

Radiotherapy may also be used for local control when wide surgical margins cannot be obtained or are inadequate (microscopic residual disease) or in surgically nonexpendable sites. There is a current trend towards lowering doses of adjuvant radiotherapy for this disease, given the risk of secondary malignancies such as osteosarcoma in the radiation field following doses of 5000 cGy or greater.[23]

During the last decade, a more aggressive approach has been taken toward the treatment of pulmonary metastasis. Lesions identified at diagnosis should be excised at the time of primary tumor-control surgery.[24]

Surgery for Local Tumor Control: Margins

There are four different kinds of surgical oncologic wound margins: intralesional, marginal, wide, and radical (Fig. 2). Intralesional margins involve removing a portion of the lesion.[10,11] With an intralesional margin, portions of the lesion, the reactive zone containing satellites, and skip lesions in the surrounding normal tissues are all left behind. Marginal margins involve removing the lesion en bloc with an extracapsular plane of dissection through the reactive zone of inflammation. Satellite and skip lesions are left behind in the normal surrounding tissue. Wide margins require en bloc excision of the lesion in a plane of dissection that is peripheral to the reactive zone through normal tissue. The distance away from the tumor required to achieve this margin has not been strictly established. With better imaging (MRI) and the development and progress of limb-salvage surgery, decreasing distances from the tumor while still maintaining a cuff of normal tissue around the tumor are being accepted. Finally, radical margins involve removing the entire compartment(s) in which the tumor has extended. An important principle in musculoskeletal tumor surgery is that the tumor itself should never be visualized or encountered at the time of

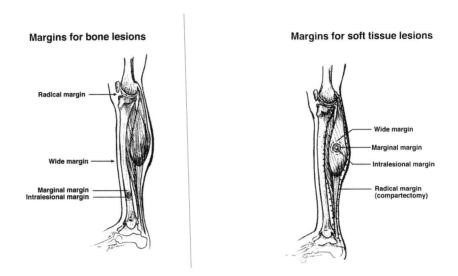

Fig. 2 *Surgical margins for bone* **(left)** *and soft-tissue* **(right)** *lesions. Wide margins are required for osteosarcomas, which are not responsive to radiation therapy. Marginal margins may be acceptable for Ewing's sarcomas when combined with adjuvant radiotherapy, although wide margins are clearly preferred. Wide margins are required for most soft-tissue sarcomas. (Reproduced with permission from Himelstein BP, Dormans JP: Malignant bone tumors of childhood.* Pediatr Clin North Am *1996;43:967–984.)*

surgery. If the surgeon does visualize or enter the substance of the tumor, he or she will no longer have a wide margin, and contamination of the tumor bed occurs; microscopic or gross residual tumor is left behind; and the likelihood of local recurrence increases.

Surgical Intervention for Local Tumor Control

Cancer surgery requires complete removal of malignant tissue. In most cases, the primary tumor is removed surgically. The tumor can be removed with wide margins through amputation or through resection, leaving uninvolved surrounding and distal parts, limb-salvage or limb-sparing surgery. The goal of surgery is to remove the tumor with a surrounding cuff of normal tissue such that the tumor is never directly seen during the operation; ie, wide margins (Fig. 2). In limb-salvage surgery, the goal is to obtain satisfactory margins with the least amount of normal tissue being removed. Better techniques are becoming available to determine the exact extent of the tumor preoperatively and to allow for better limb-salvage surgery techniques.

Historically, the success of chemotherapy in improving local control, in conjunction with improvements in surgical technique, has made limb-salvage surgery possible.[25] Several large series have shown no survival disadvantage for patients treated with limb-sparing surgery compared to those treated with amputation as long as wide margins are achieved.[26] At least for distal femoral lesions, there do not appear to be any differences in psychosocial outcome in patients treated with limb-salvage versus those treated with amputation.[26]

At our institution, over the past 5 years, 250 children with musculoskeletal tumors or tumor-like conditions have been treated. Of these, 38 have presented with primary musculoskeletal sarcomas (ranging from eight to 12 patients per year). Approximately 70% of these children have been treated using limb-sparing techniques.

Reconstruction After Resection of Extremity Sarcoma (Limb-Sparing Surgery)

After resection of the tumor with limb-sparing techniques, reconstruction of the limb is required; ie, rebuilding the extremity to accommodate the loss of the structures removed for control of the local tumor. Options include reconstruction with custom endoprosthetic devices, allograft reconstruction with or without fusion of joints, autograft reconstruction (either vascularized or nonvascularized), or combinations of endoprostheses and bone grafts. van Nes rotationplasty is another option for patients with extremity sarcoma. It allows for better function than amputation and better durability in the face of continued extremity growth than many of the endoprosthetic reconstructive options for the lower extremity. Plastic surgery procedures, such as vascularized free flaps, are often required for reconstruction of soft-tissue defects.

Reconstruction using custom endoprosthetic devices has provided surgical alternatives to children and teenage individuals with limb-threatening malignancy. Expandable prostheses may be used after resection of major growth centers of the lower extremity to address progressive leg-length discrepancies[27] (Fig. 3). The difficulties with endoprosthetic reconstruction include loosening of the prosthesis with activity and growth, difficulties with lengthening of the prosthesis, fractures, and infection. Ward and associates[28] discuss endoprosthetic bone reconstruction following malignant tumor resection in skeletally immature patients.

Allograft reconstruction (intercalary or osteoarticular) can also be used to reconstruct defects after wide resection for extremity sarcoma. The advantages are that allograft tissue is readily available. The disadvantages include the inability to account for further growth of the contralateral extremity (that is, inability to address eventual leg-length discrepancy for growing patients), joint degeneration and instability of joints for osteoarticular allografts, and higher risk of infection and fracture. Composite allograft and endoprosthesis reconstruction is another option after wide resection of extremity sarcoma, both in the lower and upper extremity.

The use of either vascularized or nonvascularized autograft for reconstruction is a reasonable option. Additionally, reconstruction of pelvic skeletal defects after resection for sarcoma can be done with these materials (Fig. 4). This is described in detail in a recent review.[29]

Rotationplasty has additionally been shown to be a practical, functional option for reconstruction after segmental limb resection as opposed to ampu-

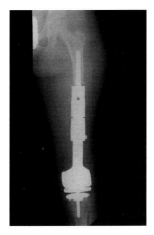

Fig. 3 Expandable endoprosthesis for reconstruction of a growing femur. This prosthesis may be lengthened in small increments to allow for growth of the younger child. (Reproduced with permission from Himelstein BP, Dormans JP: Malignant bone tumors of childhood. Pediatr Clin North Am *1996;43:967–984.)*

tation (Fig. 5). The advantages of this option include the durability of the residual limb, the observation that revision surgery is seldom needed, and the fact that the residual limb continues to grow. Discrepancies in limb length are seldom encountered, and when they do occur, they often can be addressed with prosthetic modification.[30–32] Further, patients who have had rotationplasty walk more efficiently than those with arthrodesis of the knee and those with an above-the-knee amputation.[34] The disadvantages to rotationplasty are the appearance and the need for a prosthesis.

A contraindication to limb-salvage surgery is the inability to obtain adequate wide tissue margins (for example, inability to achieve free vital neurovascular bundles). Wide surgical margins are critically important for survival. In younger children with still rapidly growing bones, the surgeon must consider the potential growth of the opposite extremity when considering limb-sparing surgery. Significant projected limb-length discrepancy is an additional obstacle for limb-sparing surgery in young children in whom tumor resection will require resection of a major growth center of the lower extremity. Athletic or active patients may be hindered with a relatively fragile endoprosthetic reconstruction compared to a rotationplasty reconstruction or an amputation and prosthesis, especially below the knee. For upper extremity lesions, durability is not as much a factor as in the weightbearing lower extremity. Limb-sparing surgery in the upper extremity is almost always preferable to amputation unless the surgeon is unable to achieve wide margins for local tumor control. Inadequate soft-tissue coverage for reconstruction is another relative contraindication to limb-sparing surgery; however, newer plastic surgical reconstructive techniques have helped bridge this obstacle. Pathologic fracture has been reported to be a contraindication to limb-salvage

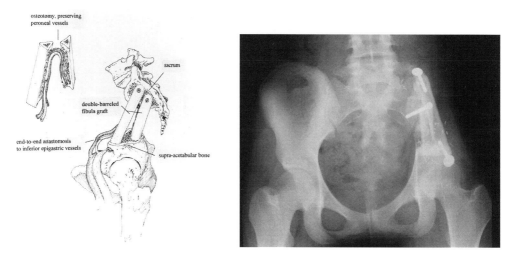

Fig. 4 *Free vascularized fibular autograft reconstruction modified internal hemipelvectomy for Ewing's sarcoma of the pelvis. Technique of double barreled reconstruction (**left**) with postoperative radiographs (**right**).*

surgery. However, with nondisplaced and carefully selected displaced fractures, limb salvage surgery may be an acceptable option, depending on extent of fracture hematoma, response to chemotherapy, and healing rate of the fracture.

Amputation

Although limb-sparing surgery is possible and indicated for most children with extremity sarcomas, amputation is still needed occasionally. Limb sparing is a worthy goal in the treatment of a child with extremity sarcoma; however, the main goal is survival. Limb-salvage surgery should be done only if wide margins are obtainable. It is foolish for the surgeon to risk local recurrence (and subsequent death) in order to do a limb-sparing surgery if a compromise in obtaining adequate margins is required. Further, limb-salvage surgery should be done only if the residual limb will have as much or better function than an amputated limb placed into a well-constructed prosthesis.[34]

Management of children with amputations after sarcoma differs significantly from the management of the traumatic amputee. Unfortunately, intensive treatment for malignant bone tumors may have a significant price for survivors. The child may or may not have been treated with radiation, and secondary osteosarcomas may occur in the radiation field of Ewing's tumors (Fig. 6). Other second malignancies outside of the radiation field, such as acute myelogenous leukemia, may also follow intensive chemotherapy. These cancers arising outside of the radiation field may be attributable to the

**Van Nes rotationplasty for reconstruction
after wide resection of tumor**

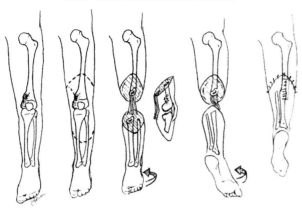

Fig. 5 *van Nes rotationplasty for malignant bone tumors of the distal femur. Following this procedure, with an appropriate prosthesis, the ankle joint serves the function of the removed knee joint.*

use of chemotherapy regimens containing high doses of alkylating agents, such as cyclophosphamide or ifosfamide, or epipodophyllotoxins, such as etoposide.[23] Additionally, rehabilitation may be affected by many other serious late effects of multimodal cancer treatment, including diminished growth, impaired sexual maturation or fertility, and potential cardiac and renal damage from chemotherapy. Many current cancer treatment trials are now being designed to more systematically study and to prevent these devastating late effects.

When amputation is used for malignancy, there is a need to proceed promptly with prosthetic fitting and rehabilitation to improve the likelihood of the child being a functional and successful prosthetic user.[35] The role of immediate postsurgical fitting of these patients is controversial.[36,37] The child with a malignant tumor who has been treated with amputation usually is fitted for a prosthesis during chemotherapy. Weight loss associated with chemotherapy may affect the fit of the prosthesis and also may affect strength and other factors involved with rehabilitation. Because of wide fluctuations in body weight, stump size, and volume, those undergoing chemotherapy often require the use of adjustable temporary sockets for a longer time.[38]

The emotional aspect of dealing with a life-threatening disease is also a factor in interacting with both the child and his or her family. Psychological and physical rehabilitation following surgery for malignant bone tumors is a lifelong process.[39] The ongoing assistance of a team of specialists who routinely deal with children with cancer may ease this burden.

Standard principles of amputation surgery for children apply to those requiring amputation for extremity sarcoma.[37,40,41] Unique problems, however, may require creative approaches to achieve satisfactory results[42] (Fig. 5).

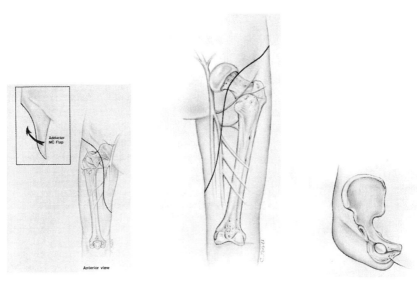

Fig. 6 *Modified adductor myocutaneous flap for wound coverage in a child who required a modified hip disarticulation for radiation-induced osteosarcoma of the femur that occurred years after radiation therapy for Ewing's sarcoma. Anterior **(left)** and posterior **(center)** views showing skin incisions used for modified hip disarticulation; **(right)** after closure. In this case, neither the commonly used posterior flap nor an anterior flap could be used because of the location of the tumor and the presence of radiation-induced skin and soft-tissue changes. The total adductor myocutaneous flap allowed for wide surgical margins and the avoidance of soft-tissue coverage using previously irradiated soft-tissue flaps, and provided excellent coverage without necessitating use of free or pedicle-based flaps. (Reproduced with permission from Dormans JP, Vives M: Wound coverage after modified hip disarticulation using a total adductor myocutaneous flap.* Clin Orthop *1997;335:218–223.)*

Summary

Although limb-sparing surgery is possible and indicated for most children with extremity sarcomas, amputation is still needed occasionally. Children requiring amputation need special attention. The potential for growth and healing are considerations that affect the process of evaluation, surgical management, and rehabilitation. Appropriate care is best undertaken with a multidisciplinary approach to ensure that the best functional outcome is achieved.

Improvements in diagnosis and treatment have increased survival for many children with malignant bone tumors. In the future, new molecular genetic discoveries will provide insights into the mechanisms of tumorigenesis and will provide novel therapeutic modalities for these children.

References

1. Tooms RE: The amputee, in Morrissy RT (ed): *Lovell and Winter's Pediatric Orthopaedics*, ed 3. Philadelphia, PA, JB Lippincott, 1990, vol 2, pp 1023–1070.

2. Heinrich SD, Scarborough MT: Preface to pediatric orthopedic oncology. *Orthop Clin North Am* 1996;27:xiii–xiv.

3. Letson GD, Greenfield GB, Heinrich SD: Evaluation of the child with a bone or soft-tissue neoplasm. *Orthop Clin North Am* 1996;27:431–451.

4. Gebhardt MC: Molecular biology of sarcomas. *Orthop Clin North Am* 1996;27:421–429.

5. Himelstein BP, Dormans JP: Malignant bone tumors of childhood. *Pediatr Clin North Am* 1996;43:967–984.

6. Vander Griend RA: Osteosarcoma and its variants. *Orthop Clin North Am* 1996;27:575–581.

7. Vlasak R, Sim FH: Ewing's sarcoma. *Orthop Clin North Am* 1996;27:591–603.

8. Conrad EU III, Bradford L, Chansky HA: Pediatric soft-tissue sarcomas. *Orthop Clin North Am* 1996;27:655–664.

9. Massengill AD, Seeger LL, Eckardt JJ: The role of plain radiography, computed tomography, and magnetic resonance imaging in sarcoma evaluation. *Hematol Oncol Clin North Am* 1995;9:571–604.

10. Enneking WF: Staging musculoskeletal tumors, in Enneking WF (ed): *Musculoskeletal Tumor Surgery*. New York, NY, Churchill Livingstone, 1983, pp 69–88.

11. Enneking WF: A system of staging musculoskeletal neoplasms, in Bassett FH III (ed): *Instructional Course Lectures XXXVII*. Park Ridge, IL, American Academy of Orthopaedic Surgeons, 1988, pp 3–10.

12. Mankin HJ, Lange TA, Spanier SS: The hazards of biopsy in patients with malignant primary bone and soft-tissue tumors. *J Bone Joint Surg* 1982;64A: 1121–1127.

13. Simon MA: Biopsy of musculoskeletal tumors. *J Bone Joint Surg* 1982;64: 1253–1257.

14. Peabody TD, Simon MA: Making the diagnosis: Keys to a successful biopsy in children with bone and soft-tissue tumors. *Orthop Clin North Am* 1996;27: 453–459.

15. Ayala AG, Ro JY, Fanning CV, Flores JP, Yasko AW: Core needle biopsy and fine-needle aspiration in the diagnosis of bone and soft-tissue lesions. *Hematol Oncol Clin North Am* 1995;9:633–651.

16. Perlman EJ, Dickman PS, Askin FB, Grier HE, Miser JS, Link MP: Ewing's sarcoma: Routine diagnostic utilization of MIC2 analysis. A Pediatric Oncology Group/Children's Cancer Group Intergroup study. *Hum Pathol* 1994;25:304–307.

17. Kruzelock RP, Hansen MF: Molecular genetics and cytogenetics of sarcomas. *Hematol Oncol Clin North Am* 1995;9:513–540.

18. Meyers PA: Malignant bone tumors in children: Osteosarcoma. *Hematol Oncol Clin North Am* 1987;1:655–665.

19. Dahlin DC, Coventry MB, Scanlon PW: Ewing's sarcoma: A critical analysis of 165 cases. *J Bone Joint Surg* 1961;43A:185–192.

20. Link MP, Goorin AM, Miser AW, et al: The effect of adjuvant chemotherapy on relapse free survival in patients with osteosarcoma of the extremity. *N Engl J Med* 1986;314:1600–1606.

21. Picci P, Sangiorgi L, Rougraff BT, Neff JR, Casadei R, Campanacci M: Relationship of chemotherapy-induced necrosis and surgical margins to local recurrence in osteosarcoma. *J Clin Oncol* 1994;12:2699–2705.

22. Frassica FJ, Frassica DA, Pritchard DJ, Schomberg PJ, Wold LE, Sim FH: Ewing sarcoma of the pelvis: Clinico-pathological features and treatment. *J Bone Joint Surg* 1993;75A:1457–1465.

23. Newton WA Jr, Meadows AT, Shimada H, Bunin GR, Vawter GF: Bone sarcomas as second malignant neoplasms following childhood cancer. *Cancer* 1991;67: 193–201.

24. Putnam JB Jr, Roth JA: Prognostic indicators in patients with pulmonary metastases. *Semin Surg Oncol* 1990;6:291–296.

25. Gherlinzoni F, Picci P, Bacci G, Campanacci D: Limb sparing versus amputation in osteosarcoma: Correlation between local control, surgical margins and tumor necrosis. Istituto Rizzoli experience. *Ann Oncol* 1992;3(suppl 2):S23–S27.

26. Rougraff BT, Simon MA, Kneisl JS, Greenberg DB, Mankin HJ: Limb salvage compared with amputation for osteosarcoma of the distal end of the femur: A long-term oncological, functional, and quality-of-life study. *J Bone Joint Surg* 1994;76A:649–656.

27. Eckardt JJ, Eilber FR, Rosen G, Mirra JM, Dorey FH, Ward WG, Kabo JM: Endoprosthetic replacement for stage II B osteosarcoma. *Clin Orthop* 1991;270:202–213.

28. Ward WG, Yang RS, Eckardt JJ: Endoprosthetic bone reconstruction following malignant tumor resection in skeletally immature patients. *Orthop Clin North Am* 1996;27:493–502.

29. Springfield D: Autograft reconstructions. *Orthop Clin North Am* 1996;27:483–492.

30. Kotz R, Salzer M: Rotation-plasty for childhood osteosarcoma of the distal part of the femur. *J Bone Joint Surg* 1982;64A:959–969.

31. Krajbich JI, Carroll NC: Van Nes rotationplasty with segmental limb resection. *Clin Orthop* 1990;256:7–13.

32. Winkelmann WW: Rotationplasty. *Orthop Clin North Am* 1996;27:503–523.

33. McClenaghan BA, Krajbich JI, Pirone AM, Koheil R, Longmuir P: Comparative assessment of gait after limb-salvage procedures. *J Bone Joint Surg* 1989;71A: 1178–1182.

34. Simon MA, Aschliman MA, Thomas N, Mankin HJ: Limb-salvage treatment versus amputation for osteosarcoma of the distal end of the femur. *J Bone Joint Surg* 1986;68A:1331–1337.

35. Aitken GT: Prosthetic fitting following amputation for bone tumor. *ICIB* 1964;3:1.

36. Burgess EM, Romano RL: Immediate postsurgical prosthetic fitting of children and adolescents following lower extremity amputations. *ICIB* 1967;7:1.

37. Herring JA, Cummings DR: The limb deficient-child, in Morrissy RT, Weinstein SL (eds): *Lovell and Winter's Pediatric Orthopaedics,* ed 4. Philadelphia, PA, Lippincott-Raven Publishers, 1996, vol 2, pp 1137–1180.

38. Watts HG, Carideo JF Jr, Marich MS: Variable-volume sockets for above-knee amputees: Managing children following amputation for malignancy. *ICIB* 1982;18:11.

39. Nicholson HS, Mulvihill JJ, Byrne J: Late effects of therapy in adult survivors of osteosarcoma and Ewing's sarcoma. *Med Pediatr Oncol* 1992;20:6–12.

40. Tooms RE: General principles of amputations, in Crenshaw AH (ed): *Campbell's Operative Orthopaedics,* ed 7. St. Louis, MO, CV Mosby, 1987, pp 597–606.

41. Rodriguez RP: Amputation surgery and prostheses. *Orthop Clin North Am* 1996;27:525–539.

42. Dormans JP, Vives M: Wound coverage after modified hip disarticulation using a total adductor myocutaneous flap. *Clin Orthop* 1997;335:218–223.

Consensus

Limb Salvage for Extremity Malignancies

Limb salvage surgery is preferable to amputation when survival is not compromised. This type of surgery requires a wide margin of resection. Upper limb salvage is more important than lower extremity salvage. Contraindications to limb salvage include inability to obtain a wide excision margin, major limb length inequality, a vigorous athletic individual, and poor soft-tissue coverage. Displaced pathologic fracture may also be a contraindication to limb salvage but needs further evaluation in light of current adjuvant treatment modes. In addition, malignant osseous lesions below the upper one third of the tibia may be better treated with amputation rather than with limb salvage. Limb salvage is complex, and complications should be anticipated. Social and cultural factors must also be considered. Management of extremity malignancies, from initial biopsy to definitive treatment, at a specialized center has significant advantages. Adjuvant therapy should not be compromised by the limb salvage procedure.

Use of endoprostheses, rotationplasties, allografts, and other reconstructive techniques may be appropriate when future growth, functional demands, individual preference, and life expectancy are considered. Preoperative education of children and families by meeting with other patients is helpful, and prior planning of the rehabilitation is helpful.

In children, the possibility of malignancy should be considered before surgery for excision of soft-tissue masses.

Section 6
Prosthetic Management of Juvenile Amputees

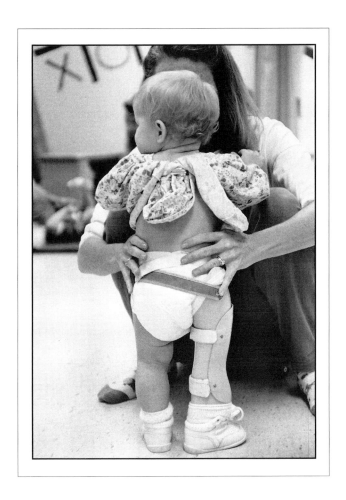

Chapter 26

Prosthetic Considerations for the Child With a Limb Deficiency (Lower Extremity)

Donald R. Cummings, CP

Unique Aspects of Pediatric Prosthetics

Growth and Development

That children with limb deficiencies grow is perhaps the most obvious statement that can be made about them. For the child who needs a prosthesis, this dynamic, ever-changing quality provides the family, the child, and the pediatric clinic team with significant challenges and unique opportunities. Like the child, the pediatric prosthesis is not a miniaturized version of the adult model. Frequently, the treatment plan, prescription, and design of the child's prosthesis have unique criteria, driven by the child's rapid ongoing development.

Growth and surgical planning can often enhance prosthetic outcomes. When the amputation is too long, for example, an epiphysiodesis at the appropriate time in the child's development can improve cosmesis, function, or both. This statement generally pertains to unilateral amputations, but there may be instances when an epiphysiodesis can aid a child with bilateral amputations. For example, a child with bilateral knee disarticulations may spend a great deal of time ambulating without prostheses, or with simple protective "stubby" sockets.[1] In this situation, unequal femoral lengths could be a significant disadvantage.

For an adult, the Syme's amputation generally results in a bulbous distal residual limb approximately 3 to 8 cm shorter than the contralateral limb. This level is usually very functional because of the resulting long lever arm, distal load-bearing tolerance, and excellent suspension. For children, the level offers the additional benefit of preserving epiphyses and avoiding bony overgrowth. In recent years, many versions of "low-profile" Syme's feet, including several dynamic-response versions, have been made available for adults, and a few have been made for children. Yet, there is generally only a small space in which to accommodate the prosthetic foot, the attachment plate, the thickness of the prosthetic socket, and a distal end pad (if any room is left).

Among young children, this challenge is even greater. Occasionally, it becomes necessary to add a shoe lift to the opposite side in order to assure the child's pelvis is level. It is important for the clinic team to monitor the child's growth and, if necessary, an epiphysiodesis should be considered to assure that when the child reaches adulthood there is adequate space for the average Syme's foot.

Knee disarticulation presents a similar challenge. For a child's knee centers to match, about 3 cm of space is required for the lowest-profile, polycentric knee-disarticulation knee. Currently, perhaps a dozen adult knees are specifically designed for the knee disarticulation level. More than 100 knee choices exist for higher levels,[2] but up to 7.5 cm of space is required for the component, attachment plate, and socket thickness. Although it is not essential that a person's knee centers match, epiphysiodesis should be considered if there will not be at least 3 cm of space with normal development. That space is needed for the person using knee disarticulation components to have a satisfactory cosmetic result. Arguably, a goal of 6 to 7 cm of discrepancy by adulthood would offer the person with a knee disarticulation all the functional benefits of the level, with the added advantage of being able to choose most knees on the market, with no discrepancy between knee centers.

When the alignment of the extremity is unsatisfactory, a hemiepiphysiodesis or corrective osteotomy may enhance prosthetic function and the cosmetic appearance of the limb. For example, severe forms of longitudinal deficiency of the fibula are often associated with a marked anterior bow of the tibia, which may require a corrective osteotomy at the time of amputation. Later, genu valgus often develops and may complicate prosthetic fitting or compromise the cosmetic appearance of the finished prosthesis. In such instances, a well-timed hemiepiphysiodesis may be necessary to correct the problem. Again, growth in combination with surgery is used to provide a better final result.

When the amputation is too short, lengthening may improve the prosthetic outcome. Because of the child's young age, exuberant healing processes, and dynamic, motivated nature, limbs that would be considered marginal or too short to be functional for an adult are often preserved following disease or trauma. In cases of a very short transverse congenital deficiency or amputation as a result of amniotic band syndrome, the child may simply present with one or more extremely short residual limbs. In such cases, limb lengthening may be a viable option. Lengthening might be considered when limb function can be converted to the next lower level. A very short transtibial amputation fit as a knee disarticulation, for example, could possibly be converted through lengthening to provide below-knee prosthetic function.

The choice to preserve and lengthen a short residual limb is often difficult and controversial. What is technically possible must be weighed against the risks and the cost to the child and family in resources and lost time during childhood. If a residual limb is to be lengthened, the ultimate result should be a stable, sensate limb with good soft-tissue coverage, free of sharp osteophytes, with adequate muscle strength and range of motion, and of sufficient length to be "fitable."

Growth Management Strategies

When designing a pediatric prosthesis, the prosthetist may choose from a number of growth management strategies.[1] The most basic method of allowing for growth is simply to fit the limb with more (or thicker plies of) prosthetic socks. As the limb grows, the socks can be substituted for thinner ones. Another traditional choice is a "slip" socket, one or more inner layers that are peeled out of the outer socket to accommodate growth.[3] Flexible inner sockets with "windowed" outer frames may be more forgiving over growing bony prominences, and they enable the flexible socket to be heat-modified or replaced with a thinner socket to accommodate growth. The TEC (Total Environmental Control) urethane gel liner seems to provide a comfortable, protective "total surface bearing" interface for active persons with amputations and may hold promise for children with amputations.[4] Suspension systems, such as silicone suction, and neoprene or silicone sleeves, are considered "growth-friendly" because they do not provide a rigid grip over growing bony prominences. Materials and components used in the prosthesis are often modular and adjustable to assist with growth adaptations, such as lengthening of the prosthesis or interchange to a larger foot. They should also be durable enough to withstand the rigors of the child who is generally as active as his or her able-bodied peers.

Patient education and frequent follow-up are just as important as any design feature. The child and family should be taught to look for signs of growth, to adjust socks when necessary, and to recognize the need for a follow-up visit for significant fitting problems. Generally, physician and clinic team follow-up should be every 6 months, and prosthetic adjustments may be required three or four times per year. Even with good follow-up and maintenance, most pediatric prostheses require replacement an average of every 12 to 18 months and then, perhaps, every 1 to 3 years during adolescence.[5]

Most growth adaptations can be combined. For example, a silicone suction socket might be fabricated to include a five-ply prosthetic sock over it. The silicone provides a form of suspension that will continue to work well during normal growth changes, and the number of socks can be reduced to prolong the fit of the socket.[6]

Appositional bone overgrowth, the most common surgical complication among juveniles with acquired amputations, requires some advanced planning during prosthetic design.[7] This complication occurs most frequently in the transected humerus, fibula, tibia, and femur (in that order).[8,9] Particularly for young children or after recent transdiaphyseal amputations, the prosthetist should provide adequate distal padding with provision for modification or replacement of the pad should overgrowth occur. Although a new distal pad, modifications to the socket, or a replacement prosthesis may relieve discomfort temporarily, surgical revision will generally become necessary, particularly when overlying skin begins to erode.[1]

Developmental Readiness

The child's developmental readiness plays a major role in a successful prosthetic prescription.[10] Lower limb prostheses, for example, are generally fit when the child begins to pull up to stand, and upper limb prosthetic fitting usually begins when the child is attempting to sit.[11,12] Components also are prescribed and fit when the child is developmentally ready to use them. For example, an articulated knee is not provided for a child with a transfemoral amputation until age 3 or 4 years when the child is more physically and intellectually ready to learn how to use it.[13]

Appropriate "staging" of the design and complexity of a child's prosthesis requires a very individualized approach. The prescription plan should be based not only on the child's physical and intellectual development, but also on demographic variables, such as the cause and level of amputation, the age at which it occurred, and the child's family and social dynamics.[14] Variances in children's psychologic adjustment to disability also play a major role. Although there is considerable variability in each child's adjustment to his or her disability, as a group, children with congenital or acquired limb deficiencies are considered at risk for psychologic and social adjustment problems.[15] Social support by friends, classmates, teachers, and parents appears to contribute significantly to the extreme variability between coping strategies and psychologic adjustment of children with limb deficiencies.[16]

This whirlwind of influences, combined with the immaturity of the child and his or her propensity for change often presents the clinic team with unique challenges. For example, a child insists he wants a camouflaged leg, but his parents are opposed. Obviously, this must be a family decision, but the child has a unique opportunity to work on his diplomacy, and the parents must grapple with the child's desire for individual expression and with their concerns regarding social implications.

How should the clinic or prosthetist respond when a new "swimming" leg has just been delivered, but the young patient now insists he or she has decided to pursue competitive skateboarding instead? This problem could have been avoided. Although sports prostheses may be important to the child's physical, and emotional well-being, a prescription for a highly specialized device is more likely to be successful when the child has demonstrated a consistent pattern of interest and participation in a certain sport.

What recommendations should be made when children's prostheses need repairs because gravel and sand constantly get in the devices, components are lost or eaten by pets, or a prosthesis is damaged because the child used it for batting practice? First, a distinction must be made between repairs resulting from the normal rigors and immature decisions of childhood and abuse or disrespect of property. Some repairs are unavoidable and simply reflect the child's active use of a prosthesis. Damage caused by intentional misuse of a prosthesis usually results in natural consequences, such as downtime or repair bills, and seldom is repeated.

Challenges Associated With Specific Amputation Levels and Conditions

Syme's Amputation

Whether due to trauma or disease of a normal limb, or for longitudinal deficiency of the fibula, Syme's amputations generally offer excellent prosthetic suspension over the malleoli and ideal rotational control. They provide the child with distal load bearing (in varying degrees) and a long lever arm, and they avoid terminal osseous overgrowth.

Length, a bulbous distal end, and any angular deformity are the greatest challenges. At least 4 cm of space is required to accommodate most "Syme's" prosthetic feet, without having to add a lift to the opposite side. If the space is not available, the prosthetist can resort to custom-made feet, external keel feet, or shoe lifts, but these are compromises. When the amputation occurs during late adolescence, or when both malleoli are present, the distal end may be bulky. Although the prominent malleoli enhance suspension, most suspension strategies, such as an internal pad, expandable inner socket, or removable medial "window," result in a bulky appearance or require visible straps or closures. Because of the long limb length, any angular deformity (varus, valgus, or flexion) will be more visible in the finished prosthesis. If the angular deformity becomes a significant functional or cosmetic problem, a hemiepiphysiodesis or corrective osteotomy should be considered.

When a Syme's amputation has been performed for longitudinal deficiency of the fibula, there often is an associated length discrepancy, which is an advantage in most cases. The extra room provides a broader choice of feet and ankle components, while retaining all the other advantages of the Syme's level. Suspension is generally good, but the absent or deficient fibula generally means the distal end is less bulbous, and occasionally the limb is so cylindrical that suspension must be provided proximally as with a transtibial prosthesis.

The more severe forms of fibular deficiency that most often result in a Syme's amputation are associated with anteromedial bowing of the tibia, a sharp tibial apex with a characteristic skin dimple, valgus deformity (partly due to a hypoplastic lateral femoral condyle), and anteroposterior (AP) knee instability.[17] Migration of the heel pad with a resulting prominent tibial malleolar tip has also been common.[18] Mild anteromedial bowing of the tibia usually does not present a problem and may actually enhance the suspension of the prosthesis. But the sharp tibia, particularly in the area of the characteristic dimple, is frequently problematic. Adequate relief in the prosthesis, padding, and frequent modifications may be necessary to prevent pressure over this area. A valgus deformity, frequently combined with internal rotation and flexion of the knee, may produce gait deviations and poor cosmesis. Often, the prosthetist may be able to accommodate the deformity through alignment and cosmetic finishing techniques, but more severe or progressive cases may require surgical intervention. Significant knee stability usually can be managed through external knee joints and a thigh corset. Finally, even though some degree of distal loading usually is well tolerated in most Syme's prostheses for fibular deficiency, a forgiving, shock-absorbent distal pad should be provided to minimize forces over the relatively small distal surface area.

The Brown procedure (fibular centralization with Syme's amputation), frequently has been performed as a treatment for children with complete longitudinal absence of the tibia. However, most have subsequently required knee disarticulation.[19,20] At best, prosthetic fitting following the Brown procedure is difficult. The child's knee usually is unstable for years, if not indefinitely, requiring limited-motion external joints. Because the absence of a patella and femoral condylar notch preclude anterior transfer of the hamstrings, active knee extension is frequently absent or minimal. Thus, the child frequently ambulates with circumduction or other compensatory patterns.[18] In the rare instance when a child presents with good quadriceps function, the procedure may be effective.[21] For partial deficiency of the tibia in which a tibial plateau is present, fusion of the proximal fibula to the tibia can provide excellent results. In such cases, the prosthesis should still provide early maximal stabilization of the knee joint and fusion site through outside joints and a thigh cuff. These children can be expected to function as well as most with transtibial level amputations.

Transtibial Amputations

The most obvious advantage over higher levels is the presence of a functional knee joint. The most common complication is osseous overgrowth. Some children have developed recurrent patellar dislocation or patella alta, possibly as a result of a valgus deformity.[22] Distal bony overgrowth can be managed for a while with appropriate, adequately soft and modifiable distal pads or, possibly, with silicone or urethane gel liners. Rigid suspension methods that grip over the femoral condyles (ie, supracondylar/suprapatellar suspension) will require more frequent modification and replacement as the femoral condyles grow. These should be provided only if indicated by a short residual limb, mild ligamentous laxity, or other appropriate justification. To minimize stretch on the tendon, deep patellar-tendon-bearing "bars" should be avoided, and principles of total contact support should be practiced. Growth may be accommodated through easily modified liners, layers of socks, and distal pads.

Knee Disarticulation

When compared to transfemoral amputation, knee disarticulation offers the child the potential prosthetic advantages of (1) preservation of the distal femoral epiphysis; (2) avoidance of bone overgrowth; (3) a load-tolerant distal end; (4) a long, powerful femoral lever arm; (5) excellent prosthetic suspension and rotational control via the wide femoral condyles and patella, if present; and (6) lower metabolic cost of walking.[23] It should be noted that these advantages depend primarily on whether or not full end weightbearing capacity is retained.

Although it is generally functionally superior to higher-level amputations and clearly is the transfemoral level of choice for children, the knee disarticulation may be somewhat less cosmetic, and the child may have fewer prosthetic knee options.[24] In recent years, specialized polycentric knees have all but eliminated most of these disadvantages. Moreover, an appropriately timed epiphysiodesis can greatly increase the patient's choice of knees by adulthood.

An important biomechanical distinction exists between the transfemoral amputation and knee disarticulation. Because the transected femur is not very load tolerant, the transfemoral prosthetic socket is designed to distribute weightbearing on load-tolerant pelvic structures, primarily the ischial tuberosity and gluteal musculature. In effect, the center of rotation of the transfemoral socket is at or near the patient's ischial tuberosity. In contrast, the center of rotation of an end-bearing knee disarticulation socket is at the distal end of the socket. During single-limb stance on the prosthetic side, the proximal brim of the knee disarticulation socket tends to press into the soft tissues in the upper medial aspect of the thigh. Thus, careful attention must be paid to this area during socket design.[25] As the child grows up out of the socket, pressures may be increased, and a painful soft-tissue overhang can develop. A wide, gradual radius at the proximal medial brim usually helps spread forces over a larger surface area. At Texas Scottish Rite Hospital, we have had success using flexible sockets with the outer rigid frame lowered in this area. The flexible socket allows the brim to remain high to spread forces over a greater area and to contain soft tissue, and the brim can be modified easily to accommodate growth.

Transfemoral Amputation

The first prosthesis for a toddler with a knee disarticulation or transfemoral amputation is usually fit when the child begins to pull to stand. In most cases, the initial system is nonarticulated or may include a manually locked knee. By 3 or 4 years of age, a child with unilateral transfemoral amputation may be able to adjust to an articulated knee. For the child with bilateral amputations, the transition to articulated knees may not be made until age 5 or 6 years, or in the case of short amputations, much later.[1]

Suspension of the transfemoral prosthesis and growth adjustability are among the greatest challenges to the pediatric prosthetist. Although active adults usually prefer ischial containment suction sockets over other systems,[26] suction suspension may be problematic among children younger than 7 years.[27]

Alternatives to traditional suction suspension include silicone suction. In this method, the child applies a thin silicone liner directly over the residual limb, followed by a sock over the liner. A distal pin or lanyard system attaches the prosthetic socket to the liner. This system provides an intimate yet growth-adjustable fit and enhances rotational control of the prosthesis. Because the liner can be torn, lost, or donned improperly, such methods require a degree of maturity and compliance on the part of the child. Therefore, children younger than 10 years are less likely to do well with suction suspension. The most common methods of suspending a trans-femoral prosthesis for young children are a traditional Silesian belt, or neo-prene alternative such as the TES belt.[28]

Femoral Deficiency

Members of a pediatric limb deficiency clinic are likely to deal with at least four manifestations of femoral deficiency that require prosthetic fitting. An equinus, or extension prosthesis, may be provided when the deficiency results in a significant leg length discrepancy, but surgery either is not indi-cated or is not planned for months or years. For children with bilateral defi-ciencies, surgery generally is not indicated, but equinus prostheses may enable the child to be the same height as his or her peers and to wear normal clothing.[29] Primarily to make wearing clothing more cosmetic and practical, the child's ankle is positioned in comfortable equinus. To reduce the piston action of the unstable hip and to reduce the typical Trendelenburg gait, the prosthetic socket generally includes the child's proximally located knee and provides ischial or gluteal weightbearing. The device is suspended by a heel strap or a waist belt.

Occasionally, Syme's amputation alone may be a realistic management option. It might be considered when the femur is more than 50% of the length of the sound side femur, but lengthening or rotationplasty are not options.[18] The prosthesis is designed and fit as a conventional, albeit long, Syme's prosthesis. Suspension is generally over the malleoli, and in most cases the child is able to bear weight distally. The biggest disadvantage of this approach, most obvious when the child sits, is that the affected knee joint is much more proximal than the opposite knee. Otherwise, these children generally function very well.

Syme's amputation with knee fusion usually is considered when the affected femur is less than 50% of the length of the sound side. This pro-cedure generally eliminates the child's hip flexion contracture and con-verts the limb to a functional transfemoral amputation, with the added advantage, in most cases, of distal end bearing. To diminish pistoning of the unstable hip and to reduce any Trendelenburg lurch, the prosthetic socket should provide some ischial or gluteal weightbearing in addition to distal loading. The prosthesis may be suspended over the malleoli if they are prominent enough, or by a waist belt. The greatest challenge to the prosthetist seems to be the maintenance of proximal weightbearing as the child grows. As soon as the limb grows in length, ischial/gluteal bearing is replaced exclusively by distal end bearing, effectively increasing forces transferred through the hip and increasing the ever-present Trendelenburg lurch. I have had some success prolonging an appropriate amount of prox-imal support by using flexible sockets and frames. The flexible socket allows greater, more comfortable proximal tissue containment, and sup-port can be adjusted by adding material between the inner flexible socket and the outer rigid frame.

The van Nes rotationplasty is the fourth surgical option that will require prosthetic fitting. The goal of this procedure is to convert the foot to a functional below-knee amputation by rotating the foot by 180°. The ankle axis of rotation should end up at about the level of the opposite knee joint center. For optimum prosthetic function, it is critical that the foot be rotated by a full 180°, and that at least a 60° arc of ankle motion is retained.[27,30]

The standard van Nes prosthesis encloses the foot in comfortable equinus, and loads the plantar aspect of the foot and calcaneus. Clearance for the toes and room for growth is provided distally, and a soft, removable socket liner usually is included. The ankle is protected from mediolateral forces by metal joints. If the hip is stable, which is often the case when rotationplasty is used to treat cancer, the joints may be attached to a thigh corset only. Generally, when rotationplasty is performed for femoral deficiency, the hip is still unstable and weak, and the joints may need to extend to a proximal brim that includes ischial/gluteal weightbearing. The prosthesis can be suspended in many cases by a strap over the calcaneus or by a Silesian waist belt.

Summary/Conclusion

In recent years, numerous innovative materials, prosthetic feet, suspension systems, and interfaces have been introduced to the adult market, and many of these products are now available for use by the child with an amputation. Modular components, dynamic-response feet, silicone suspension systems, and specialized urethane or silicone interfaces all offer the patient and the prosthetist more treatment choices. But, as with the adult population, this broad array of choices often creates confusion and uncertainty about which choice is the correct one. The patient's residual limb length, level of overall physical fitness, and age appear to play a more significant role in gait and efficiency than do the specific components used.[31] It is the prosthetist's responsibility to remain abreast of changes and to assist the clinic team and the patient's family in making appropriate prosthetic choices.

References

1. Cummings DR, Kapp SL: Lower-limb pediatric prosthetics: General considerations and philosophy. *J Prosthet Orthot* 1992;4:196–206.

2. Michael JW: Prosthetic knee mechanisms. *Phys Med Rehabil* 1994;8:147–164.

3. Gazely W, Ey M, Sampson W: Use of triple wall sockets for juvenile amputees. *Interclin Info Bull* 1964;4:1–8.

4. TEC Interface Systems: Manual: *Total Environment Control Course*. Waite Park, MN, TEC Interface Systems, 1996, 1–56.

5. Fisk JR: Introduction to the child amputee, in Bowker JH, Michael JW (eds): American Academy of Orthopaedic Surgeons *Atlas of Limb Prosthetics: Surgical, Prosthetic, and Rehabilitation Principles*, ed 2. St. Louis, MO, Mosby-Year Book, 1992, pp 731–734.

6. Fillauer C, Pritham C, Fillauer K: Evolution and development of the silicone suction socket (3S) for below-knee prostheses. *Prosthet Orthot* 1989;1:61–72.

7. Lovett R: Osseous overgrowth in congenital limb-deficient children. *J Assoc Child Prosthet Orthot Clin* 1987;22:26.

8. Aitken G: Overgrowth of the amputation stump. *Interclin Info Bull* 1962;1:1–8.

9. Speer DP: The pathogenesis of amputation stump overgrowth. *Clin Orthop* 1981; 159:294–307.

10. Michael J: Pediatric prosthetics and orthotics. *Phys Occup Ther Pediatr* 1990;10: 123–146.

11. Bochmann D: Prostheses for the limb-dfeficient child, in Kostuik JP, Gillespie R (eds): *Amputation Surgery and Rehabilitation: The Toronto Experience.* New York, NY, Churchill Livingstone, 1981, pp 293–310.

12. Kruger LM: Congenital limb deficiencies: Section II. Lower limb deficiancies, in Bowker JH, Michael JW (eds): American Academy of Orthopaedic Surgeons *Atlas of Limb Prosthetics: Surgical, Prosthetic, and Rehabilitation Principles,* ed 2. St. Louis, MO, Mosby-Year Book, 1992, pp 522–552.

13. Oglesby DG Jr, Tablada C: Prosthetic and orthotic management, in Bowker JH, Michael JW (eds): American Academy of Orthopaedic Surgeons *Atlas of Limb Prosthetics: Surgical, Prosthetic, and Rehabilitation Principles,* ed 2. St. Louis, MO, Mosby-Year Book, 1992, pp 835–838.

14. Novotny M, Swagman A: Caring for children with orthotic/prosthetic needs. *J Prosthet Orthot* 1992;4:191–195.

15. Wallander JL, Varni JW, Babani L, Banis HT, Wilcox KT: Children with chronic physical disorders: Maternal reports of their psychological adjustment. *J Pediatr Psychol* 1988;13:197–212.

16. Varni JW, Setoguchi Y, Rappaport LR, Talbot D: Effects of stress, social support, and self-esteem on depression in children with limb deficiencies. *Arch Phys Med Rehabil* 1991;72:1053–1058.

17. Gibbons PJ, Bradish CF: Fibular hemimelia: A preliminary report on management of the severe abnormality. *J Pediatr Orthop* 1996;5B:20–26.

18. Herring JA, Cummings DR: The limb-deficient child, in Morrissy RT, Weinstein SL (eds): *Lovell and Winter's Pediatric Orthopaedics,* ed 4. Philadelphia, PA, Lippincott-Raven, 1996, vol 2, pp 1137–1180.

19. Loder RT, Herring JA: Fibular transfer for congenital absence of the tibia: A reassessment. *J Pediatr Orthop* 1987;7:8–13.

20. Pattinson RC, Fixsen JA: Management and outcome in tibial dysplasia. *J Bone Joint Surg* 1992;74B:893–896.

21. Christini D, Jumar SJ: Fibular transfer in tibial hemimelia: A follow-up study. *J Assoc Child Prosthet Orthot Clin* 1981;26:8.

22. Mowery CA, Herring JA, Jackson D: Dislocated patella associated with below-knee amputation in adolescent patients. *J Pediatr Orthop* 1986;6:299–301.

23. Pinzur MS: Knee disarticulation, in Bowker JH, Michael JW (eds): American Academy of Orthopaedic Surgeons *Atlas of Limb Prosthetics: Surgical, Prosthetic, and Rehabilitation Principles,* ed 2. St. Louis, MO, Mosby-Year Book, 1992, pp 479–486.

24. Michael JW: Prosthetic management, in Bowker JH, Michael JW (eds): American Academy of Orthopaedic Surgeons *Atlas of Limb Prosthetics: Surgical, Prosthetic, and Rehabilitation Principles,* ed 2. St. Louis, MO, Mosby-Year Book, 1992, pp 487–500.

25. Hughes J: Biomechanics of the through-knee prosthesis. *Prosthet Orthot Int* 1983; 7:96–99.

26. Schuch CM: Modern above-knee fitting practice: A report on the ISPO Workshop on Above-Knee Fitting and Alignment Techniques May 15-19, 1987, Miami, USA. *Prosthet Orthot Int* 1988;12:77–90.

27. Thompson GH, Leimkuehler JP: Prosthetic management, in Kalamchi A (ed): *Congenital Lower Limb Deficiencies*. New York, NY, Springer-Verlag, 1989, pp 211–235.

28. Schuch CM: Transfemoral amputation: Prosthetic management, in Bowker JH, Michael JW (eds): American Academy of Orthopaedic Surgeons *Atlas of Limb Prosthetics: Surgical, Prosthetic, and Rehabilitation Principles*, ed 2. St. Louis, MO, Mosby-Year Book, 1992, pp 509–533.

29. Krajbich I: Proximal femoral focal deficiency, in Kalamchi A (ed): *Congenital Lower Limb Deficiencies*. New York, NY, Springer-Verlag, 1989, pp 108–127.

30. Krajbich JI, Bochmann D: Van Nes rotation-plasty in tumor surgery, in Bowker JH, Michael JW (eds): American Academy of Orthopaedic Surgeons *Atlas of Limb Prosthetics: Surgical, Prosthetic, and Rehabilitation Principles*, ed 2. St. Louis, MO, Mosby-Year Book, 1992, pp 885–899.

31. Gailey RS, Wenger MA, Raya M, et al: Energy expenditure of trans-tibial amputees during ambulation at self-selected pace. *Prosthet Orthop Int* 1994;18:84–91.

Chapter 27

Physical Therapy Management in Children With Lower Extremity Limb Deficiencies

Colleen Coulter-O'Berry, MS, PT, PCS

The role of physical therapy is obvious in the management of children with acquired lower extremity limb loss. This role is less clear in the child with congenital limb deficiencies. Traditional physical therapy skills are acutely needed and medically necessary for the child with traumatic limb loss to restore function to the presurgical/pretrauma level. In children with congenital limb deficiency, age-appropriate activities are developed by incorporating the deficiency into all functional movements. Because motor and cognitive skills are developed despite limb deficiency, learning to move with the deficiency is "normal" for the child. Regardless of the degree of the deficiency, the size, shape, flexibility, and strength of the deficient limb provide the sensory and motor input, which guides the child's motor development. The physical therapist working with children with congenital limb deficiencies and their families should be knowledgeable in all areas of gross motor, fine motor, and cognitive development, and be able to anticipate functional abilities of children with varied degrees of limb loss. In addition, a working knowledge of pediatric prosthetic and surgical options available for the different limb deficiencies is imperative. The physical therapist's role as a primary provider of treatment in the acute situation changes to that of advocate, teacher, and mentor, anticipating immediate and future needs of the children and their families. In most centers, it is the physical therapist who sees the child frequently and acts as a liaison between the physician, prosthetist, and other team members. In his/her role as teacher, the physical therapist empowers the parents to be the primary providers of therapy. Home programs are vital for the success of anticipated surgical and/or prosthetic options. The frequency of physical therapy visits is determined by multiple factors, such as the degree of limb involvement, flexibility, strength, associated neuromuscular concerns, the child's acquisition of age-appropriate developmental functions, the family's ability to follow through with a home program, and family travel distance. Videotaped therapy sessions are excellent teaching tools. Polaroid photos of therapy personalize and complement the home program. Commercially available exercise manuals for infants and children also help create excellent home therapy programs.[1,2]

One of the main goals of physical therapy is to make children with congenital limb deficiency comfortable with the surgical, prosthetic, and therapeutic decisions made by the family and the limb deficiency team. The child and the family must be prepared for future physical challenges. Maximizing a child's function within the degree of limb involvement is another important goal of physical therapy. Components of physical therapy include range of motion, strengthening, gait training, wound and skin care, edema management, and age-appropriate functional activities.

Developmental Considerations

Studies of the effectiveness of early physical therapy for the neurologically deficient and/or developmentally delayed infant and toddler are not specifically applicable to the child with limb deficiency. Assumptions can be made that would support early physical therapy intervention for a child born with a limb deficiency. According to the American Physical Therapy Association,[3] early intervention is based on seven important concepts. The rapid growth and development in the first years of life provides the foundation for later development. Infants can actively interact and form attachments, and they are capable of learning. Parents are the main providers of nurture and of early learning experiences. Parents of children with special needs may require assistance or instructions to fulfill the above role. The interaction between the biologic insult and environmental factors is a determinant of developmental outcome. Finally, "structured programming can improve the abilities of infants and children."[3] Moreover, early intervention with physical therapy is based on the following assumptions: "(1) nervous system plasticity exists; (2) young children are sensorimotor learners; (3) acquisition of motor skills is a major component of early development; (4) intervention must be started early to provide optimal outcome and prevent the development of secondary disability; and (5) family-centered services provide for maximal intervention."[3]

The child with congenital limb deficiency will benefit greatly from early intervention. Well informed and involved parents have a greater acceptance and understanding of their child's immediate and future surgical, prosthetic, and therapy needs. With positive parental input, the child is more likely to become a successful prosthetic wearer.

The following considerations should be made when developing therapy goals and home programs: (1) every child is unique and develops at his/her own rate; (2) the child with multilimb loss has special needs, and treatment interventions must be prioritized. The environment also needs to be adapted to the child to maximize function; (3) the child with a limb deficiency may have associated neurologic, medical, or orthopaedic disorders that will influence function and intervention; (4) surgical amputations and revisions may take place at any given developmental age; and (5) if an acquired amputation occurs, treatment should center on age-appropriate function (unpublished data, 1995). Exercise programs should be set up with the parents and child, when appropriate. Goals need to be age-appropriate and within limits

Table 1 Physical therapy strategies for a 6- to 9-month-old child with class C femoral deficiency and longitudinal incomplete deficiency of the fibula

Developmental Activities	Pregait/Gait Components	Physical Therapy Interventions
Prop sitting on both upper extremities.	Trunk extension down to pelvis in sitting.	Range of motion to hip, knee, and foot.
Sitting without support.	Shifting over pelvis in prone.	Instruct home progress for hip internal rotation, adduction, and extension.
Beginning to come up and down to sit.	Rolling over each hip to come up and down from sit.	Range of motion to the foot to prevent fixed contractures. Full plantarflexion desired for unconventional prosthetic fitting.
Playing in side sit.*	Gluteus maximus contract with extreme external rotation of femurs.	Home instruction to encourage coming up to sit and rolling over deficient side.
Reach with one arm.	Concentric and eccentric extension of trunk in prone.	Increases weightbearing through proximal joints and lengthens side that tends to be short.
Commando crawl.	Bouncing adds proprioceptive input to gluteals and quadriceps. Uses feet for stability.	Weightbearing activities for foot on deficient side.
Bouncing in supported stand.	Plantar flexion of ankle and toes.	Evaluate for prosthesis if beginning to pull to stand.
Into and out of sidelying.	Push off surface in prone, pivoting, and supported stand. In sidelying, the bottom hip against surface is in more extension, internal rotation, and adduction (late phase of swing).	

* Both legs turned in the same direction

of the degree of limb deficiency. Reference should be made to the biomechanical components necessary for a child to achieve an activity. Table 1 summarizes an example of a program for a specific level and degree of limb deficiency at different ages. Note the identification of age-appropriate functions and the biomechanics required to achieve function in a nonneurologically impaired child.[4–8] The therapist then creates goals that are appropriate within the limits of the deficiency. This same principle can be applied to all degrees of limb deficiency at any given age. Prosthetic interventions will also influence the treatment goals.

Physical Therapy Treatment

Birth to 12 Months
Referral to a Limb Deficiency Center should be made at the time a child with a limb deficiency is born.[9–12] The parents and family meet with the

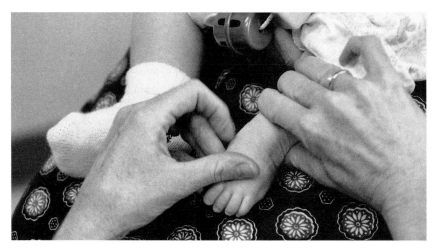

Fig. 1 *A mother learns range-of-motion exercises that will maintain the flexibility of the foot needed for optimal prosthetic fitting.*

physician and team members to identify the child's strengths and briefly outline possible future surgical, prosthetic, and therapeutic strategies that address the child's physical limitations. This is the time when a bond between the physical therapist and family should begin. Physical therapy intervention should focus on helping the child to achieve motor and cognitive milestones in context with the physical limitations. Evaluation of gross and fine motor development is necessary to establish baseline records of the infant's range of motion, strength, neurologic function, and symmetry and balance of movement patterns and to anticipate how the limb deficiency will affect the infant's development. Introducing the family to other families who have children with similar limitations is one of the most important interventions.[10] The impact of family networking is lasting and can help put to rest some of the parents' fears and concerns for their child's future. Dolls, samples of prostheses (similar to their child's first one), and photos of children in prostheses are also useful teaching tools for parents. The therapist needs to monitor the amount of information given to parents. Not every parent and family is ready for all available information at the first visit. Sensitivity to the parent's needs is imperative. Too much information can increase the parent's anxiety and fears for their child's future by focusing on the disability rather than ability.

Range-of-motion exercises (Fig. 1) are designed to minimize the development of contractures and prepare the extremity for future prosthetic fit and function. With certain levels of limb deficiency, characteristic contractures and deformities are present. Tibial and fibular deficiencies can cause foot deformities. A deformed foot can affect prosthetic and orthotic management as well as hinder gross motor development. For example, a contracted foot may rule out the future option of a rotationplasty in the infant with a congenital femoral deficiency or affect the results of future limb lengthening in an infant with fibular deficiency. The parents should be instructed in range-of-motion exercises early on. Knee flexion contractures are anticipated in an infant with a complete congenital transtibial amputation. As the infant grows, the length and mass of the extremity decrease. The foot is not present to act as an anchor for stability. Extension exercises for the hip and knee are necessary because the development of extension is limited. Prosthetic fittings as early as 6 months of age have been used to manage knee flexion stiffness in infants with unilateral below-knee limb loss (unpublished data, 1995). The benefits of early fittings are threefold. First, flexion contractures are minimized. Second, symmetric bipedal weightbearing can be achieved for early standing activities, such as during standing play while supported by a parent and in bouncer-type seats and walkers. Third, the infant receives early sensory and proprioceptive feedback, which truly prepares him/her for his/her definitive prosthesis. An added benefit is that parents are involved early in the management of their child's care (Fig. 2).

Hip flexion, abduction, and external rotation contractures are anticipated in infants with femoral deficiency or congenital complete transfemoral amputation.[13] Again, instruction is given in range-of-motion exercises, and early prosthetic fitting can be considered if the loss is unilateral.[2] Most infants with congenital femoral deficiency have marked knee instability. Maintaining mobility of the hips, knees, and ankles can be taught during simple caregiving activities, such as diapering, picking up the baby, dressing, feeding, and play.[9,10] Parents are encouraged to roll their babies to both sides and not to be afraid of further deformity. Helping the baby come up and down from sitting, kneeling, and standing on both sides is taught. Symmetric and balanced movements to both sides during early motor activities are precursors to weight shifting in standing, cruising, and ambulation[13] (unpublished data, 1995). Prosthetic fitting is recommended once the infant has pulled to stand, typically around 8 to 12 months of age.[9,13,14] The infant who has multilimb deficiencies in conjunction with neurologic and medical involvement may take longer to acquire motor skills. Monthly monitoring is recommended to update home programs and to record changes in range of motion, strength, and development.[13]

12 to 24 Months

By the first year, the child should be pulling to stand and wearing a definitive prosthesis. The therapist and prosthetist work closely on prosthetic fit and function. Instructions are given for putting on and removing the limb, monitoring the skin, and developing a schedule for wearing the prosthesis. It is not unusual for infants and toddlers, especially toddlers with congenital transfemoral loss or femoral deficiency, to reject their prosthesis because, in some cases, they are more mobile without it and can engage freely in motor activities. The initial prosthesis of an infant

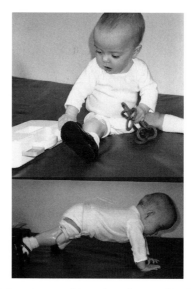

Fig. 2 *An 11-month-old infant, born at 24 weeks, who was fitted with a prosthesis at 8 months of age because of a congenital short transtibial amputation with considerable knee flexor tightness and asymmetry to all of her movements. The prosthesis acts as an anchor to assist in movement over the involved extremity and in age-appropriate weight-bearing activities. This prosthesis does not allow knee flexion and assists in managing the flexion contracture. It is used as an adjunct to treatment.*

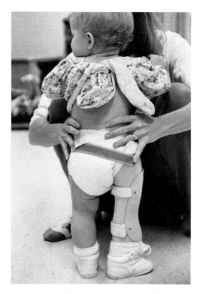

Fig. 3 *Weight shifting exercises being demonstrated in a 12-month-old infant with proximal femoral focal deficiency.*

with femoral deficiency does not have a prosthetic knee joint because of hip and knee instability and the excessive length needed to incorporate the foot inside the prosthesis.[7] The toddlers must come to sit, creep, pull to stand, cruise, and walk with a stiff knee, which will cause them to become frustrated easily. Parents need to understand the goals of the prosthesis and be supportive through this challenging time. Therapy focuses on age-appropriate upright activities.

A therapy program at this stage should stress symmetry of posture and movement and control of weight shifting over the prosthesis[13] (Fig. 3). Developmental screenings and assessment tools make excellent treatment guidelines and can assist in forming home programs.[1,2,4–7] Exercises should be fun and incorporated into a toddler's everyday play. Push toys and walkers are adjuncts to treatment. Most toddlers with single limb deficiencies do not require assistive devices, but the child with multilimb involvement may. Adaptations may be necessary to assist these toddlers in ambulation. Surgical intervention may be necessary at this age to correct deformities or perform a primary amputation. Therapy then focuses on wound healing, edema control, range of motion, and functional muscle strength to regain motor skills.

Toddler and Preschool Years

As the child masters ambulation with the prosthesis, treatment again focuses on age-appropriate activities. Toddlers with limb deficiencies should be given the same opportunities as other children. If the child is in preschool, possible activities are marching to music, climbing on tumbling equipment, riding a tricycle, and gymnastic programs. The physical therapist can educate the parents on programs appropriate for their child. Home exercise programs still include range of motion to prevent the progression of contractures. The frequency of therapy visits depends on the child's mastery of ambulation and the family's ability to follow through with the exercise program. The physical therapist can monitor a child's development during clinic visits every 4 months.[9] The prosthesis should be closely monitored for fit as the child grows. Physical therapy can be undertaken at the child's preschool and is an effective means of educating the child's teachers, classmates, and other families. The school staff is less apprehensive about having a child with special needs if they are well informed and taught strategies on managing the prosthesis and adapting the environment as needed. Toilet training is a major obstacle for a child with a lower limb prosthesis. Therapy can address this issue as well as dressing at home and at school. Surgical interventions may be introduced at this age. Following each surgical intervention, wound healing, range of motion, and functional strengthening exercises are instructed. The child may require additional physical therapy postoperatively until independent ambulation is restored.

Elementary Years

As children grow, they may receive technologically advanced prosthetic components, which may require additional gait training and balance exer-

Outline 1 Lower extremity functional outcomes in children with lower extremity deficiencies

Unilateral Syme's
No limitations in daily activities.
Able to participate in age-appropriate activities, sports, bicycle, ski, dance, gymnastics.
No assistive devices.

Unilateral Below Knee (Transtibial)
No limitations in age-appropriate daily activities.
Able to participate in sports, bicycle, ski, dance, gymnastics.
No assistive devices.

Bilateral Below-Knee (Transtibial)
Slight limitation to uneven surfaces, curbs, stairs.
Participates in age-appropriate sports with limitations.
May require adapted physical education.
Rides bicycle with adaptations.
No assistive devices.

Unilateral Above-Knee (Knee Disarticulation or Transfemoral)
No limitations to age-appropriate daily activities.
Requires adaptation to bicycle; may ride without prosthesis.
Able to participate in sports; adaptations may be required.
No assistive devices.

Bilateral Above-Knee (Knee Disarticulation or Transfemoral)
Some limitations to uneven surfaces, curbs, kneeling, stairs.
Difficulty riding bicycle; needs adaptations.
Adapted physical education.
Wheelchair sports.
Limited in sports and age-appropriate activities.
May use cane or loftstrands; most do not.

Unilateral Hip Disarticulation–Hemipelvectomy
Limitations on uneven surfaces, curbs, steps. Children with congenital deficiencies are
  quite functional; children with acquired loss have more difficulties.
Bicycle is difficult with prosthesis; may ride without prosthesis.
Limited in running and sports; requires adaptations to sports.
Wheelchair sports.
May use cane in community, school, mall.
May use crutches and no prosthesis.

Bilateral Hip Disarticulation
Wheelchair is used for primary mobility. Power mobility may be necessary if associated
  upper extremity involvement.
Prosthetic use for standing and exercise; requires assistive devices.
Wheelchair sports.

cises. At this age, amputations secondary to trauma or bone tumors are more prevalent.[9,15] Children with congenital limb deficiencies may undergo surgical revision for overgrowth or to correct deformities. Rotationplasty may be a surgical option for the child with congenital femoral deficiency. With each surgical intervention comes a period of adjustment and retraining. Edema is controlled with bandages and shrinkers. Preprosthetic range of motion and

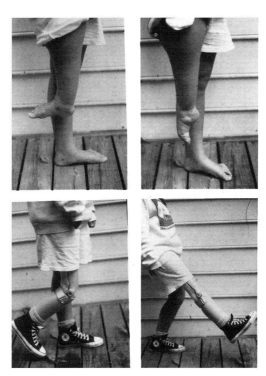

Fig. 4 *Functional relationship between the ankle and prosthetic knee in a 13-year-old girl with a rotationplasty to manage her femoral deficiency. Ankle dorsiflexion produces prosthetic knee flexion. Ankle plantarflexion produces prosthetic knee extension.*

strengthening are necessary. Gait training should begin with use of the parallel bars with weight shifts in all directions, progressing to ambulation on level surfaces with or without assistive devices, leading to functional activities. School visits by the therapist are a helpful way of acquainting the child's teachers and class with a new prosthesis.[10,13] By age 7, the child's gait pattern resembles that of an adult.[9,13] The child is able to participate actively in an exercise program and is becoming less dependent on the parents. Again, exercises focus on age-appropriate activities, sports, and recreation. Outline 1 gives examples of recreational achievements based on the accomplishments of children in the Limb Deficiency Program at Scottish Rite Children's Medical Center in Atlanta, Georgia. Although not comprehensive, this outline provides therapists and families with functional outcomes and expectations for their child within the limits of the limb deficiency.

Preadolescence and Adolescence
Malignant bone tumors are most common in preadolescents and adolescents. Children and their families are faced with surgical options for limb salvage, amputation, or rotationplasty depending on the size, location, and character-

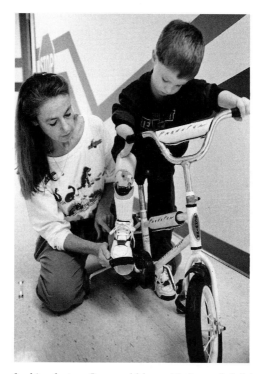

Fig. 5 *Adaptation of a bicycle to a 5-year-old boy with femoral deficiency following a Syme's amputation.*

istics of the tumor as well as the child's activity levels and cultural, psychological, and family issues. The physical therapist plays a vital role in educating the child and family as to the functional outcomes of each surgical procedure. The child who undergoes a limb salvage procedure faces numerous physical challenges. Goals of physical therapy include: (1) regaining mobility and strength; (2) progressive weightbearing; (3) improving cardiovascular endurance; (4) pain management; (5) scar mobility; and (6) independence in transfers, activities of daily living, and age-appropriate activities. Each limb salvage procedure is unique, and therapy must be under the close supervision of the orthopaedic surgeon. Usually these children receive chemotherapy, which can delay healing and rehabilitation. Amputation offers a child immediate postoperative fitting when appropriate. Activities are limited only by the child's level of limb loss. Prosthetic technology has helped these children to function with greater stability and balance. Edema control, wound healing, range of motion, strengthening, and balance exercises are necessary to move, power, and control a prosthesis.

Preteens and teenagers with congenital limb deficiency may undergo definitive surgical reconstructions to correct deformities in less than functional limbs. Most choose surgery, and improving function and cosmesis are determining factors. Surgery for overgrowth is common. It is frequently at this age that limb lengthening is begun in those with short tibiae or femorae. Physical therapy for children undergoing limb lengthening is extensive. Goals are maintaining range of motion, strengthening, weightbearing, and adequate pin care. These children should be kept as active as possible, going to school and participating in recreational activities as permitted. The child who receives a rotationplasty has unique challenges ahead. Training the foot to act as a knee in a new anatomic position requires creativity on the part of the therapist and child to develop exercises for sensory motor reeducation. Biofeedback and electrical stimulation are extremely useful modalities. Exercises are necessary at speeds, excursions, and strengths common to knee function using the foot's anatomy in the opposite orientation (Fig. 4). Phantom limb sensation is common in teenagers with acquired limb loss[13] but is less frequent in teens with congenital limb deficiencies following reconstructions or ablations. Phantom limb pain typically does not interfere with function.

Learning to drive a car is a common desire of all teenagers. The physical therapist should be knowledgeable of local resources to address age-appropriate issues such as this, which become more apparent as the adolescent goes to college and becomes independent. All children should be encouraged to participate in recreational and sport activities (Chapters 29-31). Limitations and adaptations will depend on their level of deficiency.[10]

The Child With Multilimb Loss

Children with congenital or acquired multilimb loss have special needs. They may require more intensive and regular therapy visits and are delayed in the acquisition of gross motor milestones. Special mobility aids, wheelchairs, and adaptations to the environment may be necessary. Prioritization of surgical, prosthetic, and therapeutic interventions is required in order to meet the child's and family's goals. It is important not to overburden the child with all new prostheses at the same time (Fig. 5).

Summary

Each infant, child, and adolescent is different and has expectations and goals unique for his/her needs. Age-appropriate functional activities that meet the child's and family's goals should guide the physical therapy treatments. Treatments should be fun and meaningful for the child. The therapist is a teacher, facilitator, and advocate for the child in all settings.

References

1. Jaeger L, Ascher G, Atlee J (eds): *Home Program Instruction Sheets for Infants and Young Children,* ed 3. Tucson, AZ, Therapy Skill Builders, 1987.

2. Diamant RB (ed): *Positioning For Play: Home Activities for Parents of Young Children.* Tucson, AZ, Therapy Skill Builders, 1992.

3. American Physical Therapy Association: Competencies for physical therapy in early intervention. *Ped Phys Ther* 1991;9:1–23.

4. Bayley N (ed): *Bayley Scales of Infant Development.* New York, NY, Psychological Corporation, 1969.

5. Folio MR, Fewell RR (eds): *Peabody Developmental Motor Scales* (revised experimental edition). Nashville, TN, George Peabody College for Teachers, 1974.

6. Frankenburg WK, Dodds JB, Fandal AW (eds): *Denver Developmental Screening Test: Manual* (revised 1970 edition). Denver, CO, University of Colorado Medical Center, 1970.

7. Furuno S, O'Reilly K, Hoska C, et al: *Hawaii Early Learning Profile (HELP): Activity Guide.* Palo Alto, CA, Vort Corporation, 1979.

8. Gesell A, Halverson HM, Amatruda CS (eds): *The First Five Years of Life: A Guide to the Study of the Preschool Child From the Yale Clinic of Child Development.* New York, NY, Harper & Brothers, 1940.

9. Tooms RE: The amputee, in Lovell WW, Winter RB (eds): *Pediatric Orthopaedics,* ed 2. Philadelphia, PA, JB Lippincott, 1986, vol 2, pp 979–1030.

10. Gillespie R: Principles of amputation surgery in children with longitudinal deficiencies of the femur. *Clin Orthop* 1990;256:29–38.

11. American Academy of Orthopaedic Surgeons: *Atlas of Limb Prosthetics: Surgical and Prosthetic Principles.* St. Louis, MO, CV Mosby, 1981.

12. Krebs DE, Fishman S: Characteristics of the child amputee population. *J Pediatr Orthop* 1984;4:89–95.

13. Stanger M: Limb deficiencies and amputations, in Campbell SK, Palisano RJ, Vander Linden DW (eds): *Physical Therapy for Children.* Philadelphia, PA, WB Saunders, 1994, pp 325–351.

14. Krebs DE, Edelstein JE, Thornby MA: Prosthetic management of children with limb deficiencies. *Phys Ther* 1991;71:920–934.

15. Kalamchi A (ed): *Congenital Lower Limb Deficiencies.* New York, NY, Springer-Verlag, 1989.

Chapter 28

Gait Analysis of the Child With a Lower Limb Deficiency

James A. Harder, BSc, MD, FRCSC

The Development of Normal Human Gait

The Gait Cycle

"The gait cycle" is a term used to describe a process of human movement.[1,2] It is measured by a multitude of methods, including clinical observation, force measurements (kinetics), video measurements (kinematics), and energy consumption. To understand the literature, it is important to understand the terminology used to describe gait. Therefore, I will begin by defining some commonly used words and phrases and will then proceed to a brief overview of the normal gait cycle.

Definitions

Stance phase is the portion of the gait cycle that begins with heel strike and ends with toe-off. It occupies approximately 60% of the gait cycle. The subdivisions of stance phase are initial contact, loading response, midstance, terminal stance, and preswing.[2] Swing phase is the portion that begins with toe-off and ends with heel strike. It occupies approximately 40% of the gait cycle. The subdivisions of the swing phase are initial swing, midswing, and terminal swing. The double-limb support phase is the part of the stance phase in which both feet are touching the ground. It occurs at heel strike and at toe-off. Each double-limb support phase occupies approximately one sixth of the stance phase at comforatble walking speed. Isolated single-limb stance is therefore 40% of the gait cycle (60% minus the 20% for double-limb support) at comfortable walking speed for the mature gait pattern. During running, there is no double-limb support phase. The single-limb support phase is the part of the stance phase in which only one foot is touching the ground.

A step is the distance between the two limbs contacting the floor; ie, the distance between the left foot at toe-off and the right foot at heel strike. A stride is the distance between the points where the same limb contacts the floor. Therefore, two steps equal one stride or one complete gait cycle of heel strike to toe-off equals one stride. Cadence is the number of steps per minute, and walking velocity is the distance traveled per minute. The passenger unit consists of the upper torso of the human body, and the locomotor unit consists of the pelvis and legs.

Concentric muscle contraction is the shortening of the muscle while performing work. An example would be the psoas muscle flexing or accelerating the thigh into flexion. Eccentric muscle contraction occurs when a muscle performs work while resisting elongation. An example would be the hamstrings decelerating the thigh in swing phase. In isometric muscle contraction, the muscle resists load with little or no change in length.

The first rocker is the period of the stance phase from heel strike to foot flat. The dorsiflexors contract eccentrically as the foot plantarflexes to touch the floor. The second rocker is the period during foot flat in which the tibia moves forward on the ankle joint. The gastrocnemius-soleus contracts eccentrically. The third rocker is the period from foot flat to toe-off. The gastrocnemius-soleus contracts concentrically. During midstance the knee is in 18° of flexion, and it gradually extends in terminal stance in the knee flexion wave.

The Development of Normal Gait

It is clear that normal gait is established by 5 to 7 years of age.[3] Independent sitting is present at 6 months of age, progressing to crawling at 9 months, and walking by 12 to 15 months. Sutherland and associates[3] have described the five important determinants of mature gait. These are the duration of single-limb stance, walking velocity, cadence, step length, and the ratio of pelvic span to ankle spread.

In the normal adult gait cycle, single-limb stance occupies 40% of the stance phase. Sutherland and associates[3] showed that single-limb stance was 32% at age 1 year (early walking), progressing to 38% at 7 years. Swing phase, however, remained relatively constant at 40%, indicating that there was an increased double-limb support portion of stance phase.

Walking velocity increases significantly from 1 to 3 fi years of age and then increases at a steady but gradual rate to just under 120 cm/s by age 7 years. Cadence gradually decreases with age to become stable at 7 years. Step length increases rapidly until 2 fi years of age and then slowly increases with growth and increase in leg length. The ratio of pelvic span to ankle spread increases from 1 to 7 years of age, indicating that the broad-based gait of early childhood gradually diminishes as balance improves and muscular strength increases.

The most significant determinants of gait are walking velocity, ratio of pelvic span to ankle spread, duration of single-limb stance, and cadence. Reciprocal arm swing, heel strike, and joint ranges of motion reach adult parameters very early and are not clear discriminators of the presence of an immature gait pattern. The persistence of knee flexion (or the absence of a mature knee-flexion wave) throughout the stance phase of the young child may be a function of inadequate plantarflexor power. The persistence of the knee-flexion wave has significant implications in limb deficient gait. The absence of heel strike and reciprocal arm swing by age 2 years would be considered abnormal as would the persistence of a broad-based gait by age 3 years. A number of other gross motor milestones need to be remembered when assessing the gait of children. By age 2 years, 90% of children should be able to walk on their toes; by age 3 years, they should be able to stand on one leg; by age 4 years, 90% of children are able to walk on their heels; and by age 5 years, 92% are able to hop on one leg.

The Center of Gravity and the Ground Reaction Force

The center of gravity of the passenger unit is located just anterior to the tenth thoracic vertebra and scribes a sinusoidal path in two planes during the gait cycle. It moves within a box about 2 cm high and about 4 cm wide, with the highest point at midstance and its low point at double-limb support phase.[2]

The ground reaction force passes through the center of gravity of the passenger unit. The magnitude and direction of lower limb stability are defined by the alignment of the ground reaction force to the joint centers of the lower limb. When the hip joint is in full extension, it is stabilized by the anterior hip capsule, and when the knee joint is in full extension, it is stabilized by the posterior knee capsule.

To maintain static standing ability (ie, minimal muscle forces acting and, therefore, minimal expenditure of energy), the ground reaction force must pass posterior to the hip joint and anterior to the knee joint. An extension force at the hip keeps the anterior hip capsule tight, and an extension force at the knee joint keeps the posterior knee capsule tight. No muscle action is necessary to maintain this position. There is no static stability at the ankle and foot. The ground reaction force passes just anterior to the ankle joint; therefore, a constant low level of muscle activity in the lower leg and foot is necessary to maintain static standing balance. During walking, early stance, midstance, and terminal stance, static stability does not exist and strong muscle action is necessary to keep from falling.

Walking is therefore a process of continuous forward falling and forward momentum, which is controlled and modified by muscle action about the lower limbs. Most efficient walking occurs when the center of gravity is minimally displaced from the line of progression. Additional energy is used to move the center of gravity from side to side and up and down outside the boundaries of the 2 × 4 cm box. The center of gravity is at its lowest point during the two periods of double-limb support and at its highest point in midstance.

Energy Expenditure in Normal and Limb Deficient Gait

Normal walking is a very efficient process that strives to expend the least amount of energy. The typical energy expended in normal gait is 2.5 kg-cal (10.5 kJ) per minute. Any deviation of gait from the norm will result in an increase in this value. A person with a below-knee amputation will walk using 60% more energy, while one with an above-knee amputation will walk using 100% more energy than normal at comfortable walking speed. Walking with crutches requires 300% more energy than normal walking.[1,4,5] The following terms need to be understood in order to better understand energy consumption with walking.[2] Oxygen rate is the amount of oxygen consumed over time (ml/kg•min), and oxygen cost is the amount of oxygen consumed over distance traveled (ml/kg•m). Oxygen rate at all traumatic amputation levels (below-knee, above-knee, hemipelvectomy, hip disarticulation) approximates normal because of decreased comfortable walking speed.

Movement consumes energy, which in the initial stages comes from aerobic metabolism. A simple, clinically useful method of measuring energy expenditure during gait has been to record the steady-state heart rate. A direct relationship has been shown to exist between steady-state heart rate and energy expenditure.[5] As the intensity of exercise increases, anaerobic metabolism is added to produce the required amount of ATP to sustain the activity. Exercise that requires only aerobic energy can be sustained for prolonged periods without exhaustion. With increase in exercise intensity and the addition of anaerobic metabolism, however, there is the associated development of acidosis. It is the intolerance to this acidosis that results in the development of exhaustion.

The respiratory exchange ratio (RER), the ratio of carbon dioxide production to oxygen consumption during exercise, is a simple method of quantifying this concept. For example, sustained strenuous exercise resulting in an RER greater than 0.90 indicates anaerobic activity. An RER greater than 1.00 indicates severe exercise. It has been shown that it is more efficient to walk with a prosthesis than to use crutches.[1] Higher levels of amputation, therefore, result in ever decreasing walking speeds to maintain energy expenditure within the aerobic category (RER less than 0.90) and thus maintain endurance.

Energy expended by walking is reduced by minimizing the excursion of the center of gravity, by controlling momentum (ie, the speed and direction of body movement), and by active transfer of energy between limb segments. The center of gravity excursion in a child with an amputation or a limb deficiency will be minimized by a well-fitted prosthesis. Control over momentum will be maximized by good residual limb muscle strength and control. Transfer of energy between segments of the lower limb prosthesis is not the same as energy transfer in a normal limb. It was initially hoped that energy storing terminal devices would act as an energy store, but this has not proven to be true at a comfortable walking speed. Energy can be stored in such devices at higher speed,[6,7] but energy release almost immediately follows energy storage, which may not be at the most appropriate time in the gait cycle. Double-limb support time is higher on the prosthetic side as the result of a lack of energy supplied by the plantarflexors during terminal stance and push off. Because the energy storing terminal devices are loaded with energy during midstance, this energy will be released as one uncontrolled boost almost immediately thereafter.

Studies by Engsberg and associates[8] indicate that the nonprosthetic limb is the dominant limb. More energy is expended by the amputee to walk at the comfortable walking speed of able-bodied individuals. The energy expended by the amputee during more strenuous activities, such as running, is even higher than that expended by an able-bodied individual. Concentrated exercise programs directed at specifically strengthening the residual limb may reduce the total energy levels expended for normal walking and for strenuous activities by improving control over momentum and allowing more efficient transfer of energy to the remaining normal distal segments. This concept of strengthening the residual limb is particularly important for amputees who wish to participate in sports in which they are competing with their able-bodied peers because it will decrease their total energy expenditure and increase their endurance.[4]

Methods of Evaluating Gait

Gait can be evaluated by observation, by force plate (kinetic) studies, by video recording (kinematic) studies, and by oxygen consumption studies. Observing someone walk is of utmost importance when dealing with conditions of the musculoskeletal system. I look for balance and symmetry of arm swing, stance, and swing throughout the phases of gait. Any observed deviation from the normal pattern may be described as a gait abnormality or gait deviation. Causes of gait deviations are multifactorial. I will limit my analysis to some of the gait deviations found in the child with a limb deficiency.

Common Gait Deviations

Common gait deviations found in patients who walk with a prosthetic limb are described below. Possible causes for the gait deviations are divided according to whether they are due to the prosthesis or the patient with an amputation.

Abducted gait is characterized by a wide base, with the prosthesis held away from the midline. The causes for this deviation are prosthetic based: (1) the prosthesis may be too long; (2) too much abduction may have been built into the prosthesis; (3) a high medial wall may cause the amputee to hold the prosthesis away to avoid inferior pubic ramus pressure; (4) an improperly shaped lateral wall of the socket can fail to provide adequate support for the femur, thereby resulting in the pelvis dropping on the opposite side; and (5) the pelvic band may be positioned too far away from the patient's body.

Circumducted gait, a swinging of the prosthesis laterally in a wide arc during swing phase, may be caused by a prosthesis that is too long or a prosthesis that has too much knee friction, limiting knee flexion in swing phase. It also may result from the patient having an abduction contracture of the residual limb, the patient lacking confidence to flex the prosthetic knee because of muscle weakness or fear of stubbing the toe and falling, or it may be a habit pattern.

Lateral bending of the trunk is characterized by excessive bending laterally from the midline, generally to the prosthetic side. Causes related to the prosthesis are (1) the prosthesis may be too short; (2) an improperly shaped lateral wall may fail to provide adequate support for the femur; (3) a high medial wall may cause the amputee to lean away to minimize discomfort; and (4) a prosthesis aligned in abduction may cause a wide-based gait. Patient-related causes include inadequate balance, an abduction contracture, or an overly sensitive and painful residual limb. A very short residual limb may fail to provide a sufficient lever arm for the pelvis. Finally, the defect may be due to a habit pattern.

Trunk forward flexion may result from the socket being in too much flexion, the knee being placed too far posteriorly, or a suspension belt that is too tight. Patient-related possible causes include (1) a hip flexion contracture; (2) poor balance and coordination; (3) weak hip extensors; (4) pain on the ischial seat area of the socket; and (5) degenerative spinal disease, which is painful in extension.

Excessive lumbar lordosis may be caused by a prosthesis that is too heavy, has knee friction that is too loose, or does not have enough flexion built into the socket (preflexion); or it may result from a hip flexion contracture in the patient.

Medial or lateral whip is observed best when the patient walks away from the observor. A medial whip is present when the heel travels medially on initial knee flexion at the beginning of swing phase; a lateral whip exists when the heel moves laterally or away from the midline on initial swing. There are several prosthesis-based causes. Lateral whips may result from excessive internal rotation of the prosthetic knee effectively turning the heel outward. A medial whip may result from excessive external rotation of the knee effectively turning the heel inward. The socket may fit too tightly, and the residual limb may be rotating (femoral anteversion = lateral whip; femoral retroversion = medial whip). Excessive valgus in the prosthetic knee may contribute to this defect, and a badly aligned toe-break may cause twisting on toe-off. The only patient-based cause is faulty walking habits.

Rotation of the prosthetic foot on heel strike has three prosthesis-based causes and two patient-based causes. There may be too much resistance to plantarflexion by the plantarflexion bumper or heel wedge of the prosthesis, too much toe out may have been built into the prosthesis, or the socket may be fitting too loosely. The patient may extend the limb too vigorously at heel strike or may have poor muscle control of the residual limb.

Instability of the prosthetic knee creates a danger of falling when the knee joint is too far ahead of the ground reaction force line causing the knee joint to collapse easily, when insufficient initial flexion has been built into the socket, and when resistance to plantarflexion at the ankle is too great, causing the knee to buckle at heel strike. In addition, failure to limit dorsiflexion can lead to incomplete knee control. There also are two patient-related possibilities: the patient may have hip extensor weakness, and severe hip flexion contracture may cause an inability to fully extend the knee at heel strike.

Drop-off at the end of stance phase is a downward movement of the trunk as the body moves forward over the prosthesis. Prosthesis-based possible causes include excessive dorsiflexion of the prosthetic foot, a too-short keel in a SACH-type foot or a conventional foot toe break that is too far posterior, or a socket placed too far anterior in relation to the foot. The patient may have a knee or hip flexion contracture that cannot be accommodated by a prosthesis. This situation results in a relative apparent shortening of the prosthetic side.

Uneven heel rise is characterized by the prosthetic heel rising quite markedly and rapidly when the knee is flexed at the beginning of swing phase. This occurs if the prosthetic knee joint has insufficient friction or there is an inadequate knee extension aid, or if the patient is using more power than necessary to force the knee into flexion.

Terminal swing impact is characterized by rapid forward movement of the shin piece, allowing the knee to reach maximum extension with too much force before heel strike. This defect may be caused by insufficient knee friction in the prosthesis or knee extension that is too strong. It also may result from the patient trying to assure himself or herself that the knee is in full extension by deliberately and forcibly extending the residual limb.

Inability to initiate the prosthetic knee may be caused by an overly stable knee unit (ie, friction turned up too high), a knee unit that is too far posterior, a knee joint that is too low, or a prosthetic foot that is too large. Other causes may be lack of coordination and decreased proprioception on the part of the patient.

Vaulting is characterized by a rising on the toe of the normal foot, permitting the amputee to swing the prosthesis through with little knee flexion. This may occur because the prosthesis is too long, there is inadequate socket suspension, or there is excessive stability in the alignment or some limitation of knee flexion, such as a knee lock or a strong extension aid. In the patient, possible causes are residual limb discomfort, fear of stubbing the toe, and habit.

Uneven arm swing is characterized by the arm on the prosthetic side being held close to the body during locomotion. An improperly fitting socket may cause residual limb discomfort, resulting in this defect. The patient may not have developed good balance. In addition, fear and insecurity accompanied by uneven timing will contribute to this defect, or the defect may be due to a habit pattern.

Uneven timing is characterized by steps of unequal duration, usually by a very short stance phase on the prosthetic side. Prosthetic causes are (1) an improperly fitting socket may cause pain and a desire to shorten the stance phase on the prosthetic side; (2) a weak extension aid or insufficient friction in the prosthetic knee can cause excessive heel rise and thus result in uneven timing because of a prolonged swing-through phase of gait; and (3) alignment stability with the knee too anterior may be a factor if the knee buckles too easily. Patient causes may include a weak residual limb, lack of development of good balance, and fear and insecurity.

Foot slap is a too rapid descent of the anterior portion of the prosthetic foot. It occurs when plantarflexion resistance in the prosthesis is too soft or the patient is driving the prosthesis into the walking surface too forcibly to assure extension of the knee.

Kinetics and Kinematics of Gait

Kinetics

The kinetics of gait describes the forces generated by the foot striking the ground during stance phase. The forces can be in the mediolateral, the antero-posterior, and the vertical plane. Forces usually are recorded from a force plate, which is built into the walkway and camouflaged. The patient walks along the runway and when the foot contacts the force plate, transducers record the data. The forces are measured on the Y axis and the progression of the gait cycle or time is measured on the X axis (Fig. 1). Time zero on the left is at heel strike. On the vertical force-time curve, the force is zero but quickly climbs to the first peak at midstance. The opposite limb swinging through at this time unloads the plate slightly, resulting in the valley. The forces increase again at late terminal stance to form the second peak, and then rapidly decrease to zero after toe-off. The value of the peaks are approximately 110% of body weight at a walking speed of 82 m/min. The valley is approximately 80% of body weight when measured at the same speed.

Forces generated in the anteroposterior and mediolateral planes are small compared to the vertical forces. The mediolateral forces are less than 10% of body weight and occur at midstance and terminal stance. The anteroposterior shear is less than 25% of body weight and occurs at heel strike and again at push off.[1]

Prosthetic gait will result in vertical forces that resemble the normal curve, except that the first peak will be higher than normal if the terminal device is unable to absorb the forces at heel strike.[2] The second peak will be reduced in magnitude because of the lack of push-off forces in late terminal stance.[9] Figure 2 illustrates the able-bodied gait pattern and the below-knee prosthesis pattern for the prosthetic and nonprosthetic legs. The nonprosthetic leg is vertically loaded at a greater rate than the able-bodied leg (slope of 13.4 versus 11; Table 1). The nonprosthetic leg demonstrates greater loading than the able-bodied leg ($Zmax1 = 1.51$ versus 1.28). The nonprosthetic leg has a greater stance phase or time of support than the prosthetic leg. The forces measured are related to a walking speed of 72 m/min. As the pace slows, the peak forces will diminish and the valley will disappear. In contrast, when running, there will be only one peak, which may be as high as 2.5 times body weight[1] (Fig. 3).

Kinematics

The Ankle Joint

The total range of motion necessary at the ankle joint during walking is 30°.[2] The ankle joint travels through four arcs of motion during one gait cycle (Fig. 4). Plantarflexion occurs just after heel strike (first rocker) followed by dorsiflexion through midstance to terminal stance (second rocker). Plantarflexion occurs at push off associated with strong gastrocnemius-soleus muscle contraction. The ankle remains in approximately neutral position during swing phase. The dorsiflexor muscles act primarily during swing phase. The plantarflexor muscles act primarily during stance phase. Absence of the lower leg and foot will affect gait at push off when strong concentric contraction is required by the plantarflexor muscles.

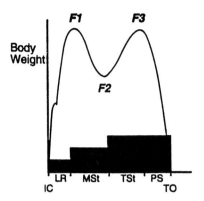

Fig. 1 *Time gait cycle. (Reproduced with permission from Perry J:* Gait Analysis: Normal and Pathological Function. *Thorofare, NJ, SLACK, 1992, p 417.*

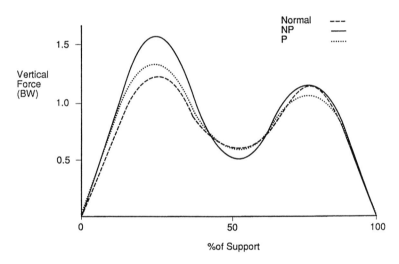

Fig. 2 *Gait patterns. (Reproduced with permission from Engsberg JR, Lee AG, Tedford KG, Harder JA: Normative ground reaction force data for able-bodied and below-knee-amputee children during walking.* J Pediatr Orthop *1993;13:171.)*

The Knee Joint

With normal walking, knee motion represents flexion from 0 to 70° (Fig. 5). This range varies with walking speed. Following almost full extension at heel strike, the knee joint begins to flex during the loading response phase of early stance. Flexion is complete with the onset of single-limb support at approximately 18° and, at this time, the knee joint is under maximum weightbearing load. More extension is obtained while passing further through midstance dur-

Table 1 Means (standard deviation) for vertical force-time variables for able-bodied, nonprosthetic, and prosthetic limbs of children during walking

Variable*	Leg		
	Able-bodied n = 450	Nonprosthetic n = 22	Prosthetic n = 22
ZImp1 BW† ratim	0.22 (0.04)	0.28† (0.07)	0.25†§ (0.07)
ZMax1 BW	1.28 (0.17)	1.51† (0.35)	1.37†§ (0.40)
ZT1 ratim	0.24 (0.04)	0.28† (0.03)	0.26† (0.03)
Slope BW/ratim	11.0 (3.6)	13.4† (6.1)	12.0 (4.9)
ZImp2 BW† ratim	0.23 (0.05)	0.23 (0.07)	0.21† (0.06)
ZMax2 BW	1.19 (0.13)	1.24† (0.30)	1.10†§ (0.28)
ZT2 ratim	0.31 (0.04)	0.30 (0.03)	0.29 (0.03)
Zmin BW	0.63 (0.13)	0.60 (0.22)	0.66 (0.23)
ZImp To BW† ratim	0.45 (0.05)	0.51† (0.11)	0.46§ (0.12)
To Time ratim	0.55 (0.04)	0.58† (0.09)	0.55§ (0.06)
DubSup ratim	0.10 (0.04)	0.13† (0.08)	0.13† (0.08)

* Ratim, ratio of total support time; ZImp1, area under vertical force–time curve from touchdown to local minimum; Zmax1, first local maximum on vertical force–time curve; ZT1, time from touchdown to ZMin; slope, slope of line from touchdown to Zmax1; ZImp2, area under vertical force–time curve from local minimum to takeoff; Zmax2, second local maximum on vertical force–time curve; ZT2, time from Zmin to takeoff; Zmin, local minimum on vertical force-time curve; ZImp To, total area under vertical force-time curve; To Time, ratio of support time for given leg to total support time; DubSup, double support time
† Significantly different from AB ($p < 0.05$)
§ Significantly different from NP ($p < 0.05$)
(Adapted with permission from Engsberg JR, Lee AG, Tedford KG, Harder JA: Normative ground reaction force data for able-bodied and below-knee-amputee children during walking. *J Pediatr Orthop* 1993;13:169–173.)

ing the second rocker. This flexion to extension is known as "the knee-flexion wave" and is a part of the mature gait pattern. The amount of knee flexion present during the knee-flexion wave will increase with increasing speed.

Progressive knee extension occurs during the later half of midstance, only to begin flexion again in the terminal stance and preswing phases of stance. The knee joint is flexed to 40° by the end of preswing as load transfer to the opposite limb takes place. Knee flexion takes place rapidly from this point on and progresses to the maximum of 60° during swing phase.

The quadriceps muscles are the dominant muscle group acting at the knee during support, beginning to act during terminal swing and reaching maximum intensity early in the loading response phase when the force vector is posterior to the knee joint. The most intense action of the hamstring muscles is during late terminal swing when they act as decelerators of the leg and stabilizers of the hip and thigh.

The Hip

The hip joint goes through a total of 40° of motion during the gait cycle2 (Fig. 6). Taking the static standing position as neutral, the hip joint arc is 10°

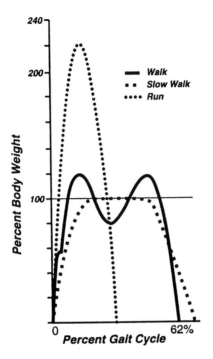

Fig. 3 *Gait cycle. (Reproduced with permission from Perry J:* Gait Analysis: Normal and Pathological Function. *Thorofare, NJ, SLACK, 1992, p 418.)*

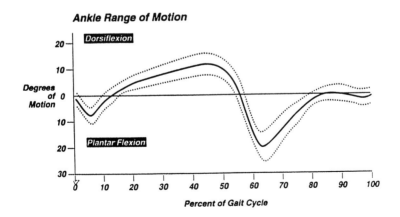

Fig. 4 *Ankle range of motion. (Reproduced with permission from Perry J:* Gait Analysis: Normal and Pathological Function. *Thorofare, NJ, SLACK, 1992, p 53.)*

341

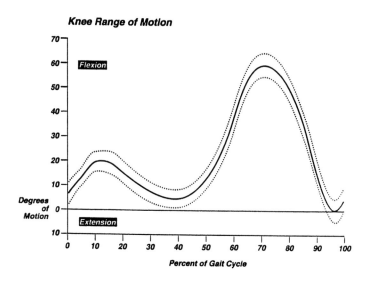

Fig. 5 *Knee range of motion. (Reproduced with permission from Perry J:* Gait Analysis: Normal and Pathological Function. *Thorofare, NJ, SLACK, 1992, p 91.)*

of extension and 30° of flexion. At heel strike, the thigh is flexed 30°. The force vector is anterior to the hip joint. At midstance, the hip progressively extends to reach the neutral position at 38% of stance phase (ie, just before the second double-limb support time). The force vector now passes behind the hip joint and the thigh reaches 10° of extension as the opposite foot contacts the floor (ie, the beginning of double-limb support). During preswing, the hip begins the flexion arc, flexing quickly and having completed flexion to 30° by midswing.

The hip extensor muscles are most active in the mid to terminal swing part of the gait cycle (approaching heel strike), diminishing their activity in midstance as the thigh reaches the neutral position and passes into extension. The ipsilateral hip abductors are very active beginning at terminal swing and increasing their activity through midstance, thus stabilizing the pelvis. The hip joint flexors must come into action in preswing, diminishing their action by midstance. A poorly fitting thigh socket will allow loss of purchase on the residual limb thigh, allowing the pelvis on the opposite side to descend. The patient will try to prevent this by leaning toward the prosthetic side, keeping the ground reaction force over the hip joint.

Prosthetic Gait in Review

Prosthetic gait is asymmetric.[8] The degree of asymmetry is related directly to the level of the deficiency. The more proximal the loss, the more asymmetric the gait pattern will be. Loss of significant muscle groups, such as the

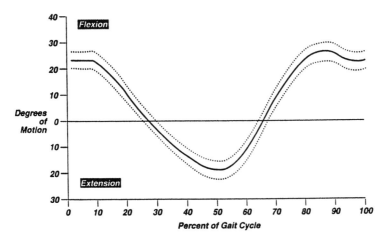

Fig. 6 Hip range of motion. (Reproduced with permission from Perry J: Gait Analysis: Normal and Pathological Function. *Thorofare, NJ, SLACK, 1992, p 113.)*

plantarflexors and dorsiflexors of the ankle, will seriously alter midstance, terminal stance, and push off. Engsberg and associates[8] make four observations that characterize the gait variations of the below-knee amputee: (1) Double-limb support time is longer on the prosthetic side. Stance phase is longer on the nonprosthetic side than on the prosthetic side. (2) Limb loading on the nonprosthetic side is significantly higher than on the prosthetic side (approximately equivalent to one fourth body weight). (3) Limb loading on the nonprosthetic limb is significantly higher than on the lower limbs of able-bodied subjects. (4) The nonprosthetic limb is dominant and accepts greater propulsive and retarding forces during the gait cycle.

Describing the gait of the above-knee amputee, Boonstra and associates[10] indicate that (1) The comfortable walking speed of above-knee amputees is reduced. (2) Swing phase time is longer on the prosthetic side than on the nonprosthetic side. (3) Energy consumption is 40% higher than in able-bodied subjects. (4) There is no clear relationship between socket design and energy expenditure.

There has been much concern about the fate of the nonprosthetic limb after years of prosthetic wear.[11] Kinetic studies have indicated that the non-amputated leg had a greater rate of loading and a greater load than the amputated side, and indeed greater than a normal limb in an able-bodied individual.[8,11] Combined kinetic and kinematic data show that there is increased stance time and a longer step length on the nonamputated side.[11] However, Lewallen and associates[12] found that the joint moments on the nonamputated side were made normal or below normal by slowing the walking speed. The step length was decreased and the double-limb support time was increased. Even though there appears to be an increase in the incidence of osteoarthritis in the nonprosthetic side, the literature has not yet shown a

343

direct relationship. Powers and associates[9] tested various terminal devices and found that peak loading forces on the nonamputated side varied with the amount of dorsiflexion available in the terminal device at terminal stance. The SACH foot showed the greatest peak loading on the nonamputated side, although the difference was not statistically significant.

Much work still remains to clearly demonstrate the gait characteristics of the person with an amputation. Age, general health, fitness, and activity level play a significant part in determining the loading characteristics of able-bodied subjects as well as of those with limb deficiencies. As the deficiencies of amputee gait are clearly defined, innovative thinking applied to modern technologies will improve prosthetic design and prosthetic devices to better "normalize" the gait and function of the child with a limb deficiency.

References

1. Gage JR, Deluca PA, Renshaw TS: Gait analysis: Principles and applications. Emphasis on its use in cerebral palsy. *J Bone Joint Surg* 1995;77A:1607–1623.

2. Perry J (ed): *Gait Analysis: Normal and Pathological Function.* Thorofare, NJ, SLACK, 1992.

3. Sutherland DH, Olshen R, Cooper L, Woo SL: The development of mature gait. *J Bone Joint Surg* 1980;62A:336–353.

4. Crouse SF, Lessard CS, Rhodes J, Lowe RC: Oxygen consumption and cardiac response of short-leg and long-leg prosthetic ambulation in a patient with bilateral above-knee amputation: Comparisons with able-bodied men. *Arch Phys Med Rehabil* 1990;71:313–317.

5. ACME Artificial Limb Co. Limited Pamphlet: *Gait Analysis*, Toronto, Ontario, ACME Artificial Limb Co.

6. Schneider K, Hart T, Zernicke RF, Setoguchi Y, Oppenheim W: Dynamics of below-knee child amputee gait: SACH foot versus flex foot. *J Biomech* 1993;26:1191–1204.

7. Gitter A, Czerniecki JM, DeGroot DM: Biomechanical analysis of the influence of prosthetic feet on below-knee amputee walking. *Am J Phys Med Rehabil* 1991;70:142–148.

8. Engsberg JR, Lee AG, Tedford KG, Harder JA: Normative ground reaction force data for able-bodied and below-knee-amputee children during walking. *J Pediatr Orthop* 1993;13:169–173.

9. Powers CM, Torburn L, Perry J, Ayyappa E: Influence of prosthetic foot design on sound limb loading in adults with unilateral below-knee amputations. *Arch Phys Med Rehabil* 1994;75:825–829.

10. Boonstra AM, Schrama J, Fidler V, Eisma WH: The gait of unilateral transfemoral amputees. *Scand J Rehabil Med* 1994;26:217–223.

11. Lemaire ED, Fisher FR: Osteoarthritis and elderly amputee gait. *Arch Phys Med Rehabil* 1994;75:1094–1099.

12. Lewallen R, Dyck G, Quanbury A, Ross K, Letts M: Gait kinematics in below-knee child amputees: A force plate analysis. *J Pediatr Orthop* 1986;6:291–298.

Chapter 29

Aspects of Sports and Recreation for the Child With a Limb Deficiency

Todd F. Anderson, CP, BS

Sports, Recreation, and the Child With a Limb Deficiency

In the 1930s, textbooks on recreation viewed it as a form of human activity that had no extrinsic purpose and was engaged in only for its own sake. Then, more and more public and private institutions began to sponsor leisure programs and the viewpoint grew that such programs could contribute significantly to society. Recreation was beginning to be viewed somewhat differently: not as an activity but as an emotional experience or condition. Gray and Greben offered this definition:

> "Recreation is an emotional condition within an individual human being that flows from a feeling of well-being and self-satisfaction. It is characterized by feelings of mastery, achievement, exhilaration, acceptance, success, personal worth, and pleasure. It reinforces a positive self-image. Recreation is a response to aesthetic experience, achievement of personal goals, or positive feedback from others. It is independent of activity, leisure, or social acceptance."[1]

Stein, in his doctoral thesis on the physically handicapped, concluded that recreation is, thus, an end product; ie, what happens to a person as a result of an activity, rather than the activity itself.[1]

Recreation can thus be defined as an activity, experience, or emotional condition brought about by an individual as a result of engaging in leisure pursuits within a framework of personal motivation and expectation.[1] It can involve a wide variety of topics. Research on enjoyment or optimal experience found "that whenever people enjoy what they are doing, they report very similar experiential states. The same dimensions are reported in the context of enjoying chess, climbing mountains, playing with babies, reading a book, or writing a poem. These dimensions are the same for young and old, male and female, American or Japanese, rich or poor."[2]

These benefits also apply to children, especially those with limb deficiencies. Research provides evidence that leisure activities benefit children in many ways. A variety of play situations is essential to maintaining optimal mental health throughout life. Numerous researchers have found that involvement in therapeutic recreation improves coping behavior of individuals with a disability. Activities include art, journal writing, day dreaming, meditation, and travel, as well as hiking, camping, and adapted sports.[3] The benefits of leisure activities are especially important for the psychological, social, and physical well being of the child with a limb deficiency.

A child's psyche can be very fragile and children's self-concepts often are determined by their reflection of how peers perceive them. Friends will often hold a child in higher regard if they are able to participate in leisure activities together. The skills that are developed through discretionary activity, leisure, and personal avocations build confidence, self-esteem, mental health, and feelings of success. Active leisure participation throughout life correlates positively with high satisfaction and happiness, and lack of opportunity results in decreased psychological well-being.[4] The benefits of regular physical activities include improved cardiopulmonary function, lowered blood pressure, increased bone mineral content, increased muscle strength and joint flexibility, and improved psychological well being.[5] A review of literature on leisure and mental health reveals that virtually all play situations provide ample testimony to the fact that once the game starts, social distinctions disappear and the status of the participants is determined by their ability to play the game.[6] This feeling of acceptance by friends is extremely important to the development of a healthy, psychologically balanced child.

The social need for leisure has been identified as an important component in the quality of life of individual citizens, particularly if their full involvement in society is limited by a disability. Recreation responds to their right to accessibility and full community participation.[7] Reports show that handicapped children who were integrated into a normal educational program showed higher scores on social play measures than those in segregated settings.[8] Youths involved in athletics tend to stay in school longer and complete their education.[9] Through integration into various leisure activities, the child with a limb deficiency develops a sense of familiarity and trust. Recreation can also serve to overcome feelings of isolation. Lack of familiarity leads to contempt and mistrust; thus, there is a need for social interaction through recreation services.[10]

Physical development of the body is enhanced through leisure activities. The undeniable benefits of physical activity are widely studied and published. Long-term physical exercise programs, that is regular swimming and gymnastic activities, were effective in reducing asthmatic symptoms, frequency of hospitalization, and use of medication for children between 5 and 14 years of age.[11] It has also been found that exercise reduced depression among individuals with physical disabilities.[12] Tennis[13] and water exercise[14] effectively reduced depression in the same population.

The ability to participate in leisure activities without regard to their limb deficiency can give children opportunities to develop psychologically, socially, and physically, regardless of the chosen leisure experience. All children deserve the opportunity to participate in their chosen recreational and athletic pursuits. Through sports and recreation, children with limb deficiencies can demonstrate competence and self-confidence that will transfer to other aspects of their lives.

The Prosthetist's Role

The prosthetist plays an important role in providing the opportunities for children to choose their leisure pursuits without being limited by a prosthetic device. Currently, health-care professionals, as well as the general public, view amputation and limb deficiency as a product of failure. Often an amputation is performed as "the last alternative" because a salvage or revascularization procedure failed. Even those who are familiar with prosthetics project nonverbal messages that the patient's life has taken an even more unfortunate turn. The same messages of catastrophic misfortune also cloud the family of the child. Practitioners need to be aware that this phenomenon can greatly affect the patient's or parents' outlook on the rest of their life.

Unfortunately, these old attitudes about life saving or last resort procedures still exist today. Although the amputation truly may be life saving and a final procedure, this is often communicated in a remorseful manner. A patient or family may become engulfed with feelings of remorse and guilt, which are very difficult to overcome. These feelings may lower the person's self-esteem, which in turn results in lowered expectations by the care givers. Health-care providers need to understand and believe that in most cases an amputation is the procedure that allows the patient to begin the rehabilitation process. From that point forward, in most cases, the patient can feel confident that he or she can build a successful future.

A survey of leading ABC (American Board for Certification in Orthotics and Prosthetics) prosthetists reveals methods and philosophies that are practiced when fitting patients involved in sports and recreation. The consensus opinion of this group is that before proceeding with fabrication, the practitioner must carefully interview the patient to find out what types of activities he or she really is interested in. The prosthetist should evaluate the fit of the current prosthesis. If the patient is not very active, the problem may be the components of the prosthesis. The prosthetist's evaluation should be objective and a full functional evaluation should be performed.

Next, it is important for the prosthetist to evaluate the patient's sports activity in detail, and often in the field if possible. This evaluation may require leaving the office to witness and videotape the activity in order to gain full familiarity. It is critical that the practitioner accompany the extremely active patient for a field trial. A field trial is to an athlete what dynamic alignment is to the average patient. At this point, the determination should be made of whether an "every day," "dual use," or "special design" prosthesis would be adequate for the patient's intended use. Economic and financial issues should not be overlooked during this discussion.

If it is determined that a new prosthetic design is warranted, several criteria need to be carefully considered. The biomechanical demand of the specific activity needs to be evaluated. What demands will be made on the prosthesis? Consulting with the engineering staff at the component manufacturer's facility can be quite enlightening. The short- and long-term durability of the components also must be considered. A minor failure during a recreational experience can be psychologically catastrophic to a child.

Comfort is another major consideration. Will a specially designed, shear force reducing interface become necessary to reduce skin breakdown? The weight, age, and level of performance of the patient are all variables that will affect the equation and the results of the practitioner's decision.

Once the practitioner has made a short list of component and design ideas, it is time to get the patient involved in the final decision-making process. Consumers today are very knowledgeable and can make significant contributions. A patient who is included feels a greater sense of ownership in his or her own care, and inclusion often results in greater effort toward reaching goals.

Striving to meet recreational goals often means an increase in activity. The active child with a limb deficiency not only has to deal with growth and physiological changes brought on by activity, but also with the additional trauma of torques and stresses far beyond normal to the skin and bone structure of the residual limb.[15] The active child also tests the limits of prosthetic design and fabrication. Because many components are computer designed to match each patient based on height, weight, activity level, and residual limb length, a change in any of these factors can affect the appropriateness or functional outcome of the prosthesis. Four areas of common problems are encountered as patients become more active: socket fit, skin trauma, stress on componentry, and multiple accessory replacements.

Socket fit is of the utmost importance to the active person with a prosthesis. An ABC certified prosthetist will make sure the initial socket fits properly. This can be done through the use of clear thermoplastic check sockets that not only help the prosthetist further customize the fit, but also help the patient understand how the prosthesis should fit. However, the residual limb of an active child is in a state of constant change due to growth, weight change, or muscle development. Although there are many strategies to accommodate these changes, there is really no way to maintain a truly intimately fitting socket in a child. Regardless of how well a prosthesis fits, there is a potential for skin breakdown of the residual limb due to overactivity.[15] Therefore, it is important that the practitioner maintain consistent regular follow-up with these patients. It is also a good idea to teach patients how to perform minor temporary adjustments or methods of dealing with skin breakdown.

Skin is the body's first line of defense against breakdown, and blisters, abrasions, pressure sores, or bruises can adversely affect the outcomes for the active amputee. Protection from damaging pressure can be provided by the use of interface materials that reduce or disperse shear forces. These include materials like silicone, urethanes, and adjustable air bladders. Multiple suspension systems or two different types of suspension used simultaneously can also reduce the likelihood of skin breakdown.

Prosthetic componentry is also prone to stress and breakdown. Active children probably generate more stress on components, pound for pound, than any other patient population. Failure of components can be dangerous and at the very least frustrating for the patient. Therefore, once again, follow-up is extremely important. Components should be checked frequently and manufacturer's recommendations should be followed.

Because so many factors affect the care of an active patient, it is especially important that these patients receive thorough education. The patient should understand (1) how his or her prosthesis works and be able to recognize component fatigue; (2) how to look for indications of early skin breakdown; and (3) how to make minor fitting adjustments using socks or skin protectants. The practitioner should be aware that these patients will be in need of multiple accessory replacements such as socks, sleeves, or covers and should be prepared to provide these items promptly.

Consensus of the ABC prosthetists surveyed is that health-care providers should concentrate on what the patient can do, rather than what he or she cannot do. The only limitations to goal-setting should be practical ones, such as starting slowly on a new prosthesis or knowing the limitations of the components for safety. Encourage, help, and support patients of all ages and performance levels in the pursuit of their chosen leisure activities.

Children become involved in sports and recreation for a variety of reasons, but the results are very similar. The practitioners noted significant improvement in the self-esteem of their patients once their patients became more involved with sports activities. The patients emitted a sense of accomplishment and achievement. Not everyone has the ability to be the best, but everyone has the ability to give their best effort, and the result is very satisfying.

Prosthetic Technology

Prosthetists have benefited from a technology bonanza over the past 15 years. Materials have been developed that are lighter and stronger than ever before. Technical knowledge from other industries, such as aerospace and electrical engineering, have trickled into the knowledge pool. New components for both upper and lower extremities have been developed that more closely mimic the human body. Orthotists and prosthetists have increased their knowledge of areas such as gait analysis. In short, recent improvements in components and methods have given children with limb deficiencies a greater opportunity than ever before to succeed in their chosen leisure pursuits.

An infinite number of prosthetic adaptations can be made for children with limb deficiencies who want to participate in sports and recreation. It might be as simple as providing additional external rotation of the foot for the transtibial runner who internally rotates when sprinting. Or it may be as complex as providing a sophisticated bow string release for the patient with multiple limb deficiencies who wants to compete in archery. Prosthetists are limited only by their creativity and ability. Specialized equipment enhances the performance and enjoyment of participation in sports and recreation activities for children with limb deficiencies.[16] However, some commonly used components are commercially available and appropriate for children.

Feet

The main functions of the anatomic foot, with respect to prosthetic foot design, could be broken down to shock absorption at heel strike, a base of support when standing, and propulsion to the next step. The goal of prosthetic foot selection is to find the foot with a combination of these functions that most appropriately accommodates the specific patient. Subjective feedback supports much of the literature that dynamic response (those that provide propulsion) feet are preferred over the SACH (Solid Ankle Cushioned Heel) foot.

In a retrospective analysis of a child's size dynamic response foot, the subjective feedback was very positive. Twenty-four feet were fit on 21 children from 2 to 12 years of age who had limb deficiencies below their knee joints, and the patients were surveyed after approximately 12 months of experience. The patients and their parents responded that the dynamic response foot improved performance, endurance, and self-esteem. The most positive response was to questions regarding cosmesis of the foot. These parents and patients felt it was very important that the artificial foot look like a real foot.

The fact that cosmesis was so important led to the question whether these patients were truly enjoying improved function or were perceiving improved function because they approved of the cosmesis. A similar retrospective analysis was run on a small number of children who had been fitted with elastic keel feet, which were not designed for propulsion, but for stability, smooth rollover, and cosmesis. The results were very positive. Foot cosmesis is very important to children and families. Therefore, cosmesis has become an additional functional consideration in prosthetic foot selection.

There is some question as to whether lightweight children can use the dynamic response properties of prosthetic feet. Young children were found to function well on either type of foot. Therefore, cosmesis and stability are the primary criteria to consider for this population.

As the patient grows, an array of cosmetic, articulated, dynamic response feet is available. New options, such as vertical shock pylons, are becoming available all the time. It is advantageous to allow an adolescent to try several feet that are designed for his or her lifestyle, whether it be active or sedate. The patient can then feel that he or she has played an active role in his or her own care, which can increase self-esteem. As children grow toward adulthood, their needs change. It is important that the prosthetic team discuss the changing needs so that the most appropriate foot is chosen at each visit.

Knees

The child's first articulating knee will probably be an exoskeletal hand-crafted "outside hinge" type of design. This design is usually necessary because the above-knee limb deficiency often presents a residual limb that approaches 50% of the child's contralateral limb length. Therefore, the outside hinge design helps to achieve the correct knee center.

As the child grows, a good option is an endoskeletal, constant friction, polycentric knee joint. These joints can be fit into a lower leg pylon that can be adjusted for length and angulation as the child's gait changes. They "fold up" nicely when flexed, which reduces the length of the thigh segment when compared to single axis endoskeletal knees. Limited models are available, but they provide good stability and their instantaneous center of rotation decreases the effort needed to initiate flexion. Even though children have various cadences, there is no need for fluid swing phase control until they require adult-size componentry.

The adolescent should be encouraged to select the knee that best meets his or her needs. At this age, young people are often able to give excellent feedback that can add to the quality of care.

Terminal Devices

Terminal devices are available for a variety of activities. Some terminal devices are versatile enough to be valuable for a multitude of activities; others are built for a specific purpose. The team approach is valuable in creating upper-extremity prostheses for sports and recreation. Often the patient has specific goals and ideas, but does not know the limitations of fabrication. The health-care team needs to be open to these ideas and work with the patient to achieve optimal results.

An ABC prosthetist has many unique devices that the patient may not be aware of. Patients should be encouraged to dream. The challenge is for the prosthetist to be able to fulfill the dream. Usually the effort to fabricate the prosthesis is less than the effort that will be necessary to master its use.

Conclusion

As discussed throughout this chapter, children have a philosophical right to live the life they choose without regard to their limb deficiencies. Through sports and recreation, children can develop psychological, social, and physical skills that will be valuable assets throughout their lives. Health-care providers, such as those on limb deficiency clinic teams, can provide the opportunity for children to set these skills in motion for the benefit of the individual and society.

References

1. Kraus RG, Bates BJ (eds): *Recreation Leadership and Supervision: The Social Context; Recreation Leadership and Supervision: Guidelines for Professional Development.* Philadelphia, PA, WB Saunders, 1975, pp 5–6.

2. Csikszentmihalyi M, Csikszentmihalyi IS: *Optimal Experience: Psychological Studies of Flow in Consciousness.* Cambridge, England, Cambridge University Press, 1988.

3. Coyle C, Kinney WB, Riley B, Shank JW: *Benefits of Therapeutic Recreation: A Consensus View*. Philadelphia, PA, Temple University, 1991.

4. DeCarlo TJ: Recreation participation patterns and successful aging. *J Gerontol* 1974;29:416–422.

5. Moore SR: Walking for health: A nurse-managed activity. *J Gerontol Nurs* 1989; 15:26–28.

6. Westland C: Leisure and mental health. *Rec Can* 1991;49:24–28.

7. Parks and Recreation Federation of Ontario and the Ontario Ministry of Tourism and Recreation: *The Benefits of Parks and Recreation: A Catalogue*. Gloucester, Ontario, Canada, Canadian Parks/Recreation Association, 1992, p 55.

8. Jenkins JR, Speltz ML, Odom SL: Integrating normal and handicapped preschoolers: Effects on child development and social interaction. *Excep Child* 1985; 52:7–17.

9. California Park and Recreation Society: *Economics of Parks and Recreation Resource Book: Institute on the Economic Impact of Parks and Recreation*. Sacramento, California, California Park and Recreation Society, 1989.

10. Lynch M, McCarney P (eds): *The Benefits and Costs of Recreation*. Toronto, Canada, Bureau of Municipal Research, 1981.

11. Szentagothai K, Gyene I, Szocska M, Osvath P: Physical exercise programs for children with bronchial asthma. *Pediatr Pulmonol* 1987;3:166–172.

12. Katz JF, Adler JC, Mazzarella NJ, Ince LP: Psychological consequences of an exercise training program for a paraplegic man: A case study. *Rehabil Psychol* 1985;30:53–58.

13. Greenwood CM, Dzewattowski DA, French R: Self efficacy and psychological well-being of wheelchair tennis participants and wheelchair nontennis participants. *Adapted Physical Activity Quarterly* 1990;7:1,12–21.

14. Weiss CR, Jamieson N: Hidden disabilities: A new enterprise for therapeutic recreation. *Therapeut Recreation J* 1988;22:9–17.

15. Riley R: The amputee athlete. *Clin Prosthet Orthot* 1987;11:109–113.

16. O'Leary HL: *Bold Tracks: Skiing for the Disabled*. Evergreen, Colorado, Cordillera Press Inc, 1987.

Chapter 30

Training the Child With Lower Limb Loss To Run

Jeanine R. Thomas, PT

Typically, rehabilitation of an individual with lower limb loss concentrates on the achievements of independent walking. However, improvements in prosthetics and the increasing popularity of organized sports for the disabled, such as paralympics, challenges the therapist to help the child achieve his or her true athletic potential.

Running is used in most sports and recreational activities, including basketball, baseball, football, and track. The benefits of running extend beyond the ability to participate in competitive sports. A recent study has demonstrated a positive association between emotional well being and sports participation in adolescents.[1]

Mastery of running required in recreational activities enhances self-esteem. Improvements in physical fitness include better cardiovascular conditioning and weight reduction. According to Enoka and associates,[2] "At the most basic level running is a 'self-preservation' skill employed in certain emergency situations." With proper training to decrease risk of injury and deter undesirable running patterns, children and adolescents with lower limb loss can reap the physical, social, and psychological benefits of running.

There has been little research on the running biomechanics of the juvenile athlete. Running gait patterns of young adults with below-knee and above-knee amputations have been described.[3,4] A study of running economy in childhood and adolescence indicates a child's running pattern is inefficient because children have a short stride and decreased oxygen consumption. Efficiency improves as the child matures. Short-term training does little to improve efficiency.[5] Running patterns have considerable variation between individuals; however, certain features are common among all able-bodied runners. A brief introduction to the biomechanics of running is necessary to understand how the amputee accommodates within the running pattern.

Biomechanics of Running

Stance Phase

At initial contact, the foot holds the body over flexed joints. All muscles crossing the joints provide stability and absorb the impact of initial ground contact. Rapid extension and adduction of the hip occurs, possibly playing a role in assisting in stability during stance phase.[6] Weight typically is shifted from the lateral border of the foot to midline; then it stays in the forefoot for the remainder of the stance phase.[7]

The talocalcaneal joint plays an important role in allowing the foot to achieve full plantigrade contact with the ground through pronation. This action also assists in the foot flat on uneven terrain and around curved pathways. In normal children, approximately 3° of frontal plane rotation of the leg occurs during running support.[8]

Midsupport to take-off is characterized by progressive hip and knee extension with plantarflexion changing the foot's function from an energy absorber to the major source of energy generation.[6] Forward propulsion of the body also occurs through the swinging arms and leg motion.[9]

Forces

Ground reaction forces change between initial ground contact and take-off. Vertical forces quickly build up to a value greater than twice the runner's body weight. They then fall off, only to be followed by increasing forces that are again two to three times body weight as the individual pushes off. The contact period is approximately one third of a second.[10]

Even larger forces (ten times body weight) result at the lower leg and talus; these forces are produced by muscle action as joint surfaces compress. Forward and backward frictional forces at the foot are described as a braking phase, then a propulsive period. A resultant force of one half body weight is applied. Therefore, a cycle of slowing down and speeding up occurs with every foot strike.[7]

Swing Phase

Normal swing phase is characterized first by rapid flexion of the hip as the iliopsoas accelerates the thigh and leg forward. The ankle dorsiflexes, and this action continues throughout the cycle to place the foot in a position of maximum stability. The knee flexes passively. However, an eccentric contraction of the knee extensors controls the posterior rotation of the lower leg as the thigh is accelerated forward. The last 25% of swing phase consists of active firing of the extensors, hamstrings, quadriceps, and gastrocnemius-soleus muscles in preparation for initial ground contract. Hip extension begins, and the knee rapidly flexes.[6]

Amputee Running

Joint Adaptations

An amputee must adapt a running pattern to a prosthesis that lacks the biomechanical function and proprioceptive feedback of a normal knee, ankle, and/or foot. The talocalcaneal joint normally plays an important role by pronating at foot strike to allow a plantigrade foot position. The absence of pronation results in an additional 16° of internal rotation of the lower leg. This rotation results in additional stresses at the knee. The amputee may adapt to these stresses through wider placement of the feet. The broader base of gait not only effects the lower extremity but also causes the upper extremity to be abducted more than usual. Perhaps this effect on running could be offset by a prosthetic talocalcaneal joint.

The above-knee amputee cannot weightbear over a flexed knee. Prosthetic knee stability is achieved by maintaining knee extension through prosthetic alignment and contraction of the hip extensors. Hi-tech prosthetic components are available to provide knee flexion control at foot strike and to absorb ground impact, improving gait symmetry. However, children with above-knee prostheses can run on basic components.

Muscle Output

In normal runners, the distal muscles of the lower extremity demonstrate the greatest amount of work during running support. In contrast, Czerniecki and Gitter[6] found that in the prosthetic lower extremity, the hip extensor muscle group becomes the major source of energy absorption at ground contact and energy generation at push-off. The large hip extensor moment produces knee flexion control at initial stance and assists in knee extension. However, below-knee amputees have been shown to have less extensor moment at the knee on the side with a prosthesis than on the intact side.[2,6] This difference may be the result of insufficient quadriceps strength or of the amputee avoiding patellar tendon pressure.[11,12] If the amputee runs with the knee straight or hyperextended, large stresses are transferred to the knee, hip, and spine.

Because the knee extensor moment is decreased and there are no motors below the knee in a below-knee amputee, total muscle work is about one half that of the intact limb.[3,11] Energy-storing prosthetic components at the feet return the distribution of muscle work to normal, thereby promoting a symmetric gait. Amputees with little or no running experience exhibit restricted range of knee flexion of the intact limb during swing. Thus, the intact foot remains closer to the ground. Normal subjects increase their running speed by increasing step length and rate. In contrast, amputees rely more on step rate to increase speed because they generally are unwilling to alter step length beyond perceived safe limits.[2] Surprisingly, during swing phase, the total amount of muscle work performed by the residual limb is close to normal. At the same time, the intact limb exhibits a 67% increase in total muscle work. The increased work occurs predominantly at the hip flexors and hamstrings in order to accelerate the thigh segment forward at initial swing and decelerate it before ground contact.[6]

Prosthetic Modifications

Running is a skill children use at an early age during play activities, and they tend to develop unique running patterns. After amputation, it is evident that not all amputees can return immediately to previous running patterns. Many factors affect running ability: the nature of the surgery, the level of amputation, the residual limb conditions, the prosthesis, the general state of physical fitness, and personal motivation.

Running is a strenuous exercise that can cause debilitating problems with the skin, muscles, ligaments, and tendons of the leg. A prosthesis should be designed with running in mind before the amputee begins intense training. A comfortably fitted and accurately contoured socket that distributes weight evenly will help prevent skin breakdown and increase tolerance to impact at initial ground contact. The weight of the below-knee running prosthesis should not exceed 3 lbs.[13]

The type of prosthetic foot is very important for both below-knee and above-knee amputees. Energy-storing feet have proven to decrease gait asymmetry by mimicking normal ground contact, response, and push-off muscle power.[11] Anterior distal tibia pressure is a common problem for the below-knee amputee during running. To control the prosthesis, the residual limb extends against the socket from initial ground contact to push-off. This increased pressure at the anterior distal tibia can result in discomfort and skin breakdown. A prosthetic foot with plantarflexion capability may alleviate this pressure. Most individuals will not be able to run or jog extended distances or time without skin irritation to the residual limb and may need to alternate aerobic activities, such as swimming and biking, with fitness training.[13]

Better suspension methods and more compliant interfaces between skin and socket improve tolerance to the shear forces placed on the residual limb. For the above-knee amputee, a prosthesis with components that absorb ground impact is recommended for foot over foot running.[13] Hydraulic knees with stance and swing control also improve running abilities.

Above-knee amputees without a proper prosthesis have difficulty in successfully performing foot over foot running. The strong prosthetic knee flexion moment during the support phase results in the transfemoral amputee running with a hop-skip style.

Hop-skip running is defined by a double stance phase by the intact leg during the prosthetic swing phase. The hop provides time to complete the prosthetic knee extension. Sometimes, undesirable circumduction of the prosthetic limb is used to increase foot clearance. Hop-skipping results in a slower running speed with an increase in energy expenditure.[4] Most transfemoral amputees use the hop-skip pattern to run long distances.

Prosthetic alignment for running with both below-knee and above-knee prostheses should be reconsidered. The foot should be toed out to compensate for greater internal rotation at the hip during running. A longer toe lever on energy-storing feet provides a stiffer spring for an increased push-off.

Training Program

Strength

A graduated training program for the child with lower limb loss should concentrate on muscle strengthening, endurance, coordination, and agility. A smooth and consistent running pattern is believed to result in greater efficiency, possibly improving a subject's ability to run greater distances. Appropriate muscle strength of the sound leg and residual limb increases the ability to control the prosthesis, stabilizes joints, and improves running symmetry. Based on research on the distribution of muscle work during running, specific muscles of the residual and intact limbs should be strengthened. The residual limb hip extensors are important during stance phase in energy absorption at ground contact and push-off, and these muscles should be conditioned. The increased work output found in the hamstrings and hip flexors during swing of the intact limb possibly functions to accelerate the trunk and stance limb forward, and they too should be strengthened.[11] Overall strengthening of the upper extremity and trunk is also recommended. Goals of the strengthening program are to improve muscle fitness, prevent sports injury, and enhance sports performance.[14] The physical therapist should incorporate resistive and open- and closed-chain exercises within the strengthening program.

Resistive exercises include partner-applied resistance and free weights. Manual resistance exercise should allow slow movement through the joints' full range of motion. To prevent injury, a child should not train with a weight he or she cannot lift for more than six repetitions. Sport cords of varying resistance can be used for children with different strength abilities. Use of both open- and closed-chain exercises is important in lower extremity strengthening. Closed-chain exercises, such as squats and step-lifts, change the mechanics of muscles that cross joints. Lower extremity muscles work in an open- and closed-chain environment during running.

With all exercises, the child should initially train at three sets of eight repetitions and gradually increase to 15 to 20 repetitions. A rest period of 60 s should be taken between each set. To increase muscular endurance, use less weight and increase repetitions to 15 to 30.

Adhering to typical principals of strength/endurance training is advised, and exercising three times a week is recommended to gain results.[14] One day of rest should be allowed between workout sessions for muscles to recover. The program should concentrate on major upper and lower extremity muscle groups unless a specific muscle weakness is identified.

Coordination and Agility

The ease with which a child can swing the prosthesis, adequately clearing his foot, then make sound, stable accurate contact with the ground at initial stance determines the degree of success the child achieves in foot over foot running. Coordination and agility can be developed through breakdown of the running pattern. Speed and precision of the prosthetic swing is improved by imitating the movement with slow repetitions. A minimum of 3 min is recommended to start. As endurance improves, the pace and time over which the exercise is performed should be increased.

Tolerance to the forces that occur at ground contact and the accuracy of prosthetic foot placement are improved by "stomping." Stomping is the act of forcefully contacting the ground in front of the body with the heel, then returning to the starting position of standing with feet slightly apart. In other words, the child pretends to be squishing a bug on the ground with the prosthesis. As with other exercises, repetitions should be gradually increased.

Running Clinic

The goals of the training program and running clinic are not to produce an elite athlete. Presently, within competitive school programs, a child with a physical disability is not encouraged to participate. Many times fear or the lack of motivation prevents the child from challenging himself or herself to attempt foot over foot running. A running clinic provides a child with basic techniques of warm-up and cool down. Building of the techniques in conjunction with supervised strength, coordination, and agility training result in the ability to run foot over foot. Foot over foot running may not be realistic for children with bilateral above-knee or even bilateral below-knee and unilateral above-knee amputations to use competitively. However, success may mean running a distance of 10 to 15 feet. All degrees of success can result in improvement of confidence and self-esteem. Aerobic and strength training have been proven to result in a greater gait velocity and decreased net energy cost during activities of daily living.[15,16] The camaraderie of children with amputations socializing and competing against each other during the clinic instills a sense of belonging, worthiness, and spirit.[17]

The running clinic consists of 3 h of fun activities. At least 30 min of warm-up, consisting of instruction in calisthenics and stretching, should be performed before running in order to prevent injury. Relays, including side stepping, braiding, and walking in a forward and backward direction, provide competition while increasing heart rate.

Stretching should concentrate on the adductors, hamstrings, hip flexors, buttocks, trunk, and major muscles of the upper extremity. Quadriceps stretching should be included for the below-knee amputee.

Training the child to run requires good weightbearing on the prosthesis. All amputees can use a hop-skip method initially until they are sufficiently confident to run foot over foot. A gradual progression from high-stepping during walking to a slow jog, then a fast jog can be achieved by increasing the speed of steps and decreasing limb support time.

The above-knee amputee may have more difficulty than the below-knee amputee in transitioning from the hop-skip method to foot over foot running. Appropriate hip flexor power is needed to throw the prosthesis forward for a solid and secure ground contact. A shorter stride length on the prosthetic side may result. During running, a relaxed and loose arm swing will aid in propelling the body forward and decrease energy expenditure. A clenched or tight jaw may actually increase the energy expended.

A record of the child's running time in the 50-yd and 100-m dash is made during the clinic. Progress can then be monitored in following clinics. Typically, a child's performance will improve when running against peers with similar levels of amputations. It is important that a prosthetist be available to make alignment adjustments as needed to promote comfort during the running clinic. Individual training can be achieved when trained staff are available. Cool down should consist of 15 min of stretching major muscle groups as previously stretched during warm-up.

Special speakers in the field of athletics, track and field, and various other recreational activities will promote participant interest. Informal reward ceremonies at the conclusion of the clinic will help motivate the child to carry out his or her training program at home. Awards are given for the "Most Improved," "Best Sportsperson," and "Most Team Spirited."

Even though there are now more nationally organized sports programs for the disabled, there are too few local programs specifically for the juvenile amputee who is a competitive runner. The Special Olympics program is not appropriate for the cognitively intact child. It is discouraging when a child who wishes to reach a higher level of athletic participation does not have a local outlet to challenge his or her running skill. Pediatric physical therapists who have an interest in training the child with an amputation to run should consider this problem and challenge specific local disabled sports organizations and the community to address and solve this issue.

A desire to function normally, including running and athletic participation, is nearly universal among children with amputations. The running clinic and training program will help them avoid injury and enable them to maximize their athletic potential. Secondary benefits, including improved self-concept and physical fitness, increase positive beliefs in general abilities and improve function.

References

1. Steptoe A, Butler N: Sports participation and emotional wellbeing in adolescents. *Lancet* 1996;347:1789–1792.

2. Enoka RM, Miller DI, Burgess EM: Below-knee amputee running gait. *Am J Phys Med* 1982;61:66–84.

3. Prince F, Allard P, Therrien RG, McFadyen BJ: Running gait impulse asymmetries in below-knee amputees. *Prosthet Orthot Int* 1992;16:19–24.

4. Mensch G, Ellis PE: Running patterns of transfemoral amputees: A clinical analysis. *Prosthet Orthot Int* 1986;10:129–134.

5. Krahenbuhl GS, Williams TJ: Running economy: Changes with age during childhood and adolescence. *Med Sci Sports Exerc* 1992;24:462–466.

6. Czerniecki JM, Gitter A: Insights into amputee running: A muscle work analysis. *Am J Phys Med Rehabil* 1992;71:209–218.

7. Cavanagh PR (ed): *The Running Shoe Book.* Mountain View, CA, Anderson World, 1980, pp 78–95.

8. Engsberg JR, Allinger TL: A function of the talocalcaneal joint during running support. *Foot Ankle* 1990;11:93–96.

9. Gailey RS (ed): *One Step Ahead: An Integrated Approach to Lower Extremity Prosthetics and Amputee Rehabilitation.* Miami, FL, Advanced Rehabilitation Therapy, 1994.

10. Herbert LM, Engsberg JR, Tedford KG, Grimston SK: A comparison of oxygen consumption during walking between children with and without below-knee amputations. *Phys Ther* 1994;74:943–950.

11. Czerniecki JM, Gitter A, Munro C: Joint moment and muscle power output characteristics of below knee amputees during running: The influence of energy storing prosthetic feet. *J Biomech* 1991;24:63–75.

12. Miller DI: Resultant lower extremity joint moments in below-knee amputees during running stance. *J Biomech* 1987;20:529–541.

13. Burgess EM, Rappoport A (eds): *Physical Fitness: A Guide for Individuals with Lower Limb Loss. A Clinical Guide.* Baltimore, MD, Department of Veterans Affairs, 1991, pp 193–205.

14. Kraemer WJ, Fleck SJ (eds): *Strength Training for Young Athletes.* Champaign, IL, Human Kinetics, 1993, pp 41–42.

15. Lane JM, Kroll MA, Rossbach PG: New advances and concepts in amputee management after treatment for bone and soft-tissue sarcomas. *Clin Orthop* 1990;256:22–28.

16. Ward KH, Meyers MC: Exercise performance of lower-extremity amputees. *Sports Med* 1995;20;207–214.

17. Burnett DJ (ed): *Youth, Sports and Self Esteem: A Guide for Parents.* Indianapolis, IN, Masters Press, 1993, pp 9–13.

Chapter 31

Sports Programs for the Child With a Limb Deficiency

Frank M. Chang, MD

Introduction

An athlete is an individual who uses body and motor skills to compete in exercises, sports, or games that require physical strength, agility, and stamina. The desire to compete has been present since the evolution of mankind, and athletic competition has been well-documented for centuries in all known cultures. Participation and viewing athletic competition continues to cross political and cultural boundaries. As our society learns to accept individuals with disabilities, opportunities are becoming increasingly available for their participation in sports and recreational activities.

Children with acquired or congenital limb deficiencies have the inherent desire to compete in sports and participate in recreational activities. Some disabled individuals have a strong desire to participate to prove something to themselves; most just want to have fun and enjoy the sport or activity. Stimulating a disabled child to participate and then watching the child succeed is a very gratifying experience (Fig. 1). The overall sense of accomplishment and rewards are great for a successful athlete with a limb deficiency or any disability.[1] Successful participation in sports increases self-confidence and improves self-esteem.[2]

Parents are often overprotective and fearful of injuries to these children. Parents, coaches, health-care professionals, and the child can be educated to prevent potential injuries. Providing access to programs supervised or recommended by health-care providers and organizations will increase parental perceptions of "safety," and provide limb deficient children with recreational and athletic experiences comparable to those of their able-bodied peers.

The spectrum of limb deficiency is very broad, and the impact on performance of athletic endeavors varies depending on the specific deficiency. Anatomic level and involvement of upper versus lower extremities will affect performance and appropriateness of participation in specific sports. An important consideration for athletes is classification of the deficiencies so competition can occur on an equal level. Almost all sports can be adapted by modifying the rules of the sport and/or using adaptive equipment to allow the disabled athlete to participate.

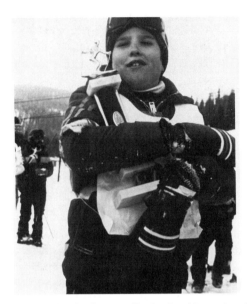

Fig. 1 *Disabled skier with cerebral palsy proudly clutches his trophy after winning a ski race. (Reproduced with permission from Chang FM: The disabled athlete, in Stanitski CL, DeLee JC, Drez D (eds):* Pediatric and Adolescent Sports Medicine. *Philadelphia, PA, WB Saunders, 1994, pp 48–76.)*

Classification of Disabilities

The classification of limb deficiencies varies according to the perspective of the responsible organization. Similar disabilities must be organized and grouped so the individuals are competing on an equal basis. From an organizational perspective, it is advantageous to group as many similar individuals together as possible so they can be organized into a league or competition with large enough groups for meaningful competition.

Classification begins by dividing the disabilities into very broad categories; eg, neuromuscular, amputees, Down syndrome, orthopaedic deformities, or physical impairments, such as hearing loss or visual impairment. Each broad category is then further subdivided to equalize the various differences. For example, amputees can be further classified according to upper and/or lower extremity and residual stump level. The neuromuscular category is further subdivided into diseases, such as cerebral palsy, myelomeningocele, spinal cord injury, brain injury, and muscular dystrophies. Myelomeningocele and spinal cord injury can be combined and then subdivided into the differing spinal cord levels or into specific vertebral levels. Cerebral palsy and brain injuries can be grouped together then categorized into hemiplegics, diplegics, and quadriplegics, or into ambulatory versus wheelchair-dependent; and ambulatory into with or without walking aids, again depending on the type of competition and the size of the group competing.

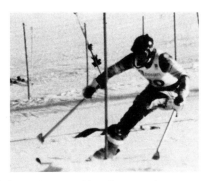

Fig. 2 *"Three track" skier using one ski and two outriggers.*

The classification must also reflect the nature of the sport under consideration. For example, although arm swing affects cadence and balance, it is unnecessary to subdivide upper extremity limb deficiency levels for running sports. Conversely, the level of the lower extremity amputation significantly affects performance in any sport requiring ambulatory skills, but makes much less difference in wheelchair sporting competitions.

The use of prostheses, wheelchairs, and other adaptive equipment must be clearly defined to deny any individual or group an advantage or disadvantage. For example, in national and international disabled alpine skiing competition, below-knee (BK) amputees must ski with their prosthesis and both skis, regardless of the stump length. An above-knee (AK) amputee must ski three-track, regardless of the level of amputation from knee disarticulation to hip disarticulation. Three-track is skiing with a ski on one leg and two short skis on forearm crutches, called outriggers, supported by the upper extremities[3] (Fig. 2).

The classification process must be consistent and fair. In most situations the classification will be obvious and easy to verify. Limb deficiencies fit this category. Other diagnoses may require physician verification.

Specific organizations also have developed classification systems.[4] Most of these organizations are advocate groups for specific disabilities (Table 1). Other classification systems have been developed by organizations responsible for organizing various competitions.

A basic and functional classification system for limb deficiencies is as follows: A, upper extremity; A1, above elbow (AE); A2, below elbow (BE); B, lower extremity, AK; C, lower extremity BK; and D, multiple extremities. In alpine ski racing, these four groups are used without distinction of upper extremity level.

For the 1996 Paralympics in Atlanta, Georgia, track and field classification began with separation into four major categories: visually impaired, cerebral palsy, amputee, and wheelchair. Each category is broken down into classes. For athletes who are visually impaired, the classes are based

Table 1 National Wheelchair Athletic Association (NWAA) junior medical classification system

Age Group*	Class I	Class II	Class III
"A" (6 to 8 years)	NWAA adult classes Ia to Ic	NWAA adult classes II and III	NWAA adult classes IV–V
"B" (9 to 12 years)			
"C" (13 to 15 years)	Cervical spinal level impairment (C1–C7)	Thoracic level impairment (T1–T10)	Impairment below T10 level includes amputees
"D" (16 to 18 years)			

*NWAA junior medical classification considers age and neurologic impairment level. Each class defined by a specific neurologic impairment level is subdivided into four age groups.
(Reproduced with permission from Chang FM: The disabled athlete, in Stanitski C, DeLee J, Drez D (eds): *Pediatric and Adolescent Sports Medicine.* Philadelphia, PA, WB Saunders, 1994, pp 48–76.)

on the athlete's ability to see. For athletes with cerebral palsy and athletes who compete in wheelchairs, the class depends on the degree of ability. For amputees, it depends on the location and degree of the amputation(s) (Table 2). The classification system in swimming is the difference between fair and inequitable competition. Functional classification groups athletes on the ability to perform certain functions, such as the movement of arms and legs (Table 3).

Medical Considerations for the Limb Deficient Athlete

Prosthetic Soft-Tissue Interface

The two special areas of concern regarding skin sensitivity are the child's awareness of skin sensibility and the additional risk at the interface of skin with an orthotic or prosthetic device or an ambulatory aid, such as a wheelchair or crutches. Children, in general, do not seem to have the same regard for their body parts as their adult counterparts, as demonstrated by the frequent bruises, cuts, and scratches visible on any active child. Children with limb deficiencies typically are not afflicted with intellectual or cognitive limitations, nor do they lack normal sensibility.

Prostheses, orthotics, crutches, and wheelchairs can all cause excessive localized pressure leading to skin irritation, blisters, skin breakdown, soft-tissue infections, and osteomyelitis. Children should be taught to become aware of their skin and its interface with prostheses, braces, chairs, and footwear. Coaches, physical education instructors, and parents also should be aware of the potential problems and check the skin periodically for erythema, callouses, blisters, and other signs of irritation. The added stress of repetitive loading with sports can cause excessive skin pressure in a child

Table 2 Track and field amputee classification

Class[*]	Description
T42	Single above the knee, combined lower and upper limb amputations, minimum disability
T43	Double below the knee, combined lower and upper limb amputations, normal function in throwing arm
T44	Double below the knee, combined lower and upper limb amputations, moderately reduced function in one or both limbs
T45	Double above the elbow, double below the elbow
T46	Single above the elbow, single below the elbow, upper limb function in throwing arm
F40	Double above the knee, combined lower and upper limb amputations, severe problems when walking, crutches may be used
F41	Standing athletes with no more than seventy points in the lower limbs[†]
F42	Single above the knee, combined lower and upper limb amputations, normal function in throwing arm
F44	Single above the knee, combined lower and upper limb amputations, normal function in throwing arm
F45	Double above the elbow, double below the elbow
F46	Single above the elbow, single below the elbow, upper limb function in throwing arm

[*] T = track; F = field
[†] The number represents the extent of the disability; the lower the number, the more extreme the disability

Table 3 Functional swimming classification

Class[*]	Description
S1	Unable to catch water; restricted range of motion; no trunk control; leg drag; assisted water start
S2	Unable to catch water; restricted range of motion; slight leg propulsion; unassisted water start
S3	Wrist control limited; limited arm propulsion; minimal trunk control; hips below water; water start
S4	Wrist control; arms not fully fluent; minimal trunk control; hips below water; better body position
S5	Full propulsion in catch phase; limited arm movement; trunk function; leg propulsion; sit or stand starts
S6	Catch phase present; arm movement efficient; trunk control; leg propulsion, push start, sit or stand
S7	Good hands; good arms; good trunk; hips level; stand or sit dive start
S8	Hand propulsion; arm cycle good; trunk good; hips and legs level; use of start blocks
S9	Full hand propulsion; full arm propulsion; full trunk control; propulsive kick; dive start from blocks
S10	Full hand and arm propulsion; full trunk control; strong leg kick; dive start and propulsion in turns.

[*] The letter indicates the stroke being performed; S = freestyle, backstroke, or butterfly

who has never before had problems. In addition, children are constantly growing, and growth-caused changes in prosthetic and orthotic fit eventually will lead to altered pressure sites.

Children wearing prosthetic limbs are at increased risk for skin breakdown. In children with prosthetic lower limbs, the weightbearing forces must be transferred to the skeleton through the skin and underlying soft tissues. At some amputation levels it is more difficult for the prosthetist to transfer these forces successfully. In the child with a well done Boyd or Syme's amputation, the stump is designed to be end bearing. There is a large surface area within the BK prosthesis to distribute the pressure forces, but more importantly, the heel pad has been preserved. The heel pad acts as a hydraulic cushion[5] to absorb and dissipate energy or force and transfer the weightbearing forces to the skeleton. For any lower extremity amputation above the level of the ankle, the skin and soft tissues transferring the weightbearing forces are more susceptible to breakdown and pressure necrosis.

An athlete with a high BK amputation will be at a disadvantage in most competitions. This athlete, for athletic classification purposes, will be grouped together with other BK amputees. A child with a Boyd or Syme's amputation externally looks the same. Both have a prosthesis that begins below the knee connected to a prosthetic foot. The child with the Boyd amputation is bearing weight through the heel pad and into the calcaneus, which approximates the normal situation. The child with a high BK stump is bearing some weight through the skin and whatever soft tissues the surgeon could cover the stump with, and the remaining pressure is distributed by friction contact to skin of the lower leg. For day-to-day normal activities, both children may do equally well. But in the arena of competitive sports, the high BK amputee is at a disadvantage, and the added stress to the end bearing skin interface may eventually provoke skin breakdown.

Stump overgrowth is another problem related to growth.[6-9] Despite the surgeon's best efforts, stump overgrowth continues to pose a significant problem for children. BK and AE prosthetic wearers are at the highest risk. Overgrowth occurs most frequently in the fibula, followed by the tibia, humerus, radius, ulna, and femur.[6,7] During this process, the bone grows through whatever soft tissues the surgeon left to cushion the end of the stump. As the child runs and jumps during athletic competition or just during normal play, the skin is at high risk for breakdown. The child, family, coaches, physical education teachers, and anyone else supervising the child should be made aware of the potential problem. If the end of the stump begins to feel more bony, or erythema and skin irritation begins, the child should be evaluated for stump overgrowth. The overgrown stump should be revised surgically to prevent the potential complications. In a young child, several stump revisions may be necessary at 2 to 3 year intervals[10] prior to skeletal maturity.

Orthopaedic Considerations

When considering participation in sports, the etiology of the deficiency should be understood. Limb deficiencies can be either congenital (present at birth) or acquired. The most dramatic and distressing to parents is a child born missing some significant parts. The missing part can be terminal (at the end of an extremity) or intercalary (somewhere in the middle of the segment).

The treatment goals for a terminal deficiency or amputation is to maximize function by providing maximum length for prosthetic suspension and control, adequate skin and soft-tissue coverage at the distal stump, and to fit an appropriate prosthesis.

Treatment for an intercalary deficiency is more challenging. The goal is again to optimize function. In the lower extremity, the foot is frequently amputated to facilitate prosthetic fitting. When indicated, this is done at about 1 year of age so prosthetic fitting can coincide with independent ambulation. The prosthesis is used to replace foot function and compensate for the difference in limb lengths. In fibular hemimelia, the foot is frequently abnormal, missing the lateral rays, and in severe cases, the ankle mortise is deficient laterally.[11–13] In proximal femoral focal deficiency the foot is usually normal, and it usually is amputated to facilitate prosthetic fitting; otherwise a nonstandard prosthetic fitting would be necessary. When considering athletic performance, an alternative is the van Nes procedure[14] in which the lower extremity is rotated 180°, and shortened appropriately so the ankle joint can substitute as an active knee joint (Fig. 3). The Brown rotationplasty with hip stabilization (Chapter 10) resects the proximal femur and hip joint, rotates the limb 180°, and fuses the femur to the pelvis. Both these procedures functionally result in a BK amputation. The ankle joint is substituted for the knee joint, allowing the patient to function as a BK amputee instead of an AK amputee. In sports, the presence of an active knee joint provides a competitive advantage. This must be weighed against the potential cosmetic disadvantages.

In the upper extremity, a similar intercalary deformity might only require therapy to improve mobility of the joints. If sensation and some functional grasp are present, the hand should be preserved. At the time of this writing, hand function cannot be satisfactorily replaced prosthetically because sensibility is a primary function of the hand that cannot be replaced. Equal upper extremity length is not nearly as important, so little attempt is made to equalize upper limb-length discrepancies, unless severe. Although normal hand function cannot be replaced prosthetically, many specialized terminal devices are available to allow participation in almost any sport.

Participation Guidelines Based on Disabilities

Limb deficiencies need not limit a child's participation in most sports. Psychologically, many children with limb deficiencies do not consider themselves disabled. Children with minor deformities will oftentimes participate and compete with able-bodied children, especially in local neighborhood and "sandlot" type games. As the organization and the level of competition increase in a given sport, the deformities and deficiencies may become relatively more of a handicap. At some point, the child or the team may decide

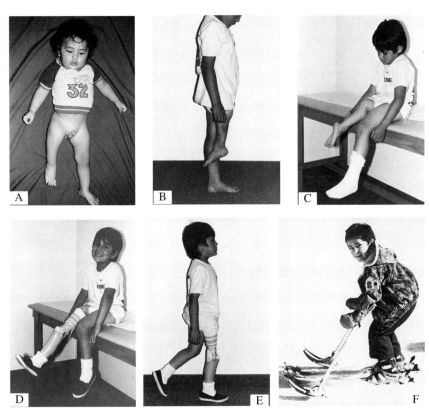

Fig. 3 A, *Child with proximal femoral focal deficiency.* ***B,*** *Postoperative van Nes turn-around procedure.* ***C,*** *Active knee extension.* ***D,*** *Active knee extension with prosthesis.* ***E,*** *Ambulaton with modified BK prosthesis.* ***F,*** *Skiing. (Reproduced with permission from Chang FM: The disabled athlete, in Stanitski CL, DeLee JC, Drez D (eds):* Pediatric and Adolescent Sports Medicine. *Philadelphia, PA, WB Saunders, 1994, pp 48–76.)*

that his or her continued participation is a handicap for the entire team and not just for the disabled individual.

Generalized participation guidelines in various sports for disabled athletes are difficult to establish. Participation guidelines must be individualized. Both the characteristics of the sport and the child's disability should be considered. A child may very much want to participate in a specific sport, but the parents may be very apprehensive and protective.

The Winter Park Seminar on Sports and Recreational Programs for the Child and Young Adult with Physical Disability[15] developed a "participation possibility chart," which includes the major physical disabilities and major sporting activities. Table 4 lists the activities pertaining to limb deficiencies.

Table 4 Participation possibility chart

Sport*	Amputations		
	Upper Extremity	Lower Extremity	
		Above knee	Below knee
Individual			
Archery	RA	R	R
Bicycling	R	R	R
Tricycling	R	R	R
Bowling	R	R	R
Canoeing/Kayaking	RA	R	R
Diving	R	R	R
Fencing	R	I	R
Field events†	R	R	R
Fishing	R	R	R
Golf	RA	R	R
Horseback riding	R	R	R
Rifle shooting	RA	R	R
Sailing	R	R	R
Scuba Diving	R	R	R
Skating:			
Roller and Ice	R	I	R
Skiing: Downhill	R	RA	R
Skiing: Cross-country	R	RA	R
Swimming	R	R	R
Table tennis	R	R	R
Tennis	R	I	R
Tennis: wheelchair		R	I
Track	R		R
Track: wheelchair		R	I
Weight lifting	R	R	R
Wheelchair poling		R	I
Team			
Baseball	R	RA	R
Softball	R	RA	R
Basketball	R		R
Basketball: wheelchair		R	I
Football: tackle	R	I	R
Football: touch	R	I	R
Football: wheelchair		R	I
Ice Hockey	R		I
Sledge hockey		R	I
Soccer	R	I	R
Soccer: wheelchair		R	I
Volleyball	R	R	R

* R = Recommended; X = Not recommended; A = Adapted; I = Individualized; and blank = No information or not applicable. "Individualized" means that, while the activity may be clearly inappropriate for some children with certain disabilities, it may well be possible for others in the same category to participate, and not contraindicated for all. Physician judgment and knowledge of the patient are important. "Adapted" means that in almost all cases, adaptations of equipment or rules are necessary. "Not Recommended" is self explanatory, suggesting the activity is not safe and has no redeeming benefits.

† Clubthrow, discus, javelin, shotput

(Reproduced with permission from Chang FM: The disabled athlete, in Stanitski C, DeLee J, Drez D (eds): *Pediatric and Adolescent Sports Medicine.* Philadelphia, PA, WB Saunders, 1994, pp 48–76.)

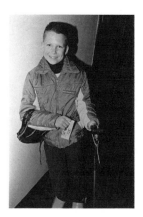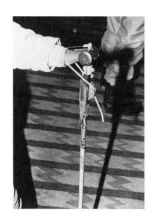

Fig. 4 *Above elbow prosthesis with All Terrain Ski terminal device, which can be used for both alpine and cross country skiing. (Reproduced with permission from Chang FM: The disabled athlete, in Stanitski CL, DeLee JC, Drez D (eds):* Pediatric and Adolescent Sports Medicine. *Philadelphia, PA, WB Saunders, 1994, pp 48–76.)*

Adaptive Equipment and Specialized Prosthetic Components

Depending on the disability and the sport, various types of adaptive equipment can be used to enhance the child's participation, performance, and enjoyment. Equipment may be as simple as the AFO (ankle foot orthosis) that the child uses every day to stabilize his or her ankle. At the other end of the spectrum are very specialized devices that facilitate athletic performance. A child that is a wheelchair ambulator, who has a very functional chair for daily use, may obtain a low profile, lightweight, sports wheelchair to participate in competitive sports.

A child's upper extremity prosthesis can be fitted with quick release wrists for interchangeable, specialized terminal devices. He or she may have several different sports-specific terminal devices. Examples include terminal devices to hold ice or roller hockey sticks, lacrosse sticks, rackets, golf clubs, bowling balls, fishing rods, and even ski poles (Fig. 4).

The same terminal device used to catch a baseball can also be used to throw for bilateral upper extremity limb deficiencies (Fig. 5) or a specialized terminal device can be fitted for a baseball glove in the unilaterally involved child. Two-handed batting can be accomplished simply with a Power Swing Ring (Fig. 6) attached to the end of the bat.

The Sport Hand (Fig. 7) is effective in assisting a child with a unilateral upper limb deficiency catch a football or basketball, or throw a soccer ball. The popularity of golf in adults has resulted in several terminal devices specifically designed to facilitate swinging a golf club (Fig. 8). Several paddle designs are available to be used with and without prosthetic upper extremities to improve swimming performance.

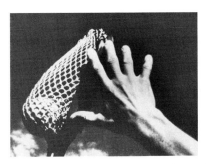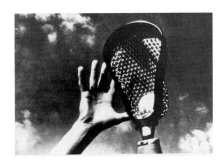

Fig. 5 *High Fly Fielder terminal device designed to catch a baseball, can also be used to throw for a bilateral upper extremity deficiency. Reproduced with permission from Bower JH, Michael JH (eds):* American Academy of Orthopaedic Surgeons Atlas of Limb Prosthetics. *St. Louis, MO, Mosby Year Book, 1992, pp 325–344.)*

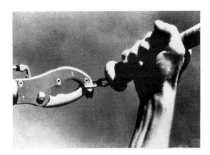

Fig. 6 *Two handed batting using a Power Swing Ring. (Reproduced with permission from Bower JH, Michael JH (eds):* American Academy of Orthopaedic Surgeons Atlas of Limb Prosthetics. *St. Louis, MO, Mosby Year Book, 1992, pp 325–344.)*

For road or mountain bicycling, many standard terminal devices can securely grip the handle bar. Additionally, the hand brake system must be modified so both front and rear brakes are activated with the hand brake on the uninvolved extremity.

Lighter and stronger materials enhance athletic performance as well as daily use for prosthetic users. Dynamic response or energy storing feet are ideal for sports. The flexible keel design improves athletic performance by providing propulsion that enhances running and jumping as well as walking. Some of the current feet with a split keel design provide some lateral mobility to simulate subtalar motion to compensate for uneven surfaces and terrain (Fig. 9). Specialized lower limbs designed exclusively for swimming are also available.

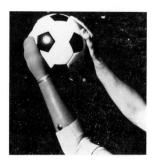

Fig. 7 *Super Sport Hand terminal device assists in throwing basketball or soccer ball and catching a football. (Reproduced with permission from Bower JH, Michael JH (eds):* American Academy of Orthopaedic Surgeons, Atlas of Limb Prosthetics. *St. Louis, MO, Mosby Year Book, 1992, pp 325–344.)*

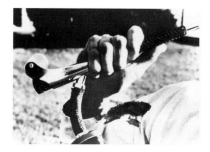

Fig. 8 *Amputee Golf Grip terminal device allows for complete wrist/club flexion and extension as well as unrestricted rotation. (Reproduced with permission from Bower JH, Michael JH (eds):* American Academy of Orthopaedic Surgeons, Atlas of Limb Prosthetics. *St. Louis, MO, Mosby Year Book, 1992, pp 325–344.)*

Children with congenital deficiencies of the lower extremities usually also lack the corresponding muscles and associated soft tissues,[16] and they may also be missing other soft-tissue structures that are not as obvious. Children with congenital short femurs or proximal femoral focal deficiency usually also have an associated anterior cruciate deficient knee[16,17] manifested by positive drawer and Lachman signs. This condition should be understood so it will not be mistaken as an acute rupture of the anterior cruciate ligament. Many of these patients are fitted in a BK prosthesis. The rigid prosthesis has less flexibility and elasticity than a normal lower leg, which will also increase the risk of an injury to the remaining knee ligaments. When participating in sports with significant potential for knee injuries, a

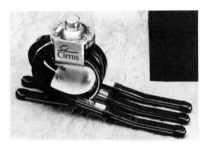

Fig. 9 *Split keel foot design simulates subtalar motion on uneven surfaces. (Reproduced with permission from Second Nature™.)*

second prosthesis with medial and lateral hinges and a thigh lacer for additional support and suspension should be prescribed to protect the knee.

Suspension for a short BK stump may pose little difficulty during normal daily activities, but for a child kicking a soccer or football, the centrifugal force may be enough to overcome the friction at the skin prosthetic interface, causing the prosthesis to fly off. This results in an embarrassing moment for the child and is potentially dangerous to others who may be hit by the flying prosthesis. The routine daily suspension can be augmented with neoprene sleeves or accessory modifications, such as a removable thigh lacer.

At The Children's Hospital in Denver, Colorado, we have had the unique experience of developing a very sophisticated and successful ski and sports program for children with many different types of disabilities. The ski program evaluates each child individually to determine the adaptive equipment that will optimize his or her performance. Depending on the specific disability, the child is categorized into the type of skier he or she will be to start with. Major skier categories are listed in Outline 1.

The child's stance is analyzed. If there is a limb-length discrepancy, lifts are incorporated between the ski and the binding (Fig. 10). If the child cannot achieve a balanced posture with weight balanced over his feet or slightly forward, then heel lifts are incorporated in the ski boot, or the binding and entire foot plate are canted forward in the more severe cases. The presence of deformed lower limbs (varus or valgus) can also be compensated by canting a foot plate appropriately. If the child has compromised balance, weakness in the lower extremities, or difficulty controlling his legs and feet, a ski bra will be used (Fig. 11). A ski bra provides a more stable platform. As the child's skills improve, a bungee cord, first with a pipe and then alone, replaces the ski bra. A bungee cord is elastic, providing some stability but more flexibility. Finally, as the child becomes more proficient and confident the bungee is removed, allowing independent control of both skis.

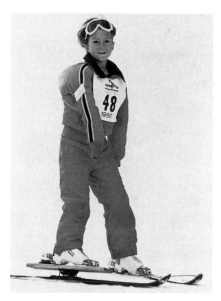

Fig. 10 *Platform mounted between ski and binding used to equalize limb lengths. (Reproduced with permission from Chang FM: The disabled athlete, in Stanitski CL, DeLee JC, Drez D (eds):* Pediatric and Adolescent Sports Medicine. *Philadelphia, PA, WB Saunders, 1994, pp 48–76.)*

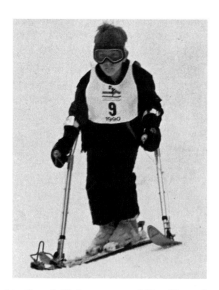

Fig. 11 *Ski bra attached to tips of skis increases stability. (Reproduced with permission from Chang FM: The disabled athlete, in Stanitski CL, DeLee JC, Drez D (eds):* Pediatric and Adolescent Sports Medicine. *Philadelphia, PA, WB Saunders, 1994, pp 48–76.)*

Outline 1 Major categories for skiers with disabilities

1. Three track: One ski and two outriggers
   a) Above-knee and higher amputees
   b) Severely deformed, damaged, weakened or fragile single lower extremity
   c) Below-knee amputee with less than 4-in stump
   d) Postpolio (monoplegia)

2. Four track: Two skis and two outriggers
   a) Mid to low lumbar level spina bifida
   b) Moderately to severely involved cerebral palsy

3. Two track: Two skis with one, two, or no poles
   a) Upper extremity amputee, unilateral or bilateral
   b) Spastic diplegic or triplegic cerebral palsy
   c) Below-knee amputee with 4-in or longer stump

4. Sit skier: Sitting in some modification of a sled device
   a) High lumbar or thoracic level spina bifida or spinal cord injury
   b) Any child dependent on a wheelchair

Intangible Benefits of Participation in Sports

The Children's Hospital Disabled Sports Program provides opportunities and programs to participate in many different sports and recreational activities for children in our community with the many physical and neurologic disabilities seen in a regional children's hospital. These include alpine and cross country skiing, wheelchair track and field, wheelchair basketball, wheelchair tennis, bicycling and mountain biking, horseback riding, golf, white water rafting, and fishing. These sports improve strength, endurance, balance, motivation, self image, and confidence. It helps the children realize that "disability is a state of mind." I truly believe this program changes the lives of the participants in a positive way and ultimately prepares them to better cope in a world of adults without handicaps.

Participants returning as adults not only have given positive feedback, but also have become volunteers in the disabled sports program. These individuals indicate that their participation meant so much to them as children, that they want to pay back and, more importantly, be a part of the joy and fulfillment they experienced as children.

Recommending and facilitating pediatric patients with limb deficiencies in a sports program certainly is appropriate. Participation in sports is safe, healthy, rewarding, exciting, and gratifying for these patients and their families. Help and encourage them to become involved. You will be glad you did!

References

1. Chang FM, Chang NS: They're reaching the highest mountain. *Sport Care Fitness* 1989;2:43.

2. Bowker JH, Michael JW (eds): American Academy of Orthopaedic Surgeons *Atlas of Limb Prosthetics: Surgical, Prosthetic, and Rehabilitation Principles,* ed 2. St. Louis, MO, Mosby-Year Book, 1992.

3. O'Leary H, Meinig MM (eds): *Bold Tracks: Skiing for the Disabled.* Evergreen, CO, Cordillera, 1987.

4. National Association of Sports for Cerebral Palsy: *Classification and Sports Rules Manual.* New York, NY, United Cerebral Palsy Associations, 1982.

5. Blum CE, Kalamchi A: Boyd amputations in children. *Clin Orthop* 1982;165: 138–143.

6. Aitken GT: Overgrowth of the amputation stump. *ICIB* 1962;1:1.

7. Aitken GT: The child amputee: An overview. *Orthop Clin North Am* 1972;3: 447–472.

8. Aitken GT, Frantz CH: The juvenile amputee. *J Bone Joint Surg* 1953;35A: 659–664.

9. Speer DP: The pathogenesis of amputation stump overgrowth. *Clin Orthop* 1981; 159:294–307.

10. Morrissy RT (ed): *Lovell & Winter's Pediatric Orthopaedics,* ed 3. Philadelphia, PA, JB Lippincott, 1990.

11. Achterman C, Kalamchi A: Congenital deficiency of the fibula. *J Bone Joint Surg* 1979;61B:133–137.

12. Coventry MB, Johnson EW Jr: Congenital absence of the fibula. *J Bone Joint Surg* 1952;34A:941–956.

13. Farmer AW, Laurin CA: Congenital absence of the fibula. *J Bone Joint Surg* 1960;42A:1–12.

14. van Nes CP: Rotation-plasty for congenital defects of the femur: Making use of the ankle of the shortened limb to control the knee joint of a prosthesis. *J Bone Joint Surg* 1950;32B:12–16.

15. American Academy of Orthopaedic Surgeons: *Sports and Recreational Programs for the Child and Young Adult with Physical Disability.* Proceedings of the Winter Park Seminar, Winter Park, CO. Chicago, IL, American Academy of Orthopaedic Surgeons, 1983.

16. Kalamchi A (ed): *Congenital Lower Limb Deficiencies.* New York, NY, Springer-Verlag, 1989.

17. Bevan-Thomas WH, Millar EA: A review of proximal focal femoral deficiencies. *J Bone Joint Surg* 1967;49A:1376–1388.

Consensus

Sports and Recreation Programs

We think sports and recreation programs are vitally important to the overall well-being of the child. The programs provide peer interaction among participants as well as actual accomplishments in the sports and recreational activities, and contribute substantially to the child's self-esteem. In addition, participation in these programs is an important learning experience for care givers.

We can promote more participation in sports and recreation in the following ways: (1) introduce parents, teachers, and anyone involved with the sports and recreation concepts to the needs of the child with limb deficiency; (2) help organize local, regional, and national programs to encourage and enable participation in competitive sports programs; and (3) make appropriate prosthetic and equipment adaptations to encourage the child's participation. We can also encourage participation in regular physical education classes at school, and when adapted physical education is necessary, make it something the child will enjoy, look forward to, and benefit from. Competition in able-bodied sports should also be encouraged whenever possible.

Section 7
Upper Extremity Deficiencies

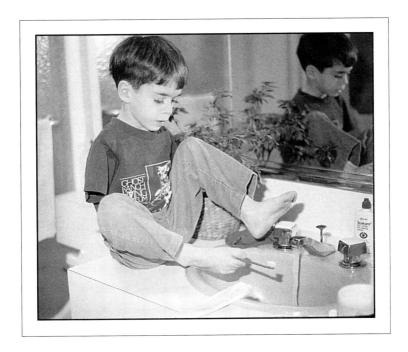

Chapter 32
Upper Extremity Deficiencies

Marybeth Ezaki, MD

Few things are as devastating to parents as having a newborn with a limb deficiency. All the expectations and dreams of what life would be with their child are shattered. Stages of shock, denial, mourning, and guilt precede and may coexist with acceptance. In one study, the support of family and grandparents was found to be a predictor of successful parental adjustment and subsequent sense of self-value on the part of the child.[1]

Parents want the best for their child and will have questions as to the best treatment. Most parents initially have unrealistic expectations for both surgical and prosthetic reconstruction. Few of the congenital upper limb differences have standard and definitive treatment protocols. Most of the anomalies are distinctive enough to require individualized treatment options. The goals of treatment must be to maximize functional independence, to minimize scarring and loss of sensation, and to do so with attention to the psychological impact on the child.

Transverse Deficiencies

Vascular Disruption

A vascular insult has been proposed as the etiology of most of these cases.[2] It is thought that premature vascular insufficiency results in a failure of normal mesodermal proliferation and in inadequate tissue substrate to allow full limb formation. Disruption of the subclavian artery supply distribution theoretically explains the pattern of limb anomaly in the diagnostic spectrum of symbrachydactyly, Poland anomaly, Möbius syndrome, and the transverse deficiencies in which there are small "nubbins." Depending on the stage of development in which the vascular insufficiency occurs, the limb abnormalities may range from minimal shortening to proximal level of absence. The characteristic finding that supports this etiology is the presence of ectoderm-derived tissues (skin, nails, and distal phalangeal tuft), which remain as a miniature reminder of the primarily mesodermal failure in these conditions.

The early decision points in treatment deal with what to do with the nubbins. Later decisions deal with reconstructive surgery to augment function. Nubbins may become ensnared by hair or strands of thread and become excoriated or dysvascular. Small nails may grow abnormally and become irritated, infected, or difficult to trim. The small nubbins are often the source of curiosity to other children and are not easily explained by the owner. Nubbins that occur on the ridge in the central part of the hand in the split hand form of symbrachydactyly are easily traumatized. Web deepening in this condition can be accomplished by local skin rearrangement and removal of the nubbins to smooth the residual commissure. Some nubbins serve a purpose. Certainly, any that have volitional control or are large enough to consider for later soft-tissue and bony augmentation should be left.

A number of surgical reconstructive options are appropriate for certain patients with transverse upper limb deficiencies. The first to consider is digital reconstruction in children who have some structures distal to the carpus. Digital remnants that lack bony support and are large enough to accept bone graft can be augmented with nonvascularized toe phalanx transfers. The timing of the procedure is controversial. The epiphysis of a nonvascularized toe phalanx transferred with its periosteum intact has a better chance of surviving and continuing its growth if the transfer is done while the child is still small.[3] Alternatively, normal growth of the phalanx will occur while it is in the foot, and only a small risk of loss of "potential" growth is incurred if the phalanx is transferred later. It is agreed that the transfer should include periosteum and ligamentous support if it is to be readily revascularized in its new position. Stability of the bone in the soft-tissue sleeve can be enhanced by suturing the ligamentous attachments of the phalanx to adjacent skeletal elements in the finger. The appearance of the donor toe will be short and telescoped, much like the finger sleeve was.

Another option for reconstruction of the digits in some cases is rearrangement of the available bony elements to a more functional position. This might mean moving an index metacarpal/ray to the middle digit position to close a defect, or moving metacarpal remnants to "stack" enough bone at a border position in preparation for later lengthening.

Distraction lengthening has a limited role in the treatment of digital insufficiency. Any lengthening procedure must be carefully planned to balance the hope of cosmetic improvement with the risk of functional loss. Digits that are longer, but also thinner, stiffer, and more scarred are not functionally better. Distraction lengthening in the hand works best where there is a normal digital tip. Lengthening against atrophic soft tissue results in ulceration and the need to augment soft-tissue coverage or shorten back to a comfortable level.

Advances in microsurgical free toe transfers provide another option for functional reconstruction of the adactylous hand.[4,5] It had long been thought that hands that lacked digits also lacked the proximal nerves for sensation, and muscles and tendons for motor function. Most of the children with these hands will have proximal structures to allow successful transfers to the hand.

It must be recognized that although the improvement in function is significant, these transferred toes will still look like toes.

Early Amnion Disruption Sequence

The other major etiology for transverse limb deficiencies is early amnion rupture with disruption of limb growth. Although there had been an "intrinsic" theory about this condition, it is accepted that the cause is breakdown of the amnion and a traumatic lesion to the limbs resulting from entanglement with strands of amnion. The fingers and toes are most often involved, with the so-called "fenestrated syndactyly" being the hallmark. Deep bands can cause distal edema, nerve injury, and impeded growth. Amputation of digits or more proximal limb can also occur. The difficulties with bony overgrowth are present in these limbs. Sensation is often impaired.

Surgery for amnion disruption sequence consists of early and late phases. Procedures in early infancy are indicated only for the rare cases in which impending tissue death requires emergency release of constriction bands. Elective release and z-plasty of the bands can wait until the child is older and better able to tolerate anesthesia. The constrictive defect around the limb can be recontoured circumferentially at one sitting if care is taken to preserve any vessels that are encountered and to carefully release impeding fascia.

The techniques available for digital reconstruction include syndactyly separation and grafting, digital lengthening, and augmentation of digits with local skeletal rearrangements or free toe transfer. Epithelialized tracts within the fenestrations, a complex bony deformity with fused, entangled digits, or poor tissue quality in the hand limit reconstructive potential in band syndactyly. Release of the transverse intermetacarpal head ligament and greater web deepening will make shorter digits seem longer. Care should be taken to preserve any normal palmar skin and its sensation.

Digital lengthening can be accomplished by distraction, but the problem of lengthening against a poor digital tip is not easily solved. Band amputation of digits, especially the thumb, is perhaps the best indication for free toe transfer, if normal donor toes are present. All the structures proximal to the injuring band are present and normal. The potential to restore motor and sensory function, as well as length, exists. Although there are a number of advantages to toe transfers, many families are reluctant to allow the surgeon to use the toe for transfer.

Late problems that occur with band amputations include diaphyseal overgrowth and instability of soft tissue at the end of the residual limb or digit. An additional problem is the development of inclusion cysts at the tip of the limb. The limb is also more susceptible to infection distal to the band where there had been disruption of the normal lymphatics.

Prosthetic fitting in the child with a transverse amputation of the upper limb is not needed for balance, crawling, or otherwise meeting developmental milestones. A prosthesis is a tool that can provide the ability to pinch or grasp an object while the intact upper limb manipulates it. An upper limb prosthesis does not provide sensory feedback.

383

Radial Deficiencies

Deficiency of the radius is a relatively common upper limb anomaly. Numerous genetic and chromosomal conditions are known to include radial deficiencies. Radial abnormalities are also known to occur in association with many skeletal, visceral, hematologic, and metabolic conditions. It appears that developmental control of radial limb formation is modulated by many different factors.

When making decisions about treatment for radial deficiencies, the surgeon must consider the prognosis of any associated conditions. New treatments are prolonging the life expectancy for previously lethal conditions, such as Fanconi's anemia. In most children who have cardiac anomalies, they are corrected within the first year of life. This leaves the radial limb deficiency and the deformity associated with it as the biggest concern for these patients on a day-to-day basis.

Radial deficiency is classified according to the amount of residual radius. Type I is a short distal radius. Type II is a small radius with both growth plates still present. Type III has a proximal radius still present. Type IV, the most common, is complete absence of the radius.

Treatment of the more severe and more common forms of radial deficiency begins with stretching and splinting of the affected infant's hand. This is often followed at an older age by centralization of the carpus on the ulna with tendon balancing or "radialization" of the ulna under the carpus. Releasing and rebalancing tendon and muscle force across the ulnocarpal articulation, and capsulorrhaphy are also done. Prolonged postoperative splinting is needed. Centralization procedures attempt to stiffen the ulnocarpal juncture to provide greater reach and stability for the function of the musculotendinous units that cross the wrist. It is extremely difficult to preserve any functional motion at this new "joint" while at the same time providing enough stability and tendon balance that subsequent growth will not redeform the limb.

The range of motion of the elbow is critical in deciding whether the carpus should be centralized. An elbow that is stiff in extension is a contraindication to any procedure that would further limit ability to reach the face. Recall that in a wrist arthrodesis, compensatory motion occurs with radioulnar joint rotation. Children with radial dysplasia lack forearm rotation; their compensatory motion is limited. Their strength, and therefore deforming force, is in flexion and radial deviation. I do not believe it is possible to restore "normal" alignment and, at the same time, preserve functional motion in these patients. With present means of treatment, preservation of motion means persistence of deformity; loss of motion accompanies realignment. Honest discussions about realistic expectations must take place frequently in order to avoid frustration and disappointment on the part of the family and the treating physician.

Reports of experience with distraction lengthening of both bone and soft tissue indicate that this technique has some application in this condition. The limiting factors are the size of the limb, the proximity of neurovascular structures, the risk of infection, and scarring. Distraction lengthening is preliminary to centralization procedures and does not obviate the need for some additional procedure.

Other options for treatment of the radial clubhand are being explored. Restoration of support for the radial side of the carpus with free metatarsophalangeal joint transfer holds promise, although it is technically demanding (SK Vilkki, unpublished data, 1996).

Late problems with radial deficiency include the inherent diminished growth potential of the ulna, the risk of injury to the distal ulnar physis and additional growth disturbance, and the significant risk of recurrence of deformity. Increased stiffness of the wrist correlates with decreased risk of recurrence of deformity. Ulnocarpal arthrodesis may be a final salvage procedure. Tendon adhesion and subluxation with resultant loss of dexterity are frequent.

Deficiency of the radial aspect of the hand includes the spectrum of thumb hypoplasia. These children will often have significant stiffness of all of the fingers as well as deformity related to the radial dysplasia. The abnormalities of the thumb range from mild hypoplasia to complete absence.

The decision points in treatment are related to the overall prognosis for the child, the condition of the forearm, and the condition of the adjacent fingers. Treatment of the hypoplastic thumbs with stable carpometacarpal joints consists of augmentation of the deficient components using adjacent tissue rearrangement, tendon transfer, and ligament reconstruction. When the basal joint of the thumb is inadequate or in the case of the floating or absent thumb, the recommended treatment is pollicization. There is no adequate prosthetic replacement for a thumb.

Summary

A brief review of the transverse and radial deficiencies of the upper limb and their treatment options shows that no treatment can adequately and predictably restore both function and cosmetic appearance to these limbs. Preservation of sensation and functional motion should remain priorities to be balanced with the desire for enhanced appearance.

References

1. Beresford BA: Resources and strategies: How parents cope with the care of a disabled child. *J Child Psychol Psychiatry* 1994;35:171–209.

2. Bavinck JN, Weaver DD: Subclavian artery supply disruption sequence: Hypothesis of a vascular etiology for Poland, Klippel-Feil, and Mobius anomalies. *Am J Med Genet* 1986;23:903–918.

3. Buck-Gramcko D: The role of nonvascularized toe phalanx transplantation. *Hand Clin* 1990;6:643–659.

4. Vilkki SK: Advances in microsurgical reconstruction of the congenitally adactylous hand. *Clin Orthop* 1995;314:45–58.

5. Lister GD: Toes to the hand, in Flatt AE (ed): *The Care of Congenital Hand Anomalies,* ed 2. St. Louis, MO, Quality Medical Publishing, 1994, pp 180–195.

Chapter 33

Ulnar Hemimelia

James B. Bennett, MD
Daniel C. Riordan, MD

Introduction

Ulnar hemimelia is a congenital musculoskeletal deficiency that primarily involves the post-axial or ulnar border of the upper extremity. Longitudinal ulnar development is deficient or absent. Ectrodactyly, carpal hypoplasia, ulnar deviation of the hand, forearm shortening with radial bowing, elbow dysplasia, and hypoplasia of the entire extremity occur.[1-4] The radius provides sufficient support and stability to the carpus in the hand. The slope of the distal radius is usually within normal limits, and as ulnar deformity increases it tends to flatten to support the carpus. The entire hand may be affected, and digital absence may be involved. Symphalangism and syndactyly have been reported by Cole and Manske[5] with abnormal involvement of the thumb and first web in 73% of ulnar hemimelia cases (Fig. 1).

Terminology includes ulnar club hand, ulnar dysmelia, para-axial ulnar hemimelia, postaxial deficiency, ulnar ray deficiency, congenital absence of the ulna, longitudinal arrest of the development of the ulna, and congenital absence of the ulna.

Ulnar hemimelia was first described by Goeller in 1683.[6] The first genetic study of this malformation was reported in 1949 by Birch-Jensen[7] who studied 19 cases with no evidence of inheritance. The role played by genetic and environment factors remains obscure.

Ogino and Kato[8] produced ulnar deficiencies in pregnant Gun-Wistar rats with the administration of busulfan teratologic agents. An ulnar ray deficiency was induced when busulfan was given on days 9, 9.5, and 10 of pregnancy. The incidence of ulnar ray deficiency also varied with dosage of busulfan administered. Comparison of ulnar ray deficiencies and radial ray deficiencies in this series showed bilaterality in nearly half the cases of radial ray deficiency while the ulnar ray deficiencies were unilateral.[8,9] Ulnar deficiencies were associated with musculoskeletal abnormalities, whereas radial deficiencies were associated with systemic abnormalities. The neurocrest theory of McCredie[10] suggests that disturbance of the C6 sclerotome results in radial aplasia and absent thumbs, disturbance of the C8 sclerotomes affects the ulnar side of the arm. The teratogenic mechanisms result in deficient mesenchymal cells in the limb bud, which cause impairment before the formation of the limb bud.

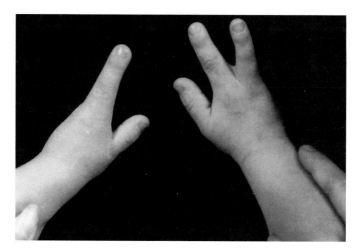

Fig. 1 *Bilateral ulnar hemimelia with thumb-index web involvement and absent ulnar digits.*

Ogden and associates[11] in laboratory experiments developed a model for ulnar absence by treating pregnant rats with acetazolamide.

Gurrieri and associates[12] have suggested that a limb deficient gene at 6q21 produces an ulnar ray defect. Reynolds and associates[13] also noted deficiency at 21q. Ulnofibular synostosis mesomelic dwarfism associated with hypoplastic ulna is reported by Langer.[14]

Congenital syndromes occurring in association with ulnar deficiency include Cornelia de Lange syndrome, Weyers ulnar ray oligodactyly syndrome, ulnar mammary syndrome, femoral fibular ulnar deficiency syndrome, and ulnar fibula dysplasia.[15,16] Vascular anomalies are noted by Di Bella and associates[17] and Inoue and Miura.[18]

Ulnar hemimelia has associated musculoskeletal abnormalities and anomalies in 55% of the 116 cases reported by Masson and associates (unpublished data, 1996). Ogino and Kato[8] found similar associations in their experimental studies and suggest that the critical period of ulnar ray deficiency is earlier than that of other abnormalities in human beings and corresponds to the period of high mortality of fetuses. It is postulated that this is why ulnar ray deficiencies are observed frequently less than other abnormalities. These anomalies may be isolated or multiple and may involve the contralateral extremities or the axial skeleton. Systemic involvement, although present, is less frequent than in cases of radial hemimelia. Radial hemimelia may include cardiac, hematologic, and renal abnormalities as well as the syndromes of thrombocytopenia-absent radius (TAR), Vater, Holt-Oram, and Fanconi.[15]

Incidence and Associated Anomalies

The incidence and prevalence of ulnar hemimelia is based on the studies by Birch-Jensen[7] published in 1949 as a review of congenital upper extremity anomalies in the Danish population. The incidence of ulnar hemimelia was felt to be 1 in 100,000. This relates to a radial hemimelia incidence in 1 in 30,000 live births. The relative incidence of ulnar deficiencies to radial deficiencies is 1 to 3.[2,19]

The clinical manifestations vary widely and include ectrodactyly, carpal hypoplasia, ulnar deviation of the hand, forearm shortening and bowing, defective elbow congruency with loss of motion, and hypoplasia of the proximal part of the extremity, including abnormalities about the shoulder girdle. Of the cases, 50% will have structural deformity of the opposite upper extremity, and 50% will have other musculoskeletal system defects throughout the body. Associated hematologic, cardiac, gastrointestinal, and genitourinary abnormalities rarely occur in association with this abnormality.[19–21]

Ulnar deficiency is also associated with three congenital syndromes. Cornelia de Lange syndrome is characterized by growth retardation, generalized hirsutism, characteristic facies, and upper limb involvement ranging from total limb agenesis to minor abnormalities. Femur-fibula-ulna syndrome involves proximal focal femoral deficiency, fibula agenesis, and ulnar defects. Schinzel syndrome involves ulnar ray deficits, hypogenitalism, and anal atresia. All three syndromes are quite rare.[15] The etiology of isolated ulnar hemimelia is unknown. Cases appear to be sporadic and nongenetic. Disorder of bone growth may result in a shortened deformed ulna, bowed radius, and dislocated radial head, but should be differentiated from ulnar hemimelia deformity.[15]

Etiology

Ogino and Kato[8] have produced ulnar deficiencies in pregnant Gunn-Wistar rats by administering busulfan at 8.5 to 10 days of gestation. The critical period for producing ulnar deficiencies is earlier than that for radial deficiencies and corresponds to a higher rate of fetal mortality. Because of this higher rate of fetal mortality, the relative incidence of this deformity may be higher than that reported for live births.[8] In a review of the gestational history, both in The Shriners Hospital for Children and in the literature, no exogenic teratogen has been identified or associated with any certainty in cases of ulnar hemimelia.

Isolated reports of familial inheritance, which were considered an autosomal dominant trait for ulnar deficiency, were found in three successive generations. Roberts in 1885, Renval in 1908, Truchi in 1960, and Blokey in 1963 report familial inheritance.[15] A recessive inheritance, or X-link recessive trait, has been reported by Bergag.[15] The 21q chromosome has been implicated.[12,13]

O'Rahilly[22] ranks long-bone deficiencies in the order of decreasing frequency: fibula, radius, femur, tibia, ulna, and humerus. Only absence of the humerus is more infrequent than ulnar deficiency as reported by Laurin and Farmer.[23]

Clinical Manifestation

The ulnar deficiencies are associated primarily with musculoskeletal defects. Fifty percent of the patients involved will have other musculoskeletal defects in addition to their ulnar hemimelia.

In ulnar hemimelia, the radius bows towards the ulnar aspect of the forearm with the apex of the bow pointing radially, creating an apparent ulnar deviation of the hand. The absence of bony development creates a rigid tethering soft-tissue and cartilaginous anlage that tethers to the radius and the ulna carpus. This structure includes the interosseous membrane, the ulna remnant as a cartilaginous structure, the ulnar-based muscles, and the ulnar neurovascular structures. Historically, significant ulnar deviation of the hand has been implicated, with the presence of the fibrocartilaginous anlage as the underlying cause, and early excision has been recommended.[3]

When severe ulnar deficiency occurs, a short proximal ulna can result with elbow instability and radial head dislocation (Fig. 2, *top*). There may be a coexisting elbow synostosis involving humeral, radiohumeral, or ulnohumeral elbow components. Involvement at the level of the elbow has created the greatest functional deficiencies in children with good hand function (Fig. 2, *bottom left*). The more complex and involved is the elbow, including radiohumeral synostosis, the more involved and deficient is the shoulder girdle (Fig. 2, *bottom right*).

Functional deficit varies with degree of involvement and bilaterality of the condition. Correctible dysfunction is a result of hand deformities that include ectrodactyly, syndactyly, hypoplasia, and malrotation of the hand, which interfere with prehension, dexterity, and hand strength. Hand deformities may involve total absence of the hand and multiple variations as outlined by Cole and Manske.[5]

Forearm, elbow, and shoulder deformity is cosmetically unacceptable and contributes to some loss of dexterity and weakness; however, if prehension is possible, excellent function is generally observed in these children. Southwood[24] reports "from the functional standpoint, therefore, the deformed limb is much more useful than its anatomic condition would lead one to accept."

Classification

Classification systems for ulnar hemimelia have been proposed by Kümmel (1895),[25] Lausecker (1954),[26] Riordan and associates (1961),[3] Ogden and associates (1996),[27] Dobyns and associates (1982),[28] Swanson (1976),[29] Miller and associates (1986),[30] and Ogino and Kato (1988).[8]

All classification systems address the ulna and elbow involvement. Lausecker,[26] Ogino and Kato,[8] and Cole and Manske[5] have included hand anomalies in the classification system. Shoulder involvement reported by Swanson and associates[22] and Masson and Bennett[19] correlates the clinical incidence of hypoplasia or dysplasia about the shoulder with elbow (radiohumeral) synostosis.

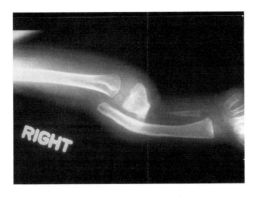

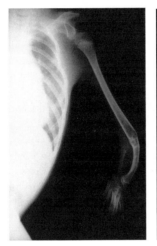 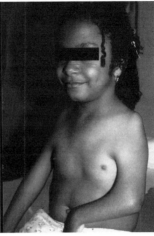

Fig. 2 Top, *Bayne type II with radial head dislocation and unstable elbow.* ***Bottom left,*** *Bayne type IV with radiohumeral synostosis.* ***Bottom right,*** *Radiohumeral synostosis, pterygium of the skin and soft tissues of the elbow, and glenohumeral shoulder deficit.*

Bayne classification of ulnar hemimelia involves four types: type I, hypoplasia of the ulna; type II, partial aplasia of the ulna; type III, total aplasia of the ulna; and type IV, radiohumerus synostosis.[28] This classification is most commonly accepted but does not address variation in hand anomalies nor does it address hypoplasia and instability of the glenohumeral joint.

International classification and nomenclature of congenital anomalies place the ulnar deficient extremity in classification I, failure of formation of parts as a longitudinal deficiency. Classification according to International Nomenclature would list Group I, L (longitudinal), L-R (left or right), UL (proximal one third), carpal partial, fifth ray.[28,29] Variations to the classification system may include a normal appearing ulna with the hand deficiencies or a complete absent hand with ulna defect.

Treatment

The goal of treatment is to maximize function. Cosmetic improvement should not be obtained at the expense of functional use. Surgical treatment has been directed at the hand, wrist, forearm, elbow, and humerus. The shoulder, although affected, has not been addressed surgically. More severe shoulder involvement is associated with more severe elbow involvement, particularly radiohumeral synostosis.

Splinting and casting techniques applied at birth and continued until surgery and throughout childhood have been recommended. The effectiveness of such splinting and casting has not been correlated clinically, and progression of deformity is rare. Surgical release of syndactyly, web deepening, metacarpal rotational osteotomy, pollicization, and lengthening procedures have all demonstrated measurable improvement in hand function.[4,29]

Resection of the distal ulnar fibrocartilaginous anlage has been recommended at an early age by many and condemned by others. Some authors state that the anlage is not a deviation force.[3,31,32] Ulnar deviation greater than 30° at the wrist has been an indication for ulnar anlage resection.[32] Ulnar anlage may be demonstrated by MRI, and resection also is indicated if simultaneous forearm or elbow procedures are performed.

Rotational osteotomies at the level of the forearm or of the humerus have been effective to position the hand in space for function. Radial head resection, because of dislocation, has not improved elbow function or corrected radial bowing. Instability of the elbow may result from radial head excision. Pterygium release has been ineffective as a means of improving function or cosmesis.

The creation of a single-bone forearm has been recommended for instability about the elbow.[33–35] Clinical results of surgically created one-bone forearms indicate that the procedure is a viable salvage option for forearm instability in selected patients.[36] Riordan[4] has recommended one-bone forearm for elbow instability. Nonunions and complications associated with this procedure are significant, and the results may be less predictable than the literature suggests (Fig. 3).

Distraction lengthening procedures, such as the Ilizarov soft-tissue and callus-distraction techniques, have been used for cosmetic improvement of unilaterally involved upper extremities.[37,38] Functional improvement from forearm lengthening has yet to be determined in a long-term clinical study.

Arthroplasty to restore elbow function or stability has been universally unsuccessful. Vascularized epiphyseal transfer using the proximal fibula has been performed experimentally, but longitudinal growth results and long-term follow-up are unknown.

Function is the most important consideration in evaluation of patients with congenital upper extremity anomalies. Blair and associates[39] report 46% of predicted normal active motion and 27% of the power grip of the contralateral extremity and state that precision tests were generally well performed. Patients performed most poorly when the ulnar hemimelia included radiohumeral synostosis or congenital absence, deformity, or contracture of the ipsilateral digits.

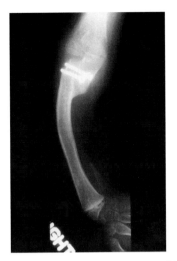

Fig. 3 Soft-tissue lengthening with the Ilizarov technique was followed by the creation of a one-bone forearm to obtain functional elbow stability and cosmetic length of the unilaterally involved extremity.

Shriners Hospital For Children Experience

Outcomes for 116 patients from seven Shriners Hospitals for Children were reviewed. A total of 75 surgical procedures were performed; 44 were related to the hand, and 31 were related to the remaining upper extremity. Three Z-plasties for elbow pterygium were performed without improvement, nine ulnar analog excisions were performed without correction of the deforming radial bow, and one distal lateral radial epiphysiodesis was performed without improvement. Procedures performed with reported improvements in either cosmesis or function included 11 radial bow corrections, four elbow rotational osteotomies, one radial head resection, one wrist fusion, and one both bone forearm creation.

The multicenter Shriners Hospitals for Children Study included 116 patients with 146 involved extremities. Of these, 30 had bilateral involvement, and 86 had unilateral involvement (47 left and 39 right extremities). Ages ranged from 2 weeks to 41 years. There were 39 females and 77 males. A total of 50 patients (43%) underwent surgery. Twenty-eight had only hand surgery, 11 had elbow and forearm surgery, and 11 had combined elbow and forearm procedures. According to Bayne's classification system, there were 11 type I, 23 type II, 40 type III, and 67 type IV findings. None of the hand findings correlated with any one type of classification system. Shoulder involvement was found in 19 patients, approximately 15%, and primarily occurred with more extensive elbow involvement, as demonstrated in Bayne type IV findings.

Surgical procedures found to be of limited or no benefit included excision of ulna anlage, pterygium correction, elbow arthroplasty, and shoulder surgery. Surgical procedures found to benefit the patient involved all hand procedures, corrective or rotational osteotomies, and stabilization of the unstable elbow with or without the creation of a one-bone forearm.

Current bone lengthening procedures for forearm and humerus with the Ilizarov technique are being used in unilateral cases. Free vascular epiphyseal transfers are being performed experimentally to correct the deformity and to provide growth. Results and functional success of these procedures are unknown at present.

Summary

Early casting or splinting have not been found to be effective. Hand procedures benefit function, and rotation osteotomy improves hand position. A single-bone forearm will create stability in cases of elbow or forearm instability.

Ulna anlage resection and pterygium correction do not improve function or cosmesis. Elbow arthroplasties are unsuccessful, and shoulder surgery is not indicated. The functional results of bone lengthening and vascularized epiphyseal fractures are unknown at this time.

The current classification systems are not useful for predicting progression of the deformity or the results of surgical reconstruction. Hand involvement and shoulder involvement are not included in the current classification systems.

References

1. Flatt AE (ed): Ulnar deficiencies, in *The Care of Congenital Hand Anomalies*, ed 2. St. Louis, MO, Quality Medical Publishing, 1994, pp 411–432.

2. Johnson J, Omer GE Jr: Congenital ulnar deficiency: Natural history and therapeutic implications. *Hand Clin* 1985;1:499–510.

3. Riordan DC, Mills EH, Alldredge RH: Abstract: Congenital absence of the ulna. *J Bone Joint Surg* 1961;43A:614.

4. Riordan DC: The upper limb, in Lovell WW, Winter RB (eds): *Pediatric Orthopaedics*. Philadelphia, PA, JB Lippincott, 1978, vol 2, pp 685–719.

5. Cole RJ, Manske PR: Classification of ulnar deficiency according to the thumb and first web. *J Hand Surg* 1997;22A:479–488.

6. Goeller DGC: Abortus humani monstros. *His Anta Misc Acad Nat* Curtos, Norimb, Decuria 2, 1683, pp 311–318.

7. Birch-Jensen A (ed): *Congenital Deformities of the Upper Extremities*. Odense, Denmark, Andelsbogtrykkeriet, 1949, pp 46–47.

8. Ogino T, Kato H: Clinical and experimental studies on ulnar ray deficiency. *Handchirurgie* 1988;20:330–337.

9. Kato H, Ogino T, Minami A, Fukuda K: Anatomical study on oligodactyly induced by myleran with special reference to the relationship between skeletal and soft tissue malformations. *J Jpn Soc Surg Hand* 1985;2:258–262.

10. McCredie J: Neural crest defects: A neuroanatomic basis for classification of multiple malformations related to phocomelia. *J Neurol Sci* 1975;28:373–387.

11. Ogden JA, Vickers TH, Tauber JE, Light TR: A model for ulnar dysmelia. *Yale J Biol Med* 1978;51:193–206.

12. Gurrieri F, Cammarata M, Avarello RM, et al: Ulnar ray defect in an infant with a 6q21; 7q31.2 translocation: Further evidence for the existence of a limb defect gene in 621. *Am J Med Genet* 1995;55:315–318.

13. Reynolds JF, Wyandt HE, Kelly TE: De novo 21q interstitial deletion in a retarded boy with ulno-fibular dysostosis. *Am J Med Genet* 1985;20:173–180.

14. Langer LO Jr: Mesomelic dwarfism of the hypoplastic ulna, fibula, mandible type. *Radiology* 1967;89:654–660.

15. Temtamy S, McKusick VA, Bergsma D, et al (eds): *The Genetics of Hand Malformations*. New York, NY, Alan R Liss, 1978, pp 48–50.

16. Goldberg MJ (ed): *The Dysmorphic Child: An Orthopedic Perspective*. New York, NY, Raven Press, 1987.

17. Di Bella D, Di Stefano G, Romeo MG, Pavone L: Abstract: Upper limb cardiovascular syndrome with ulna agenesis. *Pediatr Radiol* 1984;14:259.

18. Inoue G, Miura T: Arteriographic findings in radial and ulnar deficiencies. *J Hand Surg* 1991;16G:409–412.

19. Manske PR: Longitudinal failure of upper-limb formation. *J Bone Joint Surg* 1996;78A:1600–1623.

20. Frantz CH, O'Rahilly R: Congenital skeletal limb deficiencies. *J Bone Joint Surg* 1961;43A:1202–1224.

21. Swanson AB, Tada K, Yonenobu K: Ulnar ray deficiency: Its various manifestations. *J Hand Surg* 1984;9A:658–664.

22. O'Rahilly R: Morphological patterns in limb deficiencies and duplications. *Am J Anat* 1951;89:135–193.

23. Laurin CA, Farmer AW: Congenital absence of ulna. *Can J Surg* 1959,2:204–207.

24. Southwood AR: Partial absence of the ulnar and associated structures. *J Anat* 1927;61:346–351.

25. Kümmel W: Die missbildungen der extremitaeten durch defekt, verwachsung und ueberzahl. Kassel, Germany, Bibliotheca Medica, 1895, vol 3, pp 1–83.

26. Lausecker H: Der angeborene Defekt der Ulna. *Virchows Arch Pathol Anat Physiol Klin Med* 1954;325:211–226.

27. Ogden JA, Watson HK, Bohne W: Ulnar dysmelia. *J Bone Joint Surg* 1996;58A:467–475.

28. Dobyns JH, Wood VE, Bayne LG, Frykman GK: Congenital hand deformities, in Green DP (ed): *Operative Hand Surgery*. New York, NY, Churchill Livingstone, 1982, pp 213–450.

29. Swanson AB: A classification for congenital limb malformations. *J Hand Surg* 1976;1A:8–22.

30. Miller JK, Wenner SM, Kruger LM: Ulnar deficiency. *J Hand Surg* 1986;11A:822–829.

31. Watson HK, Bohne WH: Abstract: The role of the fibrous band in ulnar deficient extremities. *J Bone Joint Surg* 1971;53A:816.

32. Marcus NA, Omer GE Jr: Carpal deviation in congenital ulnar deficiency. *J Bone Joint Surg* 1984;66A:1003–1007.

33. Spinner M, Freundlich BD, Abeles ED: Management of moderate longitudinal arrest of development of the ulna. *Clin Orthop* 1970;69:199–202.

34. Vitale CC: Reconstructive surgery for defects in the shaft of the ulna in children. *J Bone Joint Surg* 1952;34A:804–810.

35. Lloyd-Roberts GC: Treatment of defects of the ulna in children by establishing cross-union with the radius. *J Bone Joint Surg* 1973;55B:327–330.

36. Peterson CA II, Maki S, Wood MB: Clinical results of the one-bone forearm. *J Hand Surg* 1995;20A:609–618.

37. Kitano K, Tada K: One-bone forearm procedure for partial defect of the ulnar. *J Pediatr Orthop* 1985;5:290–293.

38. Smith AA, Greene TL: Preliminary soft tissue distraction in congenital forearm deficiency. *J Hand Surg* 1995;20A:420–424.

39. Blair WF, Shurr DG, Buckwalter JA: Functional status in ulnar deficiency. *J Pediatr Orthop* 1983;3:37–40.

Chapter 34

Prosthetic Devices For Children With Bilateral Upper Limb Deficiencies: When and If, Pros and Cons

Mary Williams Clark, MD
Diane J. Atkins, OTR
Sheila A. Hubbard, PT, OT, BSc
Joanna G. Patton, BS, OTR
Julie Shaperman, MSPH, OTR

Children with bilateral upper limb differences, with or without normal lower limbs, will have many different needs depending on their age, developmental stage, cognition, presence of grasping function, usefulness of lower limbs, and length and strength of all limbs.

Age

We will consider "ages" as infancy: birth to one year; childhood: 1 to 10 years; adolescence: 11 to 17 years; and adulthood: 18 years and older.

During infancy, the gross motor functions of the child are acquired in progression, and not necessarily in the same order for all children. They include exploration of the environment, sitting, rolling, (crawling), (pulling to stand), standing, and (bimanual grasp), among others. Items in parentheses may not occur for some children missing upper limbs at a high level. The needs of the family at this time are bonding, acceptance of the child as she or he is, cosmesis, and understanding of ways to facilitate competence and independence of the child, among others.

In childhood, the child's needs extend to play, activities of daily living (ADL), interaction with others, social acceptance, communication, mobility, and learning—again, among other more detailed needs. The ADL in detail include eating, upper and lower body dressing, school and play skills, and the various aspects of personal hygiene, which include cleaning body, teeth, and hair; toileting; and feminine hygiene.

Adolescents must begin to master self-esteem and self-acceptance, extend play into recreation, sports, and other avocational activities, as well as continue with independence, prevocational activities, and the other issues noted above. In adulthood, the needs include all of the above plus vocation, financial independence, and family.

For our patients with significant limb differences, such as absence of hands or hands and elbows, some of the goals listed above will be possible only with the assistance of another person, in spite of prosthetic fitting and training. Others will be done independently, in some cases with the help of adaptations to living arrangements and equipment, with or without prostheses.

Developmental Stage

A "natural experiment" occurred over time at the Child Amputee Prosthetic Project (CAPP). In the early years (1950s and 1960s), children were fitted with equipment to replace whatever absence they had; for example, quadrimembral limb deficient babies wore shoulder caps with props, similar to stubbies for legs, to encourage crawling. That didn't work. Most of the children fitted early with lots of equipment ended up rejecting upper prostheses entirely. Starting in the late 1960s, children were provided the least amount of equipment possible, and only if necessary to meet specific needs. The second approach produced no better long-term wear acceptance than the earlier approach because parents and children demanded more and more equipment, and when they became weighed down with too much of it, they too rejected the prostheses.

Children with high level upper or multiple limb deficiencies should probably not be fitted with a prosthesis before one year of age so that they have freedom to roll on the floor, develop trunk balance, and explore with residual limbs and mouth. During the preprosthetic period, parents can become very anxious about "doing nothing." Home programs—programs taught to the parents for them to use, not home visits by the therapist—can encourage achievement of normal developmental milestones, and visits with the clinic team every 3 or 4 months can assess progress and add new information and suggestions appropriately.

Most children with limb deficiencies will not need "early intervention developmental stimulation" programs, because they have not suffered a neurologic insult and usually are normal cognitively.[1] They may alter the "normal" pattern of gross motor development; for example, rolling early, developing sitting balance late, and skipping crawling altogether. This alteration should not be interpreted as evidence of developmental delay, and will be highly individual.

Cognition

Almost all children with congenital and acquired limb deficiencies have normal cognition; the exceptions are some of the uncommon syndromes (eg, Cornelia de Lange). There may be some with traumatic loss who had preexisting impulse-control problems, or hyperactivity; these will influence training programs, but in general there will not be difficulty in understanding or being understood.

Grasping Function

If usable digits remain and can be used to grasp, they will be preferred to any prosthetic limb or device because of the sensory feedback (sensibility). If the upper limbs are long enough to meet each other, even if they have no grasping digits, they will also usually be preferred to one or two prostheses for many functions. If they meet in an area where they can't be seen well, prosthetic use on one or both limbs may offer additional function. Small digits with weak muscle may strengthen as they gain additional length with growth, and the muscle itself may be strengthened with a progressive-resistance program, using rubber bands or manual resistance. Even if grasp with these digits isn't possible, they may work switches or myoelectric controls. Surgical removal of "nubbins" or digits is usually inappropriate.

The best substitutes for hands are feet, if they are available. Children whose lower limbs are normal, or who have feet with functional toes and sufficient limb length to get them to other parts of their body, will almost always prefer using them to prostheses, although they may very well find prostheses useful for some tasks at various times (Fig. 1). They need to be encouraged from the beginning to use their feet (no socks; shoes that can be actively slipped on and off, etc).[2] Even children with acquired bilateral upper limb loss at an "older" age, even past puberty, may still have or can acquire with exercise the flexibility at hips, knees, ankles, and midfeet to use their feet and toes for grasping and manipulating, although they may never become as facile as those with congenital absence. This means that lower limb differences usually treated by "conversion" amputations, for example, fibular or tibial absence, or PFFD, should not be altered in patients with bilateral upper limb deficiency until the absence of need for foot function is clear.

Nonprosthetic grasping is also possible between shoulder and chin, limb and trunk, head and knee, in mouth, etc. These are avenues to independence and should not be discouraged. (Radios turned on by nose, balls thrown by a short, elbowless, fingerless arm and chin, etc, are definitely possible[3] [Fig. 2].)

Activities of Daily Living: Body Function "Versus" Prosthetic Fitting

"Versus" is in quotation marks because this is not an either-or dichotomy. Some tasks will be best accomplished with a prosthesis, others without, and this will vary with the particular child's anatomic situation, parents, and her or his own personality, as well as the child's particular stage in life.

Specific functional tasks need to be taught by a therapist, and the specific details very individually adapted. In general, the best success results from trying first to adapt the child's own (body movement) performance, and then to adapt the environment, including adapted equipment, and usually last to attempt prosthetic use for most ADL (unpublished data). Working with the patient and family to include their observations is usually very helpful.

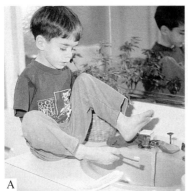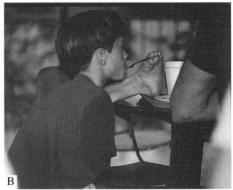

Fig. 1 *Boy with high bilateral upper limb deficiencies (longitudinal, humeral partial, rad/ulna total, carpal total, rays 1-4 total), demonstrating his independent foot function.* **A,** *Brushing teeth.* **B,** *Using fork.*

Clothing can be chosen to facilitate independence; for example, loose shirts, sweatpants, and so forth, with as few adaptive changes as possible. Make any necessary changes inconspicuous. Hygiene, including toileting and feminine menstrual hygiene, is perhaps the most challenging area. Task-specific adapted devices should be kept to the realistic minimum, to avoid the need to carry them around. Diet and routine bowel programs can establish predictable times that can be planned to be convenient; for example, at home in the morning or evening.[4]

Prosthetic options include body-powered, external powered, and hybrid systems, that is, a combination of body and external power. External power currently is battery-power, although carbon-dioxide cartridge power is again available in smaller, lighter-weight containers than those available 20 years ago. Hybrid systems are often most appropriate because they can combine lighter weight with some proprioceptive feedback, with the use of a cable to control a terminal device, or a cable-controlled elbow. Appropriate components vary with age and development. For older amputees who can tolerate the weight, powered wrist-rotators have been found to be very useful.

For those with high-level amputations, prosthetic wear should be introduced as intermittent and task-appropriate; that is, as a tool for a specific task. There need to be specific times for not wearing prostheses, to decrease sweating and heat retention. As function without prostheses develops, wear times can be modified so that the prostheses are used for appropriate functions but do not inhibit other functional options. It is also important to remember that cosmesis is a function (AB Swanson, unpublished data, 1988).

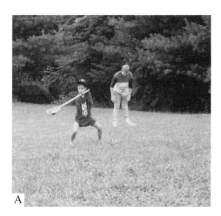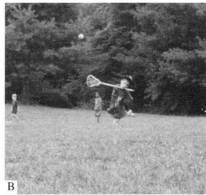

Fig. 2 *Same young man as in Figure 1, at 12 years old, catching and throwing a tennis ball during his first encounter with a lacrosse stick. He is balancing the stick with his chin and the ends of his arms. (His humeri are approximately 6 in long. He has only a single digit, originating at the side of the left humerus, with limited strength—he can support a pencil or lightweight spoon between it and the arm; a similar digit on the right arm was removed in infancy.)* **A,** *Catching a tennis ball.* **B,** *Throwing the ball.*

Relevant Experience

We reviewed children with bilateral upper limb deficiencies, excluding those with distal longitudinal deficiencies not fitted, seen by the authors in the following clinics: (1) Bloorview MacMillan Hospital, formerly Ontario Crippled Children's Centre, and Hugh MacMillan Hospital, Toronto; (2) Child Amputee Prosthetic Project (CAPP) at UCLA, Los Angeles; (3) later patients from CAPP at Los Angeles Shriners Hospital; (4) Children's Hospital of Pittsburgh; (5) Children's Hospital of New Orleans; (6) [Kluge] Children's Rehabilitation Center, Charlottesville, Virginia; and (7) University Hospital Rehabilitation Center, including the former Elizabethtown Hospital, Hershey, Pennsylvania. The numbers, respectively, were 29, 43, and 27 from the first three institutions and 11 from the last four, a total of 110 patients. Of these children, 85% (93) had congenital deficiencies, for a congenital to acquired etiology ratio of approximately 5:1.

A total of 19/38 patients (50%) were wearing their prostheses part-time or full-time at the age of 17 years or older, when last seen. The numbers of body-powered and externally powered prostheses in this group are approximately equal. Eight of these 19 patients are known to wear them primarily in public or for work only; they prefer not to use them at home.

We attempted further analysis of this apparently large number of these patients, but the number of variations, beginning with three groups for foot function: full use, partial use (requiring a prosthesis or wheelchair for mobility), or not useful; and various prostheses: body-powered, switch or myoelectrically controlled, hybrid, or cosmetic; along with age differences, brings the numbers down to small denominators with little statistical meaning to be gleaned.

Conclusion

Ironically, although the functional need increases with more anatomic absence or loss, the tolerance for wear of prostheses decreases. Perspiration, heat-dissipation problems, and energy consumption required for wear alone, not even counting energy needed for function with the prosthesis, are significant. Use of a prosthesis has been compared to learning to use a musical instrument, requiring steady and ongoing practice. Personality differences affect gadget tolerance, ability to concentrate, and ability to persevere; therefore, affecting ability to learn to use a prosthesis.

Often the benefit of fitting with external power has seemed to be primarily prestige for the child, among peers and teachers, and only secondarily task performance. The positive visibility is often countered by the discovery that the high-tech "bionic" arms are hot, heavy, and not as functional as hoped. The body-powered hooks and other non-hands, for example, CAPP terminal devices and Adept voluntary-closing terminal devices, are very often found to be more useful for grasp and manipulation than the more cosmetic terminal devices. The expectation is common that "the best"—something combining all functions—must be available somewhere else, and when something better can't be found the family and the (often by now) teenager may be frustrated and hostile, full of anger that what they are missing cannot be fully replaced.

At the same time that we have focused on restoration of function we have often, inappropriately, disparaged the need for cosmesis felt by the parents and ultimately by the children/young adults. Many individual stories emphasize the difference a hand can make to self-confidence, particularly at certain ages (and apparently well before adolescence). Counseling of patients and family (including siblings) should be made more available, as well as opportunities for children and their families to meet others in very similar situations; that is, those with similar anatomic levels, bilaterality, use of lower limbs, etc, if possible. Information about such opportunities is available from the Amputee Coalition of America.

We agree that children (and young adults) with high-level upper limb loss should have the opportunity to wear prostheses, best fitted at a time when the prostheses will help them experience developmental milestones and perform age-appropriate tasks, or selected activities. External power may be useful for situations in which body power cannot, because of lack of excursion or strength, provide the same function, but in and of itself is not better. Experienced prosthetists and therapists are essential to maximize adjustments (in cable tensioning, sensitivity of electrodes, placement and positioning, and so forth) for best function.

Decisions that children make to stop using prostheses should be respected and not seen as a negative choice; they are usually positive choices for independent function. Very often the child will wish to try one or two prostheses again, for specific functions that may vary with age. Clinics should continue to follow these patients, whether or not they are prosthetic wearers.

References

1. Rosenfelder R: Infant amputees: Early growth and care. *Clin Orthop* 1980; 148:41–46.

2. Wilke HH (ed): *Using Everything You've Got,* rev ed. Chicago, IL, National Easter Seal Society for Crippled Children and Adults, 1984.

3. Setoguchi Y, Rosenfelder R (eds): *The Limb Deficient Child*, ed 2. Springfield, IL, Charles C Thomas, 1982.

4. Friedmann L: Toileting self-care methods for bilateral high level upper limb amputees. *Prosthet Orthot Int* 1980;4:29–36.

Chapter 35

Prosthetic Principles in Fitting Myoelectric Prostheses in Children

C. Michael Schuch, BA, CPO

Introduction

Early fitting of children with upper-limb deficiency has long been an accepted objective of pediatric prosthetic clinics.[1-6] During the last 15 years, two questions have been asked. Just how early should the child be fit? What type of prosthesis is most successful and acceptable to the child, the parents, and the clinic team?[4,7-9]

When to fit is generally accepted: "fit when they sit."[4] How to fit initially is more controversial.[9-19] Some clinics first fit with passive mitts or cosmetic hands. Some fit with the intended functional device.

In 1978, the Child Amputee Prosthetics Project (CAPP) began investigating the efficacy of fitting children with myoelectric prostheses, and many children from the age of 2 years and older demonstrated the ability to use such a prosthesis. At that time, components from various manufacturers were not easily integrated, and no manufacturer made a complete system for children, so the prosthetic team had to modify components in house to provide a child-sized comprehensive system (D Blades, CPO, Torrence, CA, personal communication, 1997).

During the 1980s, interest in fitting children with myoelectric prostheses increased dramatically.[8-13,17,20-31] As a result, the ages of children fit with myoelectric prostheses began to decrease. Subsequently, reports based on the Data Acquisiton Device (DAD)[32,33] introduced by the Hugh MacMillan Medical Center indicated that many children were not functional users, but that myoelectric prostheses were accepted by children primarily on a cosmetic basis.[9,27,30] In 1984, a study involving 120 children from 11 units of the Shriners Hospital system concluded that myoelectric prostheses were not functional, but were acceptable to children cosmetically.[34] Enthusiasm for fitting younger children with myoelectric prostheses thus declined in the late 1980s.

In 1989, successful fitting was reported of infants from 1 to 6 months of age with a passive hand self-suspending prosthesis followed by a myoelectric prosthesis, usually after the infant outgrew the initial passive prosthesis.[35] The reporting group introduced the St. Anthony's circuit, also known as the "cookie cruncher," a single site, voluntary opening, automatic closing myo-electric system designed for young children who cannot comprehend the use of a dual site, dual function system.[35]

In the fall of 1989, I began to study prosthetic use in the upper-limb defi-cient population at the Shriners Hospital in Greenville, SC. At that time, children and families generally received whatever type of prosthesis they requested. They were free to experiment with new prosthetic designs, to change from one type of prosthesis to another, and, in many cases, to receive both body-powered and myoelectric prostheses. There was no pressure to accept or use any prosthesis. Those who rejected prostheses were asked to continue to be followed in clinic for educational purposes.

I initiated an observational prospective study of all the children with upper limb deficiencies seen in the clinic. I recorded demographic and clinical data as well as prosthetic choices, use patterns, and satisfaction. If a child received a new prosthesis, data included type, date received, and use patterns. Each time the child was seen, the database was updated. In addition, parents were encouraged to provide photographs and/or videos of their children using their prostheses in everyday situations or, alternative-ly, compensating without their prostheses. The study was conducted from 1989 to 1991.[7]

One hundred thirty-one children (68 girls, 63 boys) with unilateral defi-ciencies of the forearm were included in the study. Four deficiencies were traumatic, and 127 were congenital. Ages ranged from 5 months to 20 years, average age was 8 years 11 months. Eighty-four children preferred myoelectric prostheses; 32 preferred body-powered prostheses; eight pre-ferred cosmetic, passive partial hand prostheses; and seven preferred no prosthesis (Table 1). Eleven of the 84 children who preferred myoelectrics had another prosthesis for backup.

Seventeen patients were fit "early." I defined early fitting for this study as fitting at 3 years of age or under. The protocol for early fittings was a pas-sive, self-suspending prosthesis with infant hand initially, followed by a cookie cruncher myoelectric prosthesis after the passive was outgrown.

No surveys or tests were administered to study participants, nor was there any attempt to define or to measure function. However, the photographs and videos provided by the parents strongly suggested that most children really did find their prostheses functionally useful.

Subjective conclusions of the study are as follows. A child with a con-genital forearm deficiency should be provided a passive, self-suspending prosthesis during the first 3 months of life. When the child outgrows the pas-sive prosthesis, usually between 9 and 15 months of age, an acceptable pro-tocol for the next prosthesis is a voluntary opening/automatic closing/single site myoelectric prosthesis. In the study, all children fit with such a prosthe-sis spontaneously began activation or control of the hand on the first day of fitting. This is in contrast to the long delays noted in children learning to control conventional body powered/cable operated hooks or hands. Early fit children subsequently became better users than children fit later.

The choice not to use a prosthesis or to reject prosthesis use is often pre-dictable. Rejection most often occurs after a period when the child cannot

Table 1 Prostheses in Shriners Hospital study

Description of Prosthesis	Girls	Boys
Therapeutic Recreation Systems (TRS) voluntary closing, body-powered prosthesis	4	12
Split hook, voluntary opening, body-powered prosthesis	2	7
Hand, voluntary opening, body-powered prosthesis	1	0
Split hook interchangeable with hand, voluntary opening, body-powered prosthesis	2	4
Cosmetic, passive, partial hand prosthesis	6	2
Myoelectric prosthesis	51	33
Rejection or chose no prosthesis	2	5

wear a previously provided prosthesis either due to outgrowing it and un-timely delay in pursuing a new fitting, or due to excessive down time for repairs. The second most common reason for rejection was a long residual limb (wrist level or more distal), where it was felt that the prosthesis inter-fered with sensation; this reason is supported in other literature.[36]

Reliability of myoelectric prostheses was superior to that of body-pow-ered prostheses. The most common myoelectric prosthesis problems were wires disconnecting from the electrodes and hand malfunction; the most common body-powered problem was cable fraying.

Weaknesses of the study include the absence of children with bilateral limb deficiency or deficiency proximal to the forearm, the relatively short duration of the study, and the lack of statistical analysis.

Because the forearm deficient level is by far the most commonly encoun-tered upper-limb deficiency, most components, systems, and management strategies focus on the child with a forearm level deficiency.

Overview of a Typical Myoelectric System

Power Source

The power source is the muscles of the residual limb. The most common level of myoelectric fit to children is the transradial level; power sources for this level are the residual wrist extensors and flexors. Other residual limb levels capable of providing myoelectric control include the tran-shumeral level (power source, biceps and triceps) and the shoulder disar-ticulation level (power source, anterior and posterior deltoids). The higher the level of deficiency, the more complicated are the prosthesis and diffi-culty of use.

Electromyographic Surface Electrodes

The electrochemical activity of muscle contraction can be measured on the skin surface in microvolts. This output becomes the power source that will be captured and channeled into the myoelectric system. The electrode, placed over the appropriate muscle sites, receives the microvolts generated by muscle contractions, interprets these signals, and sends them down the line in the myoelectric system. Some electrodes are capable of sensitivity adjustment directly on the electrode component itself. Other electrodes merely send the signal onward to another component, which incorporates gain control.

I do not conduct surface electrode site testing in infants and small children because they do not yet have the ability to follow directions sufficiently to conduct such testing, and the electrodes are large and sensitive enough that it is easy to identify the correct location.

Batteries

The output received by the electrodes is not sufficient to run a myoelectric prosthesis. The signals captured by the surface electrodes must be supported by a more powerful electronic source, the battery. Traditional batteries in myoelectric prostheses have been nickel cadmium (NiCad) mounted either invisibly within the prosthesis or externally. Internal batteries require the availability of the entire prosthesis for the charging period, which varies from 1 to 2 hours for quick chargers to overnight for standard chargers. External batteries have the advantage of being easily removed from their housing and inserted into table-top charging components, thereby allowing the user to have one or more fully charged batteries available at all times.

A major disadvantage of NiCad batteries is decreasing memory. Unless a NiCad battery is fully discharged before the ensuing recharge cycle, battery output is reduced. In addition, it is difficult to use a myoelectric prosthesis as the battery nears full discharge because the child must exert much more effort than when the batteries are fully charged to achieve the same functional speed and response. Lithium ion batteries and their flexible cousin, lithium polymer batteries never develop decreasing memory, have greatly increased service hours, and a greatly increased total number of discharge/recharge cycles (up to ten times the total cycle lifetime of NiCad batteries).

Functional Options

In the simplest form, the function of the electric signal is a degree of hand motion. Myoelectric hand function currently includes only a basic movement of "three jaw chuck" prehension, in which the thumb opposes to the index and long fingers. The fourth and fifth digits do not move unless mechanically connected to the index and long finger, and do not move independently. The simplest hand function used for children is a format of voluntary opening with automatic closing (cookie cruncher). Myoelectric control of both opening and closing is more common. In more complicated schemes, wrist rotation control can be included. For deficiency levels above the elbow, electronic motor control of elbow flexion and extension can be included, but because of complexity, expense, and weight, these options are more for adults or older children.

Control Schemes

Control schemes are the specific methods of hand, wrist, and/or elbow control; they depend on the number of electrodes and the specific configuration of "the brains" of the myoelectric system. Early myoelectric systems controlled only hand opening and closing. Later in the evolution of systems, a wrist rotation motor was added with accompanying logic to control both hand and wrist. Even later, a special electronic circuit provided the concept of the "cookie cruncher." Until recently, control schemes have been electronic circuits or circuit boards that were programmed for a specific control scheme. Variations of control schemes often meant changing component hardware within the myoelectric system. There was no easy system of selection and instantaneous change of control schemes. The latest development is an onboard microcomputer circuit, coupled with a microcomputer prosthesis control unit (PCU), which from a remote or off-board wireless position can program any existing hardware system for any of at least a dozen different control schemes.

There are two basic types of system response to myoelectric signals: digital and proportional. Digital control is "on" or "off." Once the myoelectric signal passes a set threshold, the electronic response is constant, regardless of signal strength or speed; the signal acts as an on/off switch and the hand and/or wrist response is one speed. Proportional control is proportional to the signal strength or output. Slow or easy muscle contraction, once over a minimum threshold, provides a slow hand and/or wrist action. Fast or heavy muscle contraction provides quick response. This allows finer control of the hand or wrist speed. Most systems are either digital or proportional, not interchangeable. The latest development in myoelectric systems allows easy interchange from digital to proportional control, regardless of the other facets of the chosen control scheme.

Whenever two opposing sites are used, clear distinction of signals from each site is a must. If both muscle sites produce signal output at the same time or same rate, the signal is canceled out in most systems. Some refer to this as signal site "cross-talk." The ability to discriminate between opposing muscle site signals is sometimes the most difficult aspect of myoelectric control for the user to learn and master. The more advanced the control system, the easier it is to overcome and tune out this potential problem.

Types of Systems

Voluntary Opening/Automatic Closing/Single Site System

The cookie cruncher, the simplest of myoelectric control systems, was designed specifically for infants and small children through about 3 years. A single electrode, generally placed over the residual wrist extensor muscles, allows for voluntary myoelectric control of hand opening. When the electromyographic (EMG) signal is relaxed, the hand circuitry automatically causes hand closing. This system is quite easily learned by infants as young as 3 to 6 months. In my experience, infants from 3 to 15 months of age learn this control scheme within the first hours of initial fitting.

Dual Site/Dual Control

This control scheme was the first devised for myoelectric control of arm prostheses and remains the most common. Physiologically, it is quite natural. Two electrode sites, in opposition, control hand opening and hand closing. Opening is provided by the residual wrist extensors; closing of the hand is provided by the residual wrist flexors.

Single Site/Dual Control

This control scheme is intended for those who have only one viable muscle site. Both hand opening and hand closing are controlled from this single site. Usually, a hard muscle contraction opens the hand and a soft contraction closes it because closing of the hand requires the most delicacy.

Dual Site/Four Function Control

This control scheme is the most complicated. It is intended to control more than one set of opposing functions. In addition to hand opening and closing, the secondary function may be wrist pronation/supination or elbow control. Control of such a complex system is possible in the older child and reasonable in the teenager. With newer computerized control systems, control of both hand and wrist are becoming easier and more practical for users with transradial level amputations. Three possible options using this control scheme are presented below.

In conventional independent four-function control, there are two conventional sites. Soft contraction of the residual wrist extensors signals hand opening while hard contraction signals supination. Soft contraction of the residual wrist flexors signals hand closing while hard contraction signals pronation. Nonconventional independent four-function control uses two typical sites. Hard/soft contractions of residual wrist extensors control pronation/supination or they control hand opening/closing. Hard/soft contractions of residual wrist flexors control hand opening/closing or they control supination/pronation. In hand or wrist exclusive function, hand and wrist control are not independent, but are mutually exclusive. When the user is in wrist control mode, there is no hand control available without a conscious shift back to hand control, and vice versa. The method of shifting from one mode to the other (hand or wrist) is a small, quick cocontraction of both opposing muscles, such as forearm wrist extensors and flexors. Once the mode (hand or wrist) is selected, further muscle activity from the two sites powers either hand or wrist, not both, without cocontraction to shift modes.

Socket Design

One of the most common errors committed in fitting children with any prosthesis is to treat them as "small adults."

Various casting and socket design techniques for forearm deficiencies have been described in the literature[37-40] for adults, children, and infants. It is important for the prosthetist to understand the biomechanics and the functional attributes of these various socket designs. Each attribute depends on critical factors, such as age and anatomic development (such as epicondylar development at the elbow); length of the residual limb, which affects donning and doffing; range of motion required with the prosthesis (unilateral versus bilateral); and any desired blocking of undesirable motions, such as radial hyperextension, which is common in congenital deficiency of the forearm at a high level. The string casting technique is recommended for short residual limbs, especially congenital deficiencies; the Northwestern technique is ideal for midforearm length and longer residual limbs, because it allows for donning and doffing considerations for longer limbs; and the Bock technique works well with teenagers and adults, in whom the epicondyles are fully developed. For transhumeral deficiencies, the Utah dynamic socket technique is recommended.[41]

It is most important to design a child's socket so that growth can be easily accommodated. Total contact is not essential, and room for linear growth should be designed into any socket when allowed by such factors as distance from residual limb to wrist, components desired to be placed in the forearm section of the prosthesis, socket donning pull-hole tubes, and other space requiring considerations. When possible, the distal end of the socket should be extended for linear growth. In addition, the concept of socket layers, or "onion skin" removable layers as documented by Sauter and associates[42] should be considered. Use of this layered socket design definitely extends socket life. An additional socket modification useful with children is the open-elbow socket for children with forearm deficiency.[43]

Controversial Issues

Down Time

Myoelectric prostheses are presumed to require more repairs. However, Brenner's[44] experience with over 200 electronic fittings in 10 years is that electro/mechanical failures occur at 8-month intervals, or three failures every 2 years. In the Greenville, SC, Shriners Hospital study, there was less down time with myoelectrics than with body-powered systems. Cables fray and connections in the cable system fail more often than problems occur with myoelectric prostheses.

The weakness of any prosthesis with a hand including myoelectrics is the cosmetic glove. Brenner[44] reports glove replacement frequency averaging between two and three gloves annually.

Training

I advocate training and therapy for children who use upper-limb prostheses, whenever possible. Children may live too far away for routine sessions with the therapists at the place where the prosthesis was fit, and therapists available in the children's hometowns may lack experience in prosthetics training. Children in the study who received myoelectric prostheses and received little or no training still fared well; however, they generally did not reach the same level of performance as those who were able to receive routine, experienced training. As a minimum, parents should be provided instruction and/or literature equivalent to their ability and comprehension level to provide their children with developmental challenges and appropriate positive reinforcement.

Current Recommendations and Preferences

Age and Timing of Intervention

For the child with a congenital forearm deficiency, an initial prosthesis should be provided between 3 and 6 months of age, ideally before the infant develops visually guided reaching.[4] This initial prosthesis should be simple, self-suspending, and passive in function. Technology has led to passive hands that are quite cosmetic. I prefer flexible foam-filled passive cosmetic gloves, especially for the infant with transradial or forearm deficiency, because the flexibility is a reported aid to crawling. Many prosthetists prefer to fit the infant with a silicone roll-on liner that is strapped to the prosthesis, thereby providing self-suspension. I prefer fitting the socket directly to the skin, as will occur later with myoelectric sockets. Suspension is achieved in an anterior-posterior fashion between the upper cubital fold and the supra-olecranon area.[39]

Timing for the second prosthesis is usually determined by growth and the related fit of the initial prosthesis. With the use of layered socket designs,[42] the child should be able to use this initial prosthesis 10 to 15 months before replacement due to growth. For the second prosthesis I prefer a single-site myoelectric with a cookie cruncher control scheme and a VASI 0-3 (Variety Ability Systems, Inc, Toronto, Ontario, Canada) hand. Depending on the timing of the first prosthesis and the growth of the infant, this prosthesis is generally fit shortly after the child turns 1 year of age; however, successful fittings have occurred as early as 6 months.

Throughout childhood, growth dictates the timing of refittings. Most often, the cookie cruncher components can be reused in a third or rarely, a fourth prosthesis. Between the ages of 30 and 36 months, most normally developing children are ready for the shift to a two-site, dual-control system. The newer microcomputer control schemes with a menu of choices are ideal for this transition, because they allow the prosthetist to program the more advanced control scheme, and then, if the child is not yet ready for this change, reprogram it back to the cookie cruncher mode. For children in this age range, I prefer either the Bock System 2000 (Otto Bock Orthopedic Industry, Inc, Minneapolis, MN) or the VASI 2-6 electric hand. Two other options at this point are the VASI OMNI-Wrist, which allows friction-controlled passive flexion and extension of the hand at the wrist, and/or the VASI electric wrist rotator. The OMNI-Wrist is simple enough and allows more degrees of freedom without requiring additional muscle signal control. However, the electric wrist rotator requires significantly more sophisticated control ability and comprehension that I believe would be difficult to obtain in a child of this age without a very sensitive and easy to calibrate control system.

Children using myoelectric prostheses from 1 to 2 years of age most often continue to use them.

For the child with humeral and shoulder level deficiencies, it is recommended that the initial prosthesis also be fit early, but perhaps not so early as with the child with forearm deficiency. The increased weight and lever effect of higher level prostheses make them more difficult for an infant to tolerate. A passive type prosthesis without elbow joint should be provided before the child reaches 1 year of age. Suspension with a neoprene-fashioned chest strap harness is effective and acceptable.

Myoelectric control of the terminal device is possible with higher level deficiencies, but it is more difficult for the children to learn and master. For the child with a unilateral humeral level deficiency, a hybrid system, with myoelectric control of the hand and body-powered control of the elbow, is often advocated. For the child with bilateral humeral level deficiencies, consideration must be given to electronic elbow and hand control, either myoelectric or by switch, or a hybrid of both. Electronic control of elbow and hand is advocated at appropriate milestones for shoulder level deficiencies, because it is difficult for children to obtain enough excursion for effective body-powered control.

Choosing Candidates for Myoelectric Prostheses

The best candidates for myoelectric prostheses are children with congenital deficiencies who have previously been fit with a passive prosthesis and whose parents have a clear interest in their child receiving a myoelectric prosthesis. The parents must be able to accept the deficiency and must support and encourage early wearing and use patterns; they must arrange for the visits to the clinic and prosthetist's office; and they must recognize when a new prosthesis is needed. Most important, they must manage the early habilitation of their child.

A secondary factor in prosthetic decision making is the attitude and demeanor of the child. Unruly and unmanageable children are not candidates for myoelectrics. As the child grows and assumes more responsibility, he/she must be cooperative and realize the financial implications of a myoelectric prosthesis.

When the prosthetist must manage a child with a newly acquired amputation, information regarding prior activities, hobbies, and sports, is helpful as is the assessment of parental acceptance and support. Finally, past experiences and parental and child expectations and requests will certainly shape the care plan for an experienced prosthetic user who is a new patient to the treating practitioner.

Summary and Conclusion

Myoelectric options and protocols for children have clearly evolved over the last 25 years. While I and many practitioners affiliated with children's upper-limb prosthetic care advocate the use of and the research and development of myoprosthetics for children, the fundamental question of their ultimate long-term value remains unanswered and their use remains controversial. As is often the case in prosthetic rehabilitation, technology continues to provide new solutions. Myoelectric prostheses certainly are more user friendly to patients, prosthetists, and therapists than ever before. Perhaps the answer to the debate will lie in the future marketplace and health-care arena.

References

1. Angliss VE: Habilitation of upper-limb-deficient children. *Am J Occup Ther* 1974;28:407–414.
2. Brooks MB, Shaperman J: Infant prosthetic fitting: A study of the results. *Am J Occup Ther* 1965;19:329–334.
3. Edelstein JE: News notes. *Inter Clin Info Bull* 1970;9:15–16.
4. Fisher AG: Initial prosthetic fitting of the congenital below-elbow amputee: Are we fitting them early enough? *Inter Clin Info Bull* 1976;15:7–10.
5. Guerrero V, Epps CH: Early prosthetic rehabilitation of the child with unilateral below-elbow congenital deficiency. *Inter Clin Info Bull* 1972;11:19–14.
6. Sypniewski BL: The child with terminal transverse partial hemimelia: A review of the literature on prosthetic management. *Artific Limbs* 1972;16:20–50.
7. Schuch CM: Prosthetic management of children with upper-limb deficiencies, in Schuch CM (ed): *Journal of Proceedings, 19th Annual Meeting and Scientific Symposium of the American Academy of Orthotists and Prosthetists*. Alexandria, VA, American Academy of Orthotists and Prosthetists, 1993, p 42.
8. Sanderson ER, Caldwell RR, Wedderburn Z, Scott RN: Abstract: Myoelectric below-elbow prostheses in the very young child. *Inter Clin Info Bull* 1984;19:55.
9. Menkveld SR, Novotny MP, Schwartz M: Age-appropriateness of myoelectric prosthetic fitting. *J Assoc Child Prosthet Orthot Clin* 1987;22:60–65.
10. Dick HM, Hutnick G, Akdeniz R: Abstract: Myoelectric management of the pediatric amputee. *J Assoc Child Prosthet Orthot Clin* 1985;20:39.
11. Hubbard S, Koheil R, Heger H, Galway HR, Milner M: Abstract: Development of upper-extremity myoelectric training methods for preschool congenital amputees. *Inter Clin Info Bull* 1984;19:9.

12. Hubbard S, Galway R, Urquhart K, Mifsud M: Preschool myoelectric program: A three-year review. *J Assoc Child Prosthet Orthot Clin* 1985;20:38.
13. Kritter AE: Abstract: The Milwaukee experience with myoelectric prostheses. *Inter Clin Info Bull* 1984;19:1.
14. Kritter AE: Myoelectric prostheses. *J Bone Joint Surg* 1985;67A:654–657.
15. Lyttle D, Sweitzer R, Steinke T, Trefler E, Hobson D: Experiences with myoelectric below-elbow fittings in teenagers. *Inter Clin Info Bull* 1974;13:11–20.
16. Mendez MA: Evaluation of a myoelectric hand prosthesis for children with a below-elbow absence. *Prosthet Orthot Int* 1985;9:137-140.
17. Sauter WF: Abstract: A cost-benefit analysis of 160 patients with electrically powered limbs. *Inter Clin Info Bull* 1984;19:2–4.
18. Sörbye R: Myoelectric prosthetic fitting in young children. *Clin Orthop* 1980;148:34–40.
19. Trost FJ: A comparison of conventional and myoelectric below-elbow prosthetic use. *Inter Clin Info Bull* 1983;18:9–16.
20. Mifsud M, Al-Temen I, Sauter W, Hubbard S, Milner M, Naumann S: Variety village electromechanical hand for amputees under two years of age. *J Assoc Child Prosthet Orthot Clin* 1987;22:41–46.
21. Baron E, Clarke SD, Solomon C: Abstract: The two-stage myoelectric hand for children and young adults. *Inter Clin Info Bull* 1984;19:1–2.
22. Maiorano L: Abstract: Myoelectrics for the child below-elbow amputee. *Inter Clin Info Bull* 1984;19:56.
23. Morawa LG: Aabstract: Myoelectric program in Detroit. *Inter Clin Info Bull* 1984;19:55.
24. Kritter AE: Abstract: Myoelectric prosthesis: Current status. *J Assoc Child Prosthet Orthot Clin* 1985;20:36–37.
25. Atkins DJ, Meier RH III, Muilenburg A: Abstract: The upper-limb prosthetic prescription: conventional or electric components? *J Assoc Child Prosthet Orthot Clin* 1985;20:37.
26. Nichol W: Abstract: Control systems for high-level upper-limb amputees: Comparison of myoelectric and proportional touch control. *J Assoc Child Prosthet Orthot Clin* 1985;20:39–40.
27. Menkveld S, Novotny M: Abstract: Age-appropriateness of myoelectric below-elbow prosthetic prescription. *J Assoc Child Prosthet Orthot Clin* 1986;21:19.
28. Al-Temen I, Milner M: Abstract: New Variety Village electromechanical hand for amputees less than 2 years of age. *J Assoc Child Prosthet Orthot Clin* 1986;21:29.
29. Scott RN, Lovely DF, Hruczkowski T, Olive M, Caldwell R, Hayden J: Abstract: New myoelectric control system. *J Assoc Child Prosthet Orthot Clin* 1986;21:30.
30. Ballance R: Abstract: Review of prosthesis-wearing patterns and use in congenital unilateral below-elbow child amputees wearing a myoelectric prosthesis. *J Assoc Child Prosthet Orthot Clin* 1987;22:19.
31. Patterson DB, McMillan P, Rodriguez R: Abstract: Acceptance rate of myoelectric prostheses. *J Assoc Child Prosthet Orthot Clin* 1989;24:37.
32. Mifsud M, Galway HR, Milner M: Abstract: Current myoprosthetic development at the Hugh MacMillan Medical Centre. *J Assoc Child Prosthet Orthot Clin* 1985;20:37–38.
33. Mifsud M, Galway HR, Milner M: Current myoprosthetic developments at the Hugh MacMillan Medical Centre. *J Assoc Child Prosthet Orthot Clin* 1986;21:1–7.
34. Berger N, Edelstein JE: Abstract: Children's performance with myoelectrically controlled and body-powered hands. *J Assoc Child Prosthet Orthot Clin* 1989;24:34.
35. Williams TW III: One-muscle infant's myoelectric control. *J Assoc Child Prosthet Orthot Clin* 1989;24:53–56.
36. Scotland TR, Galway HR: Abstract: A long-term review of children with congenital and acquired upper-limb deficiency. *Inter Clin Info Bull* 1984;19:51.
37. Billock JN: The Northwestern University supracondylar suspension technique for below-elbow amputations. *Orthot Prosthet* 1972;26:16–23

38. Kay HW (ed): *A Fabrication Manual for the "Muenster-Type" Below-Elbow Prosthesis.* New York, NY, New York University School of Engineering and Science, 1965.

39. Staats TB: The string casting technique for below elbow amputations. *Orthop Prosthet* 1982;36:35–40.

40. *MyoBock Manual.* Minneapolis, MN, Otto Bock Orthopedic Industry, Inc, 1990.

41. Andrew JT: Elbow disarticulation and transhumeral amputation: Prosthetic principles, in Bowker JH, Michael JW (eds): American Academy of Orthopaedic Surgeons *Atlas of Limb Prosthetics: Surgical, Prosthetic, and Rehabilitation Principles,* ed 2. St. Louis, MO, Mosby Year Book, 1992, pp 255–264.

42. Sauter WF, Dakpa R, Galway R, Hubbard S, Hamilton E: Development of layered "onionized" silicone sockets for juvenile below-elbow amputees. *J Assoc Child Prosthet Orthot Clin* 1987;22:57–59.

43. Sauter WF: Abstract: Three-quarter-type Muenster socket. *J Assoc Child Prosthet Orthot Clin* 1985;20:34.

44. Brenner CD: Electronic limbs for infants and pre-school children. *J Prosthet Orthot* 1992;4:24–30.

Chapter 36

Powered Prosthetic Intervention in Upper Extremity Deficiency

Sheila A. Hubbard, PT, OT, BSc
Isaac Kurtz, MHSc, PEng
Winfried Heim, CP(C)
Gert Montgomery, BScN, MSW, CSW

Application of Myoelectric Technology to Children

Myoelectric prostheses for young children were first introduced in 1971. At that time, myoprosthetic components were all adult-sized and fitting/training procedures were considered too complex for application to children. Rolf Sörbye, a Swedish neurophysiologist, exploded this myth by successfully fitting a below-elbow myoelectric prosthesis to a 3-year-old girl. Although the hand used was inappropriately sized, the experiment was considered so successful that the Swedish team proceeded to supply similar prostheses to seven other young children. Needing a smaller hand, Sörbye initially converted a Canadian electric hand from microswitch to myoelectric control and then collaborated with local manufacturers to produce a new myoelectric hand and glove suitable in size for 2- to 5-year-old children. In 1977, Sörbye[1] reported his experience with 12 preschool fittings and proposed that myoelectric fitting should occur as early as possible to facilitate acceptance of the prosthesis and its integration with the child's normal psychomotor development.

The effect of Sörbye's work was soon reflected internationally. In the United Kingdom, public pressure prompted the initiation of a program of evaluation from 1978 to 1980 by the Department of Health and Social Security.[2] Three prosthetic centers were selected to run parallel programs of assessment, fitting, and training. In Canada, a 2-year (1980 to 1982) evaluation project was conducted with the specific objective of developing effective training strategies for preschool-aged children.[3] Researchers in both groups reported that their experiences supported Sörbye's claim that it was both feasible and worthwhile to provide myoelectric prostheses to young children.

These efforts attracted widespread attention and eventually other amputee clinics in Europe and North America started to prescribe myoelectric prostheses for their young clients. Although the cosmetically appealing myoelectric fittings were popular with families, their cost-effectiveness was considered contentious within the professional community. Debate was focused primarily on issues of age-appropriateness and functional benefit of myoelectric limbs versus body-powered devices. Some[4–6] were particularly critical of the trend toward myoelectric fitting for young children, whereas others[7-10] were very positive about their findings.

Unfortunately, the literature on myoprosthetic fitting of children was limited, and a number of factors made it difficult to compare one experience with another. Most of the research reported was based on case studies or small clinical reviews using nonstandard evaluation techniques. Technology and fitting techniques changed rapidly over a very short time, fitting ages differed, and variance in expertise in myoprosthetic practice meant that it was impossible to judge results without an assessment of the quality of the prosthetic fittings. Most, however, acknowledged that cosmesis was an important consideration and reported that patients and parents generally preferred the more natural, closer to normal appearance of the self-suspended myoelectric prosthesis compared to body-powered devices.

Subsequent publications by the original research groups in the United Kingdom, Canada, and Sweden produced similar results and recommendations. Mendez[11] reported that 87 children (3.5 to 4.5 years of age) had been fitted during the 3-year UK trial and that a decision had been made to continue to provide myoelectric prostheses to children through the National Health Service. Hubbard and associates[12] reviewed their experience with 89 preschool children and reported that myoelectric prostheses had become a standard option for Ontario children aged 2.5 years and older. Sörbye[13] concluded that his experience with 124 amputees indicated that early myoelectric fittings strongly correlated with positive functional and psychological outcome. He suggested that children should be fitted between 2.5 and 4 years of age.

The next breakthrough occurred in the late 1980s. Significant technological developments, including a simpler control strategy, the St. Anthony Circuit ("cookie-crusher" or single-site voluntary opening system), the production of the infant-sized VASI hand, and the availability of new smaller-sized electrodes allowed prosthetists to fabricate cosmetically appealing, self-contained myoelectric prostheses for very young children. Media reports of "bionic arms" for babies captured the imagination of the public and attracted worldwide attention and debate. Attracted by the possibility of a simpler control strategy for young children, several clinic teams decided to accept the challenge and proceeded to experiment with powered prostheses for infants on their caseloads. Many centers in the United States and Canada have all reported success with the younger-age approach.[14-18]

Current Clinical Practice at Bloorview MacMillan Centre

The Infant Amputee

Passive Prosthesis
Infants with upper-limb deficiencies are commonly fitted with a passive prosthesis between 3 and 6 months of age. The early fitting conditions the

child to wearing a prosthesis and assists gross motor development. The socket design is the same as that which will be used in the fitting of the externally powered prosthesis. Families are encouraged to gradually increase wearing time until the child is able to tolerate the prosthesis for the majority of waking hours.

First Externally Powered Prosthesis

It is possible to proceed directly to a powered fitting when the child has outgrown the passive prosthesis and is ready for activation at 10 to 15 months. Because cooperation and communication are limited, it is necessary to simplify the fitting and training process. The intent is to provide the device and then encourage the child to discover its potential in play situations.

The most effective myoelectric control system for this age group is a single-site, voluntary hand opening system. Whenever possible, the electrode is located on a wrist extensor muscle group in preparation for normal physiologic control of a two-muscle system when the child is older. If the infant has an above-elbow limb deficiency, the mid triceps area is preferred but it may be necessary to experiment with placement over biceps and triceps in order to determine which area produces the most effective control system activation.

A clear check socket is then fabricated and checked for fit, comfort, and suspension. The control system and hand are attached temporarily to determine if the electrode placement is effective in detecting EMG activity. Once any required adjustments have been completed, the prosthesis is finished and dispensed.

Young children are able to master this simple control strategy quite easily. Although the hand is activated only inadvertently at first, the noise and activity attract attention, and the child very quickly figures out how to open it intentionally. A "parental access switch" mounted externally on the forearm enables the clinician or parent to open the hand independently of the child and place toys or objects in it. The child is then encouraged to try to open the hand to release the grasped object.

The sensitivity level of the control system is initially set high for easy activation in order to attract the child's attention to the hand movement. As the child becomes accustomed to wearing the prosthesis and more conscious of the control strategy, the level is reduced and voluntary grasp and release are encouraged in play activity.

The development of bilateral prehension is a gradual process that requires ongoing assistance and encouragement by the family and other care givers. The therapist provides suggestions for encouragement of developmentally appropriate use at home. Spontaneous use of the hand for bimanual play activity is commonly observed between 18 and 24 months of age. Frequent team follow-up is essential to provide support and guidance in the progression of home training, monitor growth changes, and assess the need for socket modification or replacement.

Preschool and School Age Children

Once the children have developed improved communication skills and longer attention spans (normally 3 to 4 years of age) it becomes easier to evaluate and train them to use more advanced control strategies (voluntary control of hand closing as well as opening). Procedures used are the same as those for older children or adults.

Preprosthetic Procedures

Preprosthetic fitting/training procedures include: (1) the preliminary identification of muscles suitable for myoelectric control purposes; (2) the selection of the most appropriate control system; (3) location of the optimal site(s) for electrode placement over selected muscles; (4) socket checkout; (5) training of the selected muscles to contract and relax at will; and (6) control system calibration.

Because the child is already accustomed to using a single-muscle action for hand opening, it is necessary to determine if a second muscle group can be trained to control hand closing (Fig. 1). A myotester is used to assess the EMG response during contraction and relaxation of each muscle group. Control system selection depends on: (1) the number of muscle sites the child is able to control independently; (2) the number and type of electrical components to be used in the prosthesis; (3) the characteristics of the EMG signals generated; and (4) the degree of complexity that the child can manage.

For success with a two-muscle control system, the antagonist muscle group must be able to be contracted independently in order to close the hand. If a two-site system is selected, the choice has to be made between proportional and digital controls. The proportional system gives the child the ability to vary the speed and force of the terminal device.

If cocontraction is observed continually, and it does not appear possible to train the muscles to operate separately, the strongest muscle group is chosen and a one-muscle two-function system is considered. One-muscle systems use either the rate of muscle contraction or the level of contraction to voluntarily select hand opening or closing. Selection of the most appropriate one-muscle system is based on the ease of operation for the child and prosthetic design/space considerations. If neither of these options is possible, the child can continue to use a one-muscle voluntary opening system.

For children with amputations at the above-elbow and forequarter levels, the selection process will be limited by the number of muscle sites available. Combinations of myoelectric control with electric-switch control or body-powered control may be required to meet the individual's need to operate more than one component. For amputations at the shoulder-disarticulation level, we prefer to use push and touch controls. Scapular motion is used in a joystick fashion to operate mechanical switches or touch pads (ie, force-sensing resistors and capacitive touch controls) (F Sethna, et al, Fredericton, New Brunswick, Canada, personal communication, 1994). The hand is controlled by the site that the child finds easiest to control. The second control site, if available, is used for the elbow. Some clients can manage an additional switch for control of an electric wrist rotator.

420

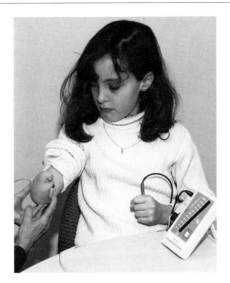

Fig. 1 *Assessment for two-site control.*

A new programmable controller (I Kurtz, et al, Frederiction, New Brunswick, Canada, personal communication, 1995) enables the clinician to experiment with a variety of control strategies to determine the optimal system and calibration for the individual client. It is also possible to reprogram the controller from a simple control strategy to a more complex one at a later time without replacing the electronic package.

After a clear check socket has been fabricated, it is evaluated for fit, comfort, range of motion, and suspension. The socket also is weighted to assess the biomechanics of dynamic loading. Electrodes are placed in the socket over the identified muscle sites to enable control training and to assure proper placement and calibration. After any required modifications have been completed and evaluated, the definitive prosthesis is completed. If the outcome of a myoelectric fitting is uncertain, the components can be temporarily attached to the socket as a preparatory prosthesis and used for a trial period until need and acceptance are established.

The first objective of voluntary control training is to train the child to be an effective operator of his/her new control system. In the case of a two-site system, the child must be able to select, contract, and relax each of the two muscle groups independently. The child also should be able to start and stop the system in large or small increments. Additional practice will be needed for the child to become proficient with a proportional system. For a one-site system, the child must learn to relax and then differentiate between two rates of muscle contraction or two levels of signal strength in the control muscle being used. The child should be able to produce control signals at will and also to relax and inhibit undesired contractions during normal activity. If an electric elbow is used, practice will be required to accurately stop and start it at will. A position chart may be mounted on a wall to aid in accuracy training.

The second objective is to increase the signal strength and tolerance for repetition. Ideally, the control training is conducted using the child's own control system and components. The hand's opening and closing operations can be used in an imaginative way for repetitive grasp and release during play activities such as construction toy assembly, block tower building, and peg boards. Older children prefer drill training in the form of games, such as checkers, dominoes, and chess.

In some cases, a new amputee may benefit from additional home training. Instructions are given to the parents and a training kit provided. The training kit consists of a control system, electrodes, battery with charger, and a hand. The family can then work with the child in a relaxed atmosphere at home until control is established.

As the child's control improves, the electrode gains are adjusted and balanced for maximum efficiency. Sensitivity levels are set high enough for ease of control without fatigue but low enough to prevent inadvertent activation. Optimal calibration depends on both the child's ability to provide feedback and the clinician's ability to analyze the EMG signals and evaluate control problems during drill training.

Final Fitting and Functional Training

The prosthetic team ensures that the prosthesis fits comfortably and that all the components are working satisfactorily before the therapist begins functional training. Initially, the amputee requires training and practice to become proficient in the control of each of the various electric or mechanical devices supplied. After the child has adapted to the fitting and is comfortable with the control strategies required for mechanical operation of the prosthesis, he or she is instructed in the use of the prosthesis for activities of daily life.

When working with children, the therapist selects activities consistent with the child's needs, interests, and developmental age level. A young child's attention span is usually short, and it may be necessary to change activities frequently to maintain interest and cooperation. Younger children respond best to the use of assembly or construction toy activity, riding toys, musical instruments, and imaginative play activities such as dressing up or playing house. Preschoolers enjoy simple crafts, coloring, cutting and pasting, lacing cards, making jewelry, and playground activity. Self-care activities are encouraged according to the age and ability of the child.

The parents, day care worker, and school teacher are encouraged to be involved in and committed to the training process. Continued facilitation of use, selection of appropriate toys and play activities, and assistance with prepositioning of the wrist (and elbow) are all essential if the child is to become an effective prosthetic user. The child's ability to operate and use the prosthesis effectively is assessed whenever the child returns to the center for socket adjustments or refitting. Additional training is provided on an "as required" basis. A child's developmental and psychosocial needs are constantly changing, and should be monitored and addressed over time.

Functional training for the older child or adult is directed more toward school or vocational needs and activities of daily living suitable to the indi-

Table 1 Type of fitting

Powered Fittings	Unilateral	Bilateral
Shoulder disarticulation	5	1
Above-elbow	18	1
Below-elbow	103	3
Wrist disarticulation	34	
AE/WD*		1
AE/SD*		1

* AE/WD, above elbow/wrist disarticulation; AE/SD, above elbow/shoulder disarticulation

Table 2 Age of fitting

Age at Fitting		Current Status	
(Months)	Number	User	Nonuser
0 to 5	32	28 (88%)	4 (12%)
16 to 23	22	17 (77%)	5 (23%)
24 to 35	30	17 (57%)	13 (43%)
36 to 47	27	14 (52%)	13 (48%)
48 to 59	18	8 (44%)	10 (56%)
60 to 72	13	6 (46%)	7 (53.8%)
	142	90	52

vidual's life-style. Training addresses self-care, communication, household activities, and leisure needs.

Bloorview MacMillan Centre Preschool Experience

From 1978 to 1996, the Bloorview MacMillan Centre has provided externally powered prostheses to 167 children (87 girls, 80 boys) who were younger than 6 years of age at the time of their first powered fitting. Of these children, 164 had congenital limb deficiencies and three had acquired deficiencies; 96 deficiencies were on the left side; 64 were on the right side; and seven were bilateral. Fittings are described in Table 1, and ages of the children at the first powered fitting are in Table 2.

A parent telephone survey was conducted in 1997. Results indicate that 89 children continue to wear their powered prostheses and 53 are known to have discontinued use. The user status of the remaining 25 is unknown. Current ages and status of the known 142 are in Table 3.

Although the differences in prosthetic acceptance between the groups might suggest a greater tendency for rejection with age, it is important to remember that it is an 18-year experience. The older children in this sample were fitted later in age; received heavier, less suitable, or less reliable componentry; and participated in a variety of experimental regimes. Several of the children also came to us from out of province and had difficulty continuing

Table 3 Current ages and status of Bloorview Macmillan patients

Age (years)	No. of Children	Active User	Nonuser
1 to 7	50	86%	14%
8 to 10	25	64%	36%
11 to 21	67	45%	55%

Table 4 Parent satisfaction with prosthetis scale 1 (very unsatisfied) to 5 (very satisfied)

	Mean	Standard Deviation
Appearance	4.34	0.81
Function	4.19	0.90
Comfort	3.84	1.05
Durability	3.87	1.21
Large grasp	3.10	1.58
Small grasp	3.96	1.33
Grip strength	4.43	0.91

service closer to home. In contrast, the younger children have been fitted earlier with improved, age-appropriate technology, and have benefited from established fitting/training practices.

Separate questionnaires were used to evaluate parent satisfaction of myoelectric fitting for both the active and nonuser groups. Eighty-two (92%) parents responded to the questionnaire for active users. Reasons cited for prosthetic wear were primarily for appearance value (12.2%), primarily for functional value (29.3%), and appearance and function of equal value (58.5%). Satisfaction is described in Table 4. Of the parents, 41% found the prosthesis very useful for day-to-day activities; 54% found it somewhat useful; and 5% found it not at all useful. Most (78.1%) thought the age of the child at fitting was just right; 6.1% thought the child was too young; 13.4%, too old; and 2.4% didn't know. Ninety-one percent reported that they had received sufficient guidance and assistance. Parents were also asked to rate the amount of time their children wore their myoelectric prostheses at home, at school, and for social activities. High patterns of wear were reported for school and social use, Monday to Friday. On weekends the majority still reported high use for social activities, but only part-time wear at home.

Thirty-six (68%) parents responded to the questionnaire for parents of nonusers. Most commonly cited reasons for rejection included too heavy (81%); not useful, child could do more without it (78%); child was more comfortable without it (75%); too uncomfortable (72%); child did not like to wear it (69%); preferred other type of prosthesis (31%); too far to travel (17%); stopped working (13%); and breakdown too frequent (9%). However, 81% agreed that their children should have been fitted, 47% felt that their children would likely reconsider a myoelectric fitting again in the future, and 72% felt that the age of fitting was just right.

Recommendations

Questions commonly asked of specialized centers such as ours include: at what age should myoelectric fitting begin; what is the acceptance rate of myoelectric prostheses; how much will the child wear the prosthesis; what function will the child gain using the prosthesis; how often does it break down; and ultimately, is it cost-effective? Unfortunately, it is difficult to provide simplistic answers because there is a lack of objective data. Technology and fitting/training techniques have changed so frequently over the years that it is impractical to compare results of earlier experiences with those of present day practice or to consider collective long-term results as representative. There has not been any systematic collection of data across prosthetic centers because of the lack of standardized outcome measures. Few scientific studies have been conducted, and the terminology and operational definitions of reported experiences have been ambiguous.

What then have we learned as a result of our 18 years of experience with myoelectric fittings for children and how would we respond to these inquiries?

Fit Young

The age of fitting is an important consideration (Table 2). Critics have long maintained that it is too expensive to fit early and that there is no functional benefit. Advocates propose that early fitting is essential if a prosthesis is to be incorporated into body image.

Perhaps we should consider our goal in providing any prosthetic device to a young child. Many would cite enhanced function as the rationale. Although we know that congenital amputees can perform many activities of daily living extremely well without any prosthesis, prosthetic users tell us that a prosthesis provides body symmetry, balance, and some functional benefit. It is necessary then to determine what type of functional gain the user should achieve. Is the goal natural use or tool use? Natural use implies smooth, spontaneous, integrated use of the prosthesis in normal bilateral activity whereas tool use suggests gross grasp or stabilization assist for a specific purpose.

The developmental literature indicates that hand use patterns begin very early. The normal baby progresses from asymmetry to symmetry to differentiated asymmetric movements in bilateral hand use. The mature stage of bilateral hand use, which is the ability to use opposing hand and arm movements for highly differentiated activities such as scissor use, begins to emerge at about 2.5 years. The development of visual perception and eye-hand coordination skills in conjunction with cognitive and social development allow the child to engage in increasingly complex activities.[19] Why then would we wish to delay fitting until compensatory patterns have been adopted and body image established and then introduce a prosthetic device and expect the child to engage in new patterns of learning?

Our experience indicates that a child who is fitted young and wears the prosthesis regularly will demonstrate spontaneous use in daily activities and

Table 5 Affect of degree of limb deficiency on prosthesis use

Amputation	Fitting*	No.	Accepted	Rejected
UNILATERAL	SD	1	100%	
	AE	9	67%	33%
	BE	83	70%	30%
	WD	29	48%	52%
BILATERAL		4	50%	50%
MULTIPLE		16	50%	50%

*SD, shoulder disarticulation; AE, above-elbow; BE, below-elbow; WD, wrist disarticulation

use the prosthesis more naturally. For example, these children are likely to reach out and grasp with the prosthetic hand and to pass objects back and forth between hands. In contrast, the children fitted at later ages are less spontaneous and more inclined to use the prosthesis passively.

Hand skill development is a gradual process. If the child is fitted early, the prosthesis will be integrated with use of the sound limb. The child will have had practice doing things like crossing the midline, bringing the hands together, knowing where the hand is in space, and using the hand to grasp objects so that by the time two-handed tasks are required at preschool and kindergarten, the child will be ready to use the prosthesis to thread beads, cut and paste, and assemble construction toys. This skill acquisition will also allow the child to keep up with peers and to integrate more easily in the classroom situation.

Acceptance Results Are Very Individual

We have found that myoelectric fitting can be very successful for some children and of little benefit to others. We believe that a number of factors influence the outcome of any individual fitting. These include the attitude of the family; age at time of fitting; the level of limb deficiency; the quality and location of the prosthetic practice; and possibly, hand dominance predisposition.

An enthusiastic family commitment is essential for success. Family attitudes significantly affect a child's acceptance of a disability and related assistive devices. Attitudes toward disability are determined by a complex and dynamic interplay of each child's unique family, culture, and social milieu. Parents and extended family members' emotional reactions and attitudes to limb deficiency and their expectations regarding present and future social acceptability and life choices, all influence how they perceive and value treatment, training, and prosthetic wear. Responsibility for encouraging use, monitoring growth changes, and attending to repair needs demands heavy involvement. Parents who see the tangible benefits of prosthetic wear in terms of function, comfort, and ease of use and who also like the appearance find it much easier to reinforce and reward their child's prosthetic learning and to carry through with treatment/training goals.

The degree of limb deficiency is also a key factor to consider in predicting long-term outcome. Our experience would suggest that the child with a unilateral, below-elbow amputation/limb deficiency, mid-forearm level, is the most likely candidate for successful fitting (Table 5). A myoelectric prosthesis provides cosmesis, function, and freedom from harnessing. The unilateral amputee uses the prosthesis primarily to grasp or stabilize objects to enable the sound limb to perform fine motor or manipulative skills. The myoelectric prosthesis performs this function relatively well, providing a strong grasp with ease of operation in any body position. Results generally have been less positive for the longer, through-wrist or partial hand level amputees. Minimal functional gain and questionable cosmetic value at the expense of loss of sensation have commonly resulted in less wear and a high rate of rejection. However, it should be noted that we generally did not fit these children as young as the others, and this may have influenced the outcome.

Above elbow, long to midhumeral limb deficiency is the ideal length to accommodate the need for adequate muscle sites, shoulder motion, and sufficient leverage to bear the weight of the prosthetic components. Although the numbers in our experience have been small, six of the nine children with unilateral deficiencies continue to be active users. Because restorative function becomes increasingly difficult to achieve at higher levels (ie, through shoulder, forequarter) or for bilateral limb deficiencies, electric prostheses are not likely to be any better accepted than conventional devices long term by these individuals.

The experience and expertise of the clinical team is fundamental to the success of any myoelectric program. Myoelectrics is a specialized practice and it requires experienced, multidisciplinary teamwork to make it successful. Team members need to enjoy working with children and to know how to assess and prescribe appropriate systems and componentry; how to fit a comfortable, well-suspended, lightweight, cosmetic prosthesis; how to apply age-appropriate training strategies; and finally, how to be sensitive to psychosocial issues and willing to provide the support and encouragement required. Flexibility in appointment scheduling is necessary to accommodate the needs of working parents.

Consistency of wear is critical to the development of bilateral patterns of usage. Therefore, the amount of "down-time" experienced will have a significant impact on the outcome of a myoelectric fitting. A child cannot be expected to become a natural user if the prosthesis breaks down frequently and is unavailable for use. It is equally important that a comfortable fit be maintained. Sockets should be modified frequently to accommodate minor growth changes and then replaced quickly when it becomes obvious that refitting is necessary. Distance from the prosthetic facility, efficiency of the repair service, choice of reliable components, conscientiousness of parents in attending to repair/maintenence needs, and financial restrictions or considerations will undoubtedly influence results.

The influence of hand dominance is largely unknown. Therapists[17] and parents have questioned whether there might be a correlation between a dominance predisposition and prosthetic proficiency. Further study is required in this area.

To summarize, it would appear that it is the interplay of family dynamics and strengths with the other factors of age, length of limb, and quality of practice that determines the outcome for each individual child. A measure of family functioning and acceptance of disability in combination with these other elements could be extremely useful in predicting long-term value of myoelectric fitting.

Variation in Wearing Patterns

We have found that there is great variation in wearing patterns among children. It is difficult to determine if these patterns are characteristic or if they have been influenced by the variation in technology over time. It is also too early to judge whether the high percentage of reported most or full-time wear associated with the younger age fittings will continue to remain as positive as the children become older. We assume that if a regular pattern of wear and functional use is established in infancy, children will be more likely to continue to be good prosthetic users in their later childhood years. However, as they advance through the school and teen-age years, numerous other influences can affect wear.

For example, although bilateral hand use is an important feature of preschool play and early school-age functional activities, it becomes less of a requirement in the older grades, and the children may find they have less need to use their prostheses in the classroom. However, psychosocial factors may influence the children to continue to wear their prostheses for cosmetic value. In addition, older children tend to become involved in sports, music, part-time jobs, or other activities that may require the removal of the myoelectric in favor of other prosthetic devices or even a preference for use of their residual limbs instead.

An examination of wear patterns for children fitted before 24 months of age in the years 1989 to 1996 (newer technology and methodology) indicates that even for this group, overall wear of the powered prosthesis begins to decrease as the children become school-aged. Associated use of recreational devices has not yet been evaluated.

It is also not uncommon for children to abandon use of their prostheses for a few years and then request to be refit again for cosmetic and/or changed functional needs. In some cases, rejection of the prosthesis may be used as a temporary means of establishing autonomy or self identity.

Functional/Psychological Benefit

We have found that it is very difficult to scientifically evaluate the outcome of external powered fittings for children. How do you define success? Whose perception is most important: the child, the parent, the clinician, or the funding agency? How do you evaluate without any standardized measurement tools?

Myoelectric prostheses are commonly purported to provide functional benefit to the child. In some cases, the prosthetic use is very bimanual and the child is at a loss when the prosthesis is not available. For others it may be more task specific but considered requisite for the particular activity. How then do you develop a single measure of its functional value? Is it used primarily for active grasp or more often for passive stabilization, which could be achieved with a simpler prosthetic device?

In order to resolve some of these functional issues, a new instrument, the Prosthetic Upper Extremity Functional Index (PUFI) (V Wright, et al, Dallas, Texas, personal communication, 1997), has been developed for use with parents and older children. This self-report measure has been designed to analyze use, passive versus active elements, value of a prosthesis for daily bimanual activities, and ability to use the residual limb.

Preliminary results of a reliability study are positive. Parents and older children have found the questionnaire easy to follow and have only required an average of 30 minutes to complete it. Results indicate that the respondents are able to differentiate between active and passive use of the prosthesis and are quite candid and discerning in their task-specific evaluation of the value of the prosthesis. Test-retest scores indicate that the instrument will prove to have acceptable reliability. Funding is being sought for a multicenter validation study.

A second study[20] explored the issue of the cosmetic benefit of a myoelectric fitting. This research assessed multidimensional self-concept in a homogeneous sample of 39 children fitted with myoelectric limbs and compared them to a sample of 98 school children. Results of this study revealed that the children with congenital limb deficiencies had overall levels and developmental patterns of multidimensional self-concept similar to those of their limb-intact peers. Further testing is planned to determine if results are the same for children wearing other types of prostheses and for those children who choose not to wear any prosthesis.

Financial Implications

Improved methodology and technology have made it easier and less costly to fit, manufacture, and service powered prostheses for children. Increased reliability of components have also resulted in fewer repairs. Glove durability and water/sand damage to hands continue to be the biggest repair problems. It is possible to institute some measures to keep costs from being prohibitive. For example, components such as hands and electrodes can be refurbished and re-used, growth allowances can be built into sockets, and adjustments can be made to prolong the life of a socket for months at a time. However, there is still a need to seek cost reduction measures to make it economically feasible to continue to provide the technology.

Summary

There are no simple ways to predict long-term results or to judge the cost-effectiveness of myoelectric fitting for children. However, we do believe that myoelectric limbs provide an acceptable combination of cosmesis and function for many children. Although individual outcome cannot be predicted with absolute certainty, it is possible to identify and assess important indicators. Successful outcome is most likely when all influencing factors are positive. Better patient selection would help to ensure that funding is available for those children who are most likely to benefit. Objective, standardized outcome measures are required to assist this process.

There is also a need for continued research and development. Hands with greater prehensile capabilities, gloves that do not tear or stain, improved cosmesis, softer coverings, systems that are more impervious to sand and water damage, and reduction in weight of components are all required. Funding problems need to be addressed, and solutions sought to reduce costs.

Psychosocial benefits of a cosmetically attractive prosthesis should not be trivialized. Our society places a high value on appearance, and it is important that a child develops a positive self-image in the formative years. It has been aptly stated that "myoelectric prostheses help the interaction of the amputee with family, friends and school acquaintants in our current social environment. Should that environment change and parents cease to demand that each child appear whole, friends accept limb deficiency without pity and acquaintances cease to overreact to the appearance of a missing limb, then the needs of the young amputee might be different."[21]

References

1. Sörbye R: Myoelectric controlled hand prostheses in children. *Int J Rehabil Res* 1977;1:15–25.

2. Day HJB: The United Kingdom trial of the Swedish myoelectric hand for young children: An interim report. *Inter Clin Info Bull* 1980;17:5–8.

3. Hubbard S, Galway HR, Milner M: Myoelectric training methods for the preschool child with congenital below-elbow amputation: A comparison of two training programmes. *J Bone Joint Surg* 1985;67B:273–277.

4. Trost FJ: A comparison of conventional and myoelectric below-elbow prosthetic use. *Inter Clin Info Bull* 1983;18:9–16.

5. Kruger LM, Fishman S: Myoelectric and body-powered prostheses. *J Pediatr Orthop* 1993;13:68–75.

6. Menkveld SR, Novotny MP, Schwartz M: Age-appropriateness of myoelectric prosthetic fitting. *J Assoc Child Prosthet Orthot Clin* 1987;22:60–65.

7. Kritter AE: Abstract: The Milwaukee experience with myoelectric prostheses. *Inter Clinic Info Bull* 1984;19:1.

8. Baron E, Clarke SD, Solomon C: Abstract: The two-stage myoelectric hand for children and young adults. *Inter Clin Info Bull* 1984;19:1–2.

9. Weaver SA, Lange LR, Vogts VM: Comparison of myoelectric and conventional prostheses for adolescent amputees. *Am J Occup Ther* 1988;42:87–91.

10. Crone N: A comparison of myo-electric and standard prostheses: A case study of a pre-school aged congenital amputee. *Can J Occup Ther* 1986;53:217–222.

11. Mendez MA: Evaluation of a myoelectric hand prosthesis for children with a below-elbow absence. *Prosthet Orthot Int* 1985;9:137–140.

12. Hubbard S: Hugh MacMillan Rehabilitation Centre pre-school myoelectric experience, in Scott RN (ed): *UNB Monographs on Myoelectric Prostheses: Myoelectric Prostheses for Infants.* New Brunswick, Canada, University of New Brunswick, 1984, pp 21–29.

13. Sörbye R: Upper-extremity amputees: Swedish experiences concerning children, in Atkins DJ, Meier RH III (eds): *Comprehensive Management of the Upper Limb Amputee*. New York, NY, Springer-Verlag, 1989, pp 227–239.

14. Hubbard S, Bush G, Kurtz I, Naumann S: Myoelectric prostheses for the limb-deficient child. *Phys Med Rehabil Clin North Am* 1991;2:847–866.

15. Hubbard S: Myoprosthetic management of the upper limb amputee, in Hunter JM, Mackin EJ, Callahan AD (eds): *Rehabilitation of the Hand: Surgery and Therapy*, ed 4. St. Louis, MO, Mosby-Year Book, 1995, vol 2, pp 1241–1252.

16. Brenner CD: Electronic limbs for infants and pre-school children. *J Prosthet Orthot* 1992;4:24–30.

17. Jacobs R: Fitting young children with myoelectric prostheses, in Scott RN (ed): *UNB Monographs on Myoelectric Prostheses: Myoelectric Prostheses for Infants*. New Brunswick, Canada, University of New Brunswick, 1984, pp 31–37.

18. Meredith JM, Uellendahl JE, Keagy RD: Successful voluntary grasp and release using the cookie crusher myoelectric hand in 2-year-olds. *Am J Occup Ther* 1993;47:825–829.

19. Exner CE: Development of hand functions, in Pratt PN, Allen AS (eds): *Occupational Therapy for Children*, ed 2. St. Louis, MO, CV Mosby, 1989, pp 235–259.

20. Hubbard J: *The Self-Concept of Children with Congenital Upper Limb Deficiencies*. Toronto, Ontario, Canada, York University, 1996. Thesis.

21. Lyttle D: The proper age for fitting a myoelectric prosthesis. in Scott RN (ed): *UNB Monographs on Myoelectric Prostheses: Myoelectric Prostheses for Infants*. New Brunswick, Canada, University of New Brunswick, 1984, p 45.

Consensus

Prosthetic Use in Children With Upper Limb Deficiency

Prosthetic wear and use varies among individuals and between different centers and clinics. Some centers achieve 70% prosthetic use while others have a 20% use rate. The value of a prosthesis for upper limb deficiency may be more related to the ability to perform specific tasks than to the total time of wear. Body-powered and externally powered devices are both useful in various circumstances. In some centers, a low rate of prosthetic use leads to the belief that patients are more functional with their residual limb than with a prosthesis. In other centers, a much higher rate of use and a lower rate of rejection suggests that there are significant functional advantages for prosthetic use.

For patients with transradial (below elbow) or transhumeral, unilateral amputations, very early prosthetic fitting and training produce higher rates of prosthetic use. Early fitting means a passive fitting when the child is as young as 3 to 6 months of age. Fitting with an active terminal device between 12 and 24 months of age is also part of the early fitting program. As far as possible, all of these children should have the opportunity for prosthetic fitting; however, many children will and many will not become long-term prosthetic users. Aggressive training programs requiring significant commitment by the child and family may result in higher rates of usage. Going without a prosthesis is also a reasonable alternative that may lead to a successful outcome. Outcome studies that measure not only function, but also use tools such as the Health Related Quality of Life instrument are important for evaluating prosthetic use. **Success should be defined as a happy child who has reached his or her maximum potential.**

Children with congenital bilateral upper extremity deficits at the high transhumeral level are unlikely to use prostheses. The higher the level of deficit, the less likely is prosthetic use. Children with bilateral below elbow absence, or one above and one below elbow congenital absence may or may not use prostheses. While some centers recommend that children who are missing both hands be fitted with prostheses, others believe that prostheses should be prescribed when there are specific functional needs to address. Those children and families who are highly motivated to use prostheses should have that opportunity. Children with long forearms and wrist disarticulation levels are less likely to use prostheses in the experience of some centers but not in that of others.

We encourage research on sensory feedback and see that as a major need in prosthetic design.

Surgical intervention may be useful in lengthening existing structures, providing prehension, and allowing the arms to reach the midline. The Krukenberg procedure should be reconsidered for its functional sensory and motor advantages, although it does have cosmetic disadvantages. Removal of rudimentary digits should be discouraged.

Section 8
Multiple Amputations

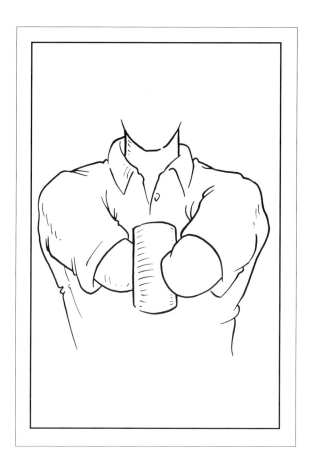

Chapter 37

Functional Assessment and Management of Multilimb Deficiency

John A. Herring, MD

Introduction

The management of a child born without two, three, or all four extremities is one of the most challenging and, at the same time, most rewarding experiences in the practice of medicine. Management is really not the correct word, because the real duty of those involved in the care of the child is to accompany that person through life, being as helpful as possible when the opportunities arise. Each of these children has a unique configuration of anomalies, a concerned and often frightened family, and a lifetime of opportunities and limitations of their own. Yet, within this uniqueness, certain patterns of adaptation emerge, and the broad palate of these patterns will paint the pictures of this discussion.

Etiology

What caused this to happen? This persistent question is foremost in the minds of parents of children with these deficiencies. Unfortunately, congenital absence of several extremities is still a poorly understood event. The only known cause of a large number of cases of congenital limb deficiency is the use of the drug Thalidomide. Current lack of knowledge limits us, the child's physicians, to informing most parents that we simply do not know the cause of their child's limb deficiency. We do know, however, the approximate fetal age at which the insult occurred. Virtually all major deficiencies originate as a developmental failure within the first 7 weeks of gestation. One exception, amputation by amniotic bands, occurs considerably later in development. The commonest cause of acquired multiple limb deficiency is meningococcemia. The management of the younger child after meningococcemia is similar to that of a child with congenital deficiency, with some exceptions that will be noted.

The First Priority

Our most important encounter with a child and family is the very first one, no matter what the presenting problem. Simple though it sounds, we should begin by making friends with the child and the family. We must let them know that we can help, that we have information and services that will help them. At that time we also should show them that we care about them and that to some degree we understand their problems. We realize that they are upset, as well as disappointed and afraid. We know that they must grieve a loss, even though that loss is of something hoped for. This foundation of empathy, while necessary in any setting, is of utmost importance in working with a child with multiple limb deficiencies.

There are some specific things to impart to the young child and his or her family on the first meeting. Some may be unnecessary when meeting an older child.

This child has great potential. Emphasize the child's potential and do not focus on the missing body parts. Remember that even a child with total quadrimelic limb absence has a remarkable intellectual and emotional potential.

We can predict many functional abilities. We understand certain patterns of limb deficiency and can anticipate many future accomplishments within the child's range.

We can predict certain functional limitations. We can explain some of them and describe ways in which they can be mastered.

We can intervene successfully in specific ways. For example, we know how a child will use lower extremity prostheses; we know that some extremities will need to be lengthened or altered surgically. We know when to do these things in order to maximize function. We also know that it is unwise to intervene too often. Our interventions will be carefully timed to the child's development.

There are limitations in what we can accomplish. We do not have any upper extremity prostheses with sensory feedback, and most children with bilateral upper extremity absence will not find currently available prostheses very useful. We can lengthen an extremity only a certain amount and only if the joints above and below the lengthened segment are relatively normal. We cannot create a joint when the child is born without one. We cannot transplant an extremity from one person to another. We cannot impart growth where there is none.

Some of these things, which are impossible today, may be feasible tomorrow. We have some idea of likely innovations and likely future limitations, and beyond that we cannot predict.

Going down this fascinating path of great adaptation with this child should be a remarkable adventure that, in spite of many obstacles, will be more emotionally rewarding than any other experience the parents have ever had, and we will help make this happen.

Everything we do will be a learning process for us. We will learn what works best for a child by watching and listening to that child at each step along the way. The child's responses will always be the barometer of our success or failure. We hope the parents will be good observers as well, and we will always consider their evaluation of our efforts.

The single most helpful step for most parents is to meet another family whose child has a similar deficiency. A clinic setting is ideal for developing a parental support network, and every clinic should keep a list of parents willing to participate. (Most are more than willing.)

Patterns

Young children have remarkable abilities to adapt to limb absences as they mature. Although each child has a unique set of limb abnormalities, children with similar anomalies adapt in similar ways. This uniquely human adaptability is possible because of the developmental immaturity of the infant's nervous system. It is this immaturity that allows the developing nervous system to arrange itself to match the child's specific limb structure. For example, when a child who has no arms begins to use the feet for manual activities, the brain becomes programmed to repeat and refine that function, just as it would had the child used the hands instead. Most fascinating is the fact that the substitution patterns a child chooses are invariably the most efficient for that child's limb anatomy. When we understand these patterns, we can anticipate future functional abilities and needs of the child.

One Upper and One Lower Limb Deficiency

Children with a deficiency of one upper limb and one lower limb can be managed as if the deficiencies were single, with minor additional considerations. The child will certainly use a lower limb prosthesis. The only difference in management will be if the child needs walking support. The child may use an adapted crutch for the abnormal upper extremity (or the upper extremity prosthesis) when learning to use the lower extremity prosthesis. Many of these children, however, may not choose to use an upper extremity prosthesis.

Bilateral Upper Limb Deficiency

The child with partial or complete absence of both upper extremities adapts in quite predictable ways. We can understand these adaptations more easily when we consider both the motor and sensory needs of the child. For example, a child with missing hands and mobile wrists will use the two wrists together for most prehension. These children will almost never use prostheses for major functional activities. I believe that they do not use prostheses for three reasons. First, the devices cover and block the sensory surfaces of the arms. Second, current prostheses have very simple and limited functions, and are poor substitutes for the complexity of function of the human hand. The third reason is probably the most important. The child's nervous system develops most of its motor and sensory pathways postnatally and makes the best functional adaptations for that child's anatomy. These adaptations are highly efficient and result in function that is almost as sophisticated as that of normal hands and arms. Prosthetic attempts to improve on these functional adaptations are inadequate when compared to the child's motor and sensory abilities with the residual limbs. Although, at times, physicians and

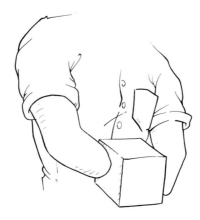

Fig. 1 *The child with absence of both arms at the midforearm level will hold larger objects with both arms together.*

prosthetists become enamored with our devices, the child will perceive the functional advantages of his or her sensate limbs at a very young age.

The child with absence of the structures below the mid forearms will hold objects with the two arms at once (Fig. 1). The child will also grasp objects with each elbow. Even those with very short forearms have good elbow prehension. There may be a role for the Krukenberg procedure in some of these individuals, but I have no experience with the procedure.[1]

The child with one functional elbow and one distal humeral level of absence will use the side with the elbow as the dominant extremity. Elbow prehension will be the major functional unit for writing and other fine motor activities, while both arms will be used together if possible to handle large objects (Fig. 2). The child will also hold objects against the body with one or both limbs (Fig. 3, *left*). Alternatively, with a very short limb, the child may hold objects against the cheek (Fig. 3, *right*).

The child with bilateral upper extremity absence above the elbow will likely use the feet for some functional activities and the arms for others, depending on the length of the residual upper limbs. The short upper limbs will be used together to hold an object (Fig. 4). Shorter limbs can only hold large objects in this manner. With very short upper limbs, the child will hold things against the face with the arm (Fig. 3, *right*). Although these children can write and do some other activities with the arm against the cheek, they are much more efficient in using their feet for most functions. For social reasons, they may use the arm against the face for writing while in school, but will write more efficiently with their feet in private (Fig. 5).

The child with complete absence of the upper extremities will use the feet for all upper extremity functions (Fig. 5). The ability of a child to adapt to foot use is amazing. Writing, typing, using a computer, brushing the teeth, handling a knife and fork or a pool cue, putting a worm on a hook,

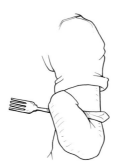

Fig. 2 The child with one functional elbow and absence of the other arm at the distal humeral level will use elbow prehension for fine motor activities.

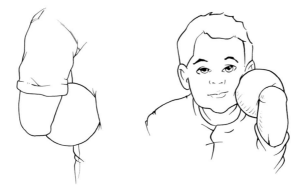

Fig. 3 Left, The child with absence of the arm at the transhumeral level will often hold objects against the body with that extremity. Right, The child with absence of the arm at the transhumeral level will also hold objects against the cheek with the residual limb. These children frequently write with this maneuver.

and driving a car all can be done with the feet. The child will learn to do all these things just as other children learn their tasks.

How does a parent fit into this picture? The answer is the same as with any other child, and is just as complicated. The parent should facilitate but not direct, help just enough but not too much, and protect without overprotecting. As one mother said, "I couldn't have taught a child who has no arms to do any of these things, he just seemed to know how to do it."

The two major limits for these children are reaching above the head and toileting. Reach with the feet will always be limited, but will not diminish with age. Toileting can usually be done with the feet with special adaptations that will need to be taught to the child. These children usually do not benefit from prostheses and should not be forced to "try" them. I have been told

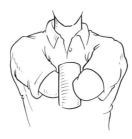

Fig. 4 *The child with bilateral absence of the arms at the transhumeral level will hold objects with both residual limbs if they are long enough.*

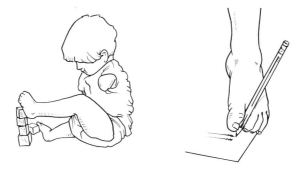

Fig. 5 Left, *The child missing most or all of both upper extremities will use the feet for play activities as well as for all activities of life.* ***Right,*** *The child with upper amelia will learn to write, type, and use utensils with the feet. The "footwriting" of such children often exceeds that of their peers and should be encouraged and enabled by teachers and parents.*

by several adults with upper limb amelia that they are bitter and disturbed because they were made to use a prosthesis that reduced their function. Forcing the use of a prosthesis in this situation is a serious mistake that may have strong emotional consequences.

Often the challenge in the management of these children is to convince the family that the child should be encouraged to use the feet as hands. If a parent is repulsed by the sight of the child using the feet, it is important to devote as much time and discussion as necessary to show the parent why this ability must be promoted. As a first step, the child should be allowed to be barefoot whenever possible. The child must be able to easily put on and take off his or her shoes, and the child should wear socks as often as the rest of us wear gloves, that is only when outside in the cold. It may be helpful to place schoolwork on the floor beneath the child's seat. On the other hand, the child may prefer to sit on the floor and work. Sports participation should be encouraged, and once again the parents will be surprised at the sports these children can master.

Bilateral Upper Limb and One Lower Limb Deficiency

The child missing both upper limbs with an additional deficient lower limb presents some tough challenges in the management of the lower extremities. The most vexing problem is the fact that the lower limb must function both as a hand and as a limb for ambulation. Certain conventional approaches, such as amputation for fibular deficiency, are out of the question because the child uses the feet as hands, and a physician would certainly not consider amputating a functional hand. Prosthetic intervention must be planned carefully to maximize function. For example, a child with no upper extremities, a proximal femoral deficiency on one side, and a normal leg on the other can probably use an equinus prosthesis to equalize leg lengths, provided that entry and exit from the prosthesis is quick and easy. If it is difficult to get the prosthesis off in order to use the feet as hands, then the child will reject the prosthesis, because "hand" function takes priority over lower limb function.

When the upper extremities and an entire lower extremity are absent, the child will have a difficult time using a prosthetic leg without the upper limbs for support. The child will find it difficult to remove the prosthesis with the single lower limb because the foot is the only functional "hand." Some such children will ambulate by hopping on the leg, while others will use a prosthesis.

Quadrimelic Limb Deficiency

The function of a child with quadrimelic extremity absence depends on the length of the residual limbs. If both the arms are present below the elbows and both legs are present below the knees, independent ambulation with lower extremity prostheses is almost certain. A young child will use very short lower extremity prostheses, or "stubbies." The older children will use relatively longer lower prostheses.

When the child has long above elbow residual limbs and long above knee or knee disarticulation levels, ambulation is usually possible. At first, very short lower prostheses are useful, followed at a later age by longer, nonarticulated prostheses. Some teenagers will use articulated knees, while others will prefer the stability of stiff knees, depending on the levels of absence and the child's body size and motivation. Getting up from a chair without forearms to push up with and quadriceps to extend the knees is difficult, but can usually be done with a pivot maneuver. When the residual limbs are short, the likelihood of independent ambulation with prostheses decreases, and the child will probably use a motorized wheel chair.

Bilateral Lower Extremity Deficiencies

A child with bilateral lower extremity deficiencies at the transtibial level is managed in the same way as one with a unilateral deficiency. For bilateral deficiencies at the knee disarticulation level or higher, we usually start the child with stiff knees. As the child matures, one or both knees may be articulated. We tend to lose sight of the fact that even though the child may walk well with articulated knees in the hospital, the child's outdoor world is filled with rough terrain and many obstacles. In this arena, the locked knees enable the child to run and play with abandon and vigor. An adolescent will usually prefer articulated knees, but some type of locking knee or stance phase stabilizer may still be needed.

The ability of the child with bilateral transfemoral limb deficiencies to ambulate depends upon the length of the residual limbs. Shorter residual limbs are associated with greater energy consumption in gait.[2] Most children and adolescents will ambulate well with bilateral above knee prostheses, but many will rely upon other means of locomotion as they reach adulthood.

Prostheses for Upper Extremities

Several published works suggest that children with multiple limb deficiency will use upper extremity prostheses with much functional benefit. Aitken's[3] classic article on bilateral upper limb deficiency describes a program of early fitting with passive devices and progressive "motoring" of the prostheses. He does not document rates or types of usage of these prostheses. Many clinics adopted this approach and for many years most children were fitted with one or two prostheses. Scotland and Galway,[4] in 1983, reviewed 131 children who used upper extremity prostheses at the Ontario Crippled Childrens Center. They found only 42 who had abandoned their prostheses.[4] Most surprisingly, four of six children with bilateral upper extremity absence were still using prostheses. This work noted the duration of prosthetic wear (a common lack in other papers) and found that most used their devices more than 8 hours a day.

Why then am I reluctant to prescribe prostheses while other authors have reported successful prosthetic use in bilateral upper extremity absence? The answer lies in my clinical experience. For many years the staff at Texas Scottish Rite Hospital vigorously fit passive devices at the age of independent sitting and followed that with cabled and motorized prostheses. We used state of the art myoelectric terminal devices. We used both powered and passive elbows. Patients would demonstrate adept use of the devices in a therapy setting but would quickly discard the prosthesis at home. The only exception in my experience was a boy who had quadrimelic amputations from meningococcemia. Although he used bilateral below elbow prostheses for a number of years, he stopped using them as an adult and stated that he was more functional using his arms without prostheses. As I mentioned earlier, several patients in adulthood expressed their frustration and anger with the fitting and training process. All patients clearly stated that either the sensory surfaces of their arms or their feet were more functional than prostheses. They often noted that the prostheses blocked function by covering sensory surfaces and were hot and uncomfortable. The Texas Scottish Rite Hospital lack of prosthetic success is common but not universal in the community of prosthetic clinics.

Summary and Conclusion

The child with multiple limb deficiencies can enjoy a rich and functional life, and our job is to work knowledgeably and helpfully with the child and family to achieve this goal. A team approach is essential, and each member of the team must be prepared to learn with and from the children in order to help them adapt to their own unique anatomy.

References

1. Swanson AB: The Krukenberg procedure in the juvenile amputee. *J Bone Joint Surg* 1964;46B:1540–1548.

2. Waters RL, Perry J, Antonelli D, Hislop H: Energy cost of walking of amputees: The influence of level of amputation. *J Bone Joint Surg* 1976;58A:42–46.

3. Aitken GT: Management of severe bilateral upper limb deficiencies. *Clin Orthop* 1964;37:53–60.

4. Scotland TR, Galway HR: A Long-term review of children with congenital and acquired upper limb deficiency. *J Bone Joint Surg* 1983;65B:346–349.

Chapter 38

Surgical Treatment of Meningococcal-Induced Purpura Fulminans

William P. Adams, Jr, MD
P. Craig Hobar, MD

Introduction

Purpura fulminans, a thromboembolic condition that results in high rates of extremity gangrene and amputation, is an uncommon but potentially life-threatening sequela of sepsis-induced viral, rickettsial or bacterial infections. Although the precise incidence of purpura fulminans in the various infectious disorders is unknown, patients with meningococcemia are at greatest risk for developing the condition, especially in endemic regions including Texas, the Pacific Northwest, and the Southeast.[1,2] The clinical course of fulminating meningococcemia may be characterized by rapid progression from nonspecific initial symptoms of fever, headache, lethargy, and vomiting to hemodynamic collapse and death in less than 12 hours.

In 1971, Toews and Bass[3] reported a 10% incidence of purpura fulminans in patients with meningococcemia; the mortality rate in those patients was 44% compared with 3% for patients who did not develop purpura. In a more recent report of 113 patients with meningococcal C disease, purpura fulminans occurred in 25% of patients, and their mortality rate was substantially higher (50%) than in the nonpurpuric patients (1%).[4] In a review of children treated for meningococcal-induced purpura fulminans at our institution, 16 (11%) of the 139 patients with meningococcemia treated over a 10-year period developed purpura fulminans during the course of their infection.[5] Ten patients (62%) were male and six (38%) were female; their ages ranged from 3 months to 10 years (mean, 3.5 years). Four children were younger than 1 year of age, five were from 1 to 3 years, and seven were from 4 to 10 years of age.

Soft-Tissue Injury

The precise biologic mechanisms for the microvascular disease that invariably accompanies meningococcal-induced purpura fulminans have not been fully identified. It has been hypothesized that site specific differences in cytokine release by endothelial cells may be responsible for the damage that occurs in specific tissues, such as the skin and adrenal medulla.[6] Recently, Powars and associates[4] demonstrated decreased concentrations of protein C in patients with severe purpura fulminans caused by *Neisseria Meningitides.* These authors speculated that the depletion of this naturally occurring anticoagulant is the major factor causing the microvascular thrombosis that is a hallmark of purpura fulminans. Furthermore, they speculated that children who are younger than 4 years of age would be those at greatest risk for developing meningococcal-induced purpura fulminans because their naturally occurring production of protein S and protein C is less than that of older children and adults. Whether the precipitous decline in protein C concentrations that occur in patients with meningococcal purpura is responsible for the microvascular injury or is a secondary phenomenon remains to be determined. Adjunctive treatment of purpura fulminans with protein C concentrate has demonstrated encouraging results in reducing thromboembolic complications and warrants further study.[7]

Management

Little information is available on the sequelae in infants and children who survive meningococcal-associated purpura fulminans. In a review of 86 infants and children with meningococcal disease, Edwards and Baker[6] reported that 16 of 20 (80%) patients with purpura survived and 11 (69%) of these survivors were normal. They mentioned no patient who required skin grafting or amputation. In contrast, ten of 14 (71%) patients reported by Powars and associates[4] had gangrene that resulted in autoamputation, and there have been other isolated reports of limb amputations in patients who survived purpura fulminans. Our experience indicates that children with purpura fulminans who survive the initial acute phase of the disease are at risk for serious complications that are the result of endotoxin-induced microvascular injury. Treatment of these patients requires an interdisciplinary approach between pediatricians, plastic surgeons, psychiatrists, psychologists, and rehabilitation experts.

Our treatment algorithm is outlined in Figure 1. Early in the course of meningococcal-induced tissue injury, we recommend conservative treatment of affected tissues until a clear line of demarcation between viable and nonviable tissue is apparent. Fasciotomies should be performed when indicated, although the nature of injury usually does not make this a useful treatment regimen.

All limbs should be carefully examined. Usual assessment for compartment syndrome may be difficult in the severely septic patient. The clinical hallmark of pain on passive extension of the involved compartment usually is not feasible in the acute setting. Direct measure of compartment pressures may be useful. Magnetic resonance imaging is also a valuable adjunct for delineating deep muscle and bone involvement; however, it is often impractical in the acute intensive care unit setting.

Initially, a period of demarcation is granted, and silvadene dressing changes are begun once the soft-tissue progression is stable and the patient is a surgical candidate. Serial debridement of all necrotic tissue is essential and may require extensive excision of nonviable skin, subcutaneous tissue, and muscle. We will leave any questionable tissue to be assessed at the next debridement to maximize soft tissue for reconstruction.

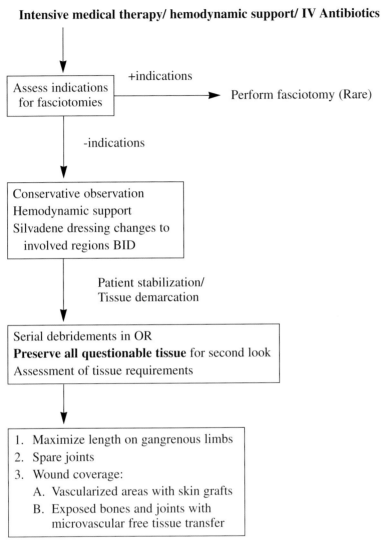

Intensive medical therapy/ hemodynamic support/ IV Antibiotics

Assess indications for fasciotomies

+indications → Perform fasciotomy (Rare)

-indications

Conservative observation
Hemodynamic support
Silvadene dressing changes to
  involved regions BID

Patient stabilization/
Tissue demarcation

Serial debridements in OR
Preserve all questionable tissue for second look
Assessment of tissue requirements

1. Maximize length on gangrenous limbs
2. Spare joints
3. Wound coverage:
    A. Vascularized areas with skin grafts
    B. Exposed bones and joints with
        microvascular free tissue transfer

Fig. 1 *University of Texas Southwestern management algorithm for management of purpura fulminans.*

Reconstruction with skin grafts and local, regional, and free flaps is performed in a timely fashion. Skin grafts are used over all areas with well-vascularized beds. Areas with exposed bone and joints require extremely well-vascularized tissue for coverage. The use of local random or pedicled axial subcutaneous or fasciocutaneous flaps usually is not useful. We find that these flaps fail to adequately cover the defects. Free tissue transfer is an important option in these patients and should be used without hesitation when indicated. Microvascular free flaps provide the hypervascularity needed to control the wound types produced by this disease process. We have successfully used free flaps to preserve limb length and joints. We have not found it necessary to obtain a preoperative arteriogram.

Whenever useful function of an affected limb can be preserved, amputation should be avoided. Although 5 cm of tibia is adequate for an adult below knee amputation, any tibial length should be preserved in a growing child. Residual limb lengthening may provide useful below-knee function at a later date.

Surgical Outcomes and Prognosis

Despite the overall improvement in outcome for patients with meningo-coccal disease since intensive care has been added to the therapeutic regimen, the prognosis for patients with meningococcal-induced purpura fulminans remains poor.[4] Although the 27% mortality rate for patients who developed purpura fulminans at our institution during the period of study was smaller than has been reported in several previous studies, 54% of the survivors had major morbidity and permanent sequelae. Forty-six percent of the children who survived their disease required amputations of two or more limbs; 30% of these had high-level quadruple limb amputations. It is likely that the improved medical care of these acutely ill patients has improved survival, resulting in more patients with nonviable limbs that require surgical reconstruction.

Our experience has resulted in a near 50% incidence of amputation of two or more limbs.[5] Purpuric lesions were present in all patients at the time of admission or within the first 12 hours of hospitalization. All children had purpuric lesions on at least one of their extremities, and the majority had lesions on the chest, back, face, and abdomen. Skin necrosis was first observed in all patients within 18 hours after admission; the largest number of necrotic lesions were in areas of distal circulation, such as the extremities, the digits, and the nose. All children required multiple surgical procedures and extensive rehabilitation.

Four patients (24%) died within the first 36 hours after hospital admission. Each of the surviving patients required multiple soft-tissue debridements and skin grafts, principally to the legs, arms, and chest. Soft-tissue involvement of the extremities is often extensive (Fig. 2). Radiographs of the affected limbs demonstrated bone irregularities and destruction of the distal metaphyses. Six patients required amputations of at least one limb; three patients required high-level quadruple amputations at the proximal humeri and proximal femurs (Fig. 3), one patient had bilateral midtibia amputations, and one underwent disarticulation at the left knee and right ankle. A 6-month-old female patient with a severely affected foot with exposed medial malleolus and calcaneus required microvascular free latissimus dorsi flap to save the extremity (Fig. 4). A 4-year-old male patient required bilateral above-knee amputations, a left midhumerus amputation, and a right trans-metacarpal amputation and proximal row carpectomy with extensive debridement of the triceps muscle compartment. On this same extremity, an open elbow joint required a rectus abdominus free flap and a groin flap to

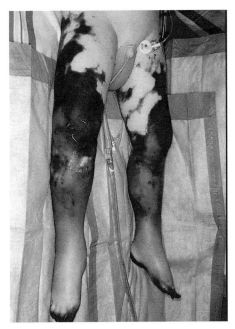

Fig. 2 *Severe bilateral lower extremity involvement in a 2-year-old patient with purpura fulminans.*

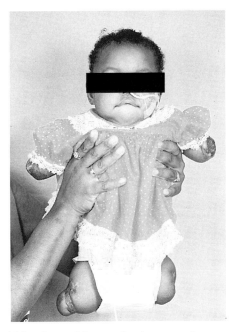

Fig. 3 *Five-month-old female requiring quadruple amputations.*

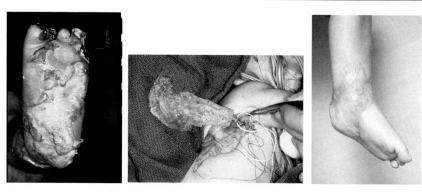

Fig. 4 Left, *Extensive medial malleolar and calcaneal exposure in 6-month-old patient requiring a free flap for coverage.* **Center,** *Free lattissimus dorsi flap harvested in situ.* **Right,** *Long term follow-up with stable coverage.*

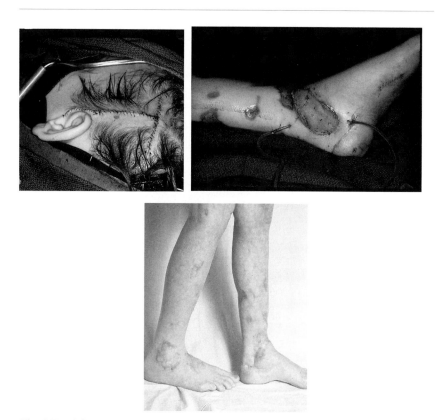

Fig. 5 Top left, *Free temporoparietal fascial flap donor site.* **Top right,** *Free temporoparietal flap inset over lateral malleolus with skin graft.* **Bottom,** *Long-term follow-up with stable coverage over right lateral malleolus.*

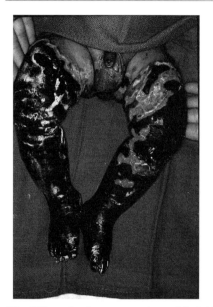
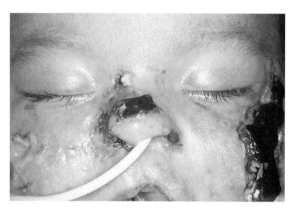

Fig. 6 *Extensive lower extremity and facial involvement in 1-year-old patient.*

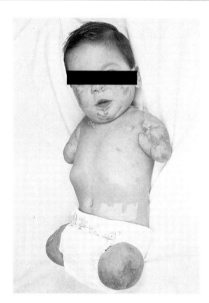

Fig. 7 *Same patient requiring four extremity amputation. Note facial wounds healed with only conservative management.*

cover an exposed wrist joint. The initial groin flap never adhered to the wound bed, and a repeat procedure with resection of the distal ulna was required to obtain stable wrist coverage. A 10-year-old male with exposed lateral malleolus was treated with a free temporoparietal fascia flap (Fig. 5, *top left* and *right*). The patient obtained an excellent result (Fig. 5, *bottom*). We discourage the use of pedicled fasciocutaneous or regional flaps for coverage of these wounds because of complications secondary to lack of robust vascular supply; however, we have had excellent success with free fasciocutaneous flaps when indicated as a result of the added vascularity afforded to the flap as a free flap. The 1-year-old patient depicted in Figure 6 demonstrates severe involvement of the lower extremities and the face. The 2-month follow-up demonstrates healing of the facial wounds with only conservative care (Fig. 7), compared to the more severe sequelae with extremity involvement. We have found the overall recovery of these patients remarkable. The diligent efforts to maximize limb length and joints have resulted in functional recovery far surpassing our expectations as demonstrated in one of our 10-year-old patients with bilateral below-knee amputations who plays football among a host of other activities.

Summary

Menigococcemia-associated purpura fulminans is a devastating condition often resulting in severe soft-tissue loss and amputation. The hallmark of treatment is conservative initial management followed by multiple serial debridement and coverage of soft-tissue deficits using our reconstructive algorithm (Fig. 1). Attempts to preserve maximal limb length and joint function should be the reconstructive goals and will maximize outcome in these patients.

References

1. Gedde-Dahl TW, Bjark P, Hoiby EA, Host JH, Bruun JN: Severity of meningococcal disease: Assessment by factors and scores and implications for patient management. *Rev Infect Dis* 1990;12:973–992.

2. Kirsch EA, Barton RP, Kitchen L, Giroir BP: Pathophysiology, treatment and outcome of meningococcemia: A review and recent experience. *Pediatr Infec Dis J* 1996;15:967–978.

3. Toews WH, Bass JW: Skin manifestations of meningococcal infection: An immediate indicator of prognosis. *Am J Dis Child* 1974;127:173–176.

4. Powars D, Larsen R, Johnson J, et al: Epidemic meningococcemia and purpura fulminans with induced protein C deficiency. *Clin Infect Dis* 1993;17:254–261.

5. Herrera R, Hobar PC, Ginsburg CM: Surgical intervention for the complications of meningococcal-induced of purpura fulminans. *Pediatr Infect Dis J* 1994;13:734–737.

6. Edwards MS, Baker CJ: Complications and sequelae of meningococcal infections in children. *J Pediatr* 1981;99:540–545.

7. Rivard GE, David M, Farrell C, Schwarz HP: Treatment of purpura fulminans in meningococcemia with protein C concentrate. *J Pediatr* 1995;126:646–652.

Section 9

Outcome Measures

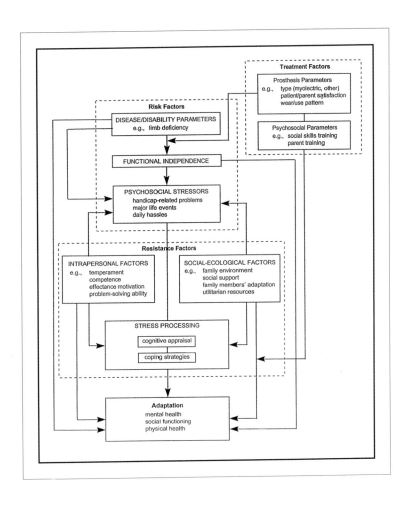

Chapter 39

Health-Related Quality of Life in Pediatric Limb Deficiency

James W. Varni, PhD
Sheri D. Pruitt, PhD
Michael Seid, PhD

Introduction

Most of the older literature on pediatric limb deficiencies focused on the problems of the adolescent amputee, whether traumatic or disease-related.[1] However, the vast majority of limb deficiencies in children are congenital.[2] Children with limb deficiencies are at increased risk for psychological and social adjustment problems, and the range of these problems varies among individuals. We have systematically investigated the degree of risk for these adjustment problems and have sought to identify risk and protective factors that may explain why some children adapt better than others.

Health Outcomes

Health outcome assessment seeks to determine whether surgical techniques, therapeutic interventions, or medical devices really cure disease, relieve symptoms, or prevent future health problems.[3] Broadly, health outcomes assessment answers the question: "Does the health-care intervention work as it is intended?"

The study of health outcomes, particularly in pediatrics, is in its early stage of development. Regulation of health care focuses largely on structure, on the characteristics of the health-care system necessary for service to be delivered (eg, licensure, hospital facilities, safety procedures). However, most health-care services and procedures are unregulated, and there are few empiric data to guide clinicians and policy makers to the most efficacious medical interventions.

One problem in the evaluation of health care is the current state of methodologies and outcome measurement.[4,5] For most health-care services, the desired outcome is not clearly evident, and it can range from specific symptom relief to reduced mortality or improved health-related quality of life (HRQOL). Thus, the simple task of determining whether a medical treatment is "effective" quickly becomes a complicated endeavor. Effective in what way and from whose perspective are pertinent questions. In addition, there is a dearth of empirically derived instruments for evaluating outcome. Few psychometrically sound measures are available to evaluate benefits associated with health-care services.

The measurement of outcomes associated with a given intervention is not a new concept; however, outcomes assessment currently is highlighted because of the growing emphasis on health-care reform and medical-cost reduction. Third-party payers have become ubiquitous in their application of cost-containment strategies; no populations or health-care services are protected from inquiry or accountability. In pediatric limb deficiency, the expense of prosthetic components has come under scrutiny. For example, there is an increasing reluctance by state crippled children's funds and private insurance companies to cover the expense associated with myoelectrically-operated hand prostheses.[6] What once were considered customary prosthesis prescriptions (even for toddlers as young as 15 months), now require substantial justification before third-party payers will cover costs that may be in excess of $10,000. Empirically based outcome assessments, designed to measure potential health benefits derived from prosthetic components, may allow an accurate assessment of the need for costly prostheses.

Health-Related Quality of Life

Accurate measurement of outcome in chronic pediatric physical disorders requires a multidimensional approach. Quality of life, functional status, or health status are terms frequently used interchangeably in the assessment of the impact of disease, although quality of life is the more comprehensive concept. There is a general consensus that the term HRQOL is an accurate and concise measure of outcome for many diverse chronic physical disorders in children.[7-8] Similar to screening for biologic disease, screening for HRQOL in a patient population requires a standardized test with established reliability and validity.[9] An HRQOL measurement instrument that can be used with a broad range of pediatric patients would be of great value for evaluation of both direct clinical service at the individual level and cost-effectiveness at the system level.

HRQOL measures typically include as a minimum the physical, mental, and social health dimensions originally delineated by the World Health Organization in 1948. In sharp contrast to the myriad of well-developed HRQOL measures for adult patients, multidimensional pediatric HRQOL measures are just now being developed.[7-8]

As medical technologies advance and health-care resources tighten, the need for multidimensional health-related outcomes assessment becomes increasingly necessary in clinical decision making, policy development, and program evaluation.[10] Because traditional outcome measures of mortality and morbidity are of little use for patients with nonfatal chronic disorders, more comprehensive and sensitive outcome measures are needed to evaluate the effect of medical care on HRQOL in pediatric chronic physical conditions, such as limb deficiency. Linking clinical variables, such as degree of limb loss, or biomechanical interventions, such as a well-designed prosthesis, with pediatric health outcomes requires not only HRQOL standardized measurement, but also a conceptual model or theoretical framework that specifies possible algorithms or clinical pathways to selected health outcomes. Wilson and Cleary[11] have described a conceptual model that proposes specific causal pathways to adult patient HRQOL outcomes.

Theoretical Framework

Wallander and Varni[12–14] have developed a well-accepted technique for evaluating factors that affect a child's adaptation to chronic physical disorders. Their model considers pediatric chronic physical disorders to be chronic stressors that produce an ongoing strain for both the children and their parents.[12–14] Chronic strains are defined as persistent objective conditions that require continual readjustment and interfere repeatedly with the performance of ordinary activities.[15] Thus, limb deficiency would be considered a chronic strain for the pediatric patient and his/her family.

Identification of modifiable risk and resistance factors provides data-based guidance for the development of new ways to treat children and adolescents with chronic physical disorders.[12–14] Risk factors in the model include disease/disability parameters (eg, disease diagnosis, handicap severity, medical problems, bowel/bladder control, visibility, cognitive functioning, brain involvement), functional independence in the activities of daily living (ADL), and psychosocial stressors (handicap-related problems, major life events, daily hassles). Resistance factors in the model are delineated into three categories (Fig. 1). An algorithm has been developed that tests components (detailed microanalytic models) of the integrative multifactorial model using multivariate data-analytic strategies. We will illustrate the use of this framework in pediatric limb deficiencies.

Risk Factors

Disease/Disability Parameters

We have not found the degree of limb loss to be directly associated with depressive symptoms, anxiety, or behavior problems in children and adolescents with limb deficiencies.[9,16,17] Although degree of limb loss was not significantly correlated with general self-esteem in children,[18] it was in adolescents.[16] A comparison of congenital and acquired limb deficiencies in adolescents showed no differences for depressive symptoms, anxiety, or general self-esteem.[16]

Functional Status

Children and adolescents with upper or lower extremity limb deficiencies face a lifetime of functional limitations. Almost all of them are fitted with prosthetic components to enhance their ability to participate in ADL. Functional status has long been recognized as an important outcome of clinical care.[19–21] In pediatric limb deficiency, the functional benefits asso-

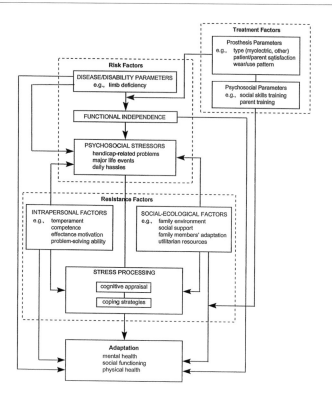

Fig. 1 *Theoretical Model.*

ciated with different prosthetic devices have been described.[22–24] Body-powered limbs with a hook have been compared with myoelectric components, and clinically observed improvements in functional abilities and psychosocial functioning were noted with the myoelectric devices.[22–24] However, because the measurement strategies used were not empirically validated, previous clinical findings of functional and psychological benefits may be unreliable. For example, most assessments of function in children with limb deficiency relied on observation of task performance in a clinic setting. Clinical observations are important, but they are not necessarily reliable evaluations of the child's performance of ADL.

Third-party payers want "hard evidence" of the functional benefits of expensive prostheses and surgical procedures. We believe that outcome assessments based on empiric research can best provide this evidence. The Child Amputation Prosthetics Project-Functional Status Inventory (CAPP-FSI)[25] is a recently developed standardized measure designed specifically for children (ages 8 to 17) who have either upper or lower limb deficiency. It is a 40-item inventory of behavioral manifestations of limb deficiency that interfere with childrens' daily self-care and developmentally relevant activities. Parents rate their child's behavior on two dimensions: "Does the Activity," which is the frequency of the child's independent performance of a specific task, and "Uses a Prosthesis," which is the frequency of the child's use of a prosthesis to perform the task. Items on the CAPP-FSI include separate upper and lower extremity activities such as "put toothpaste on brush and brush teeth," "put on and remove shoes," "hold a sandwich and eat," "turn pages in a book," "walk up and down a flight of four steps," and "cross the street before the traffic light turns red."

Initial psychometric properties of the CAPP-FSI have been reported.[25] Internal consistency reliability (alpha = 0.96) is more than adequate for the two scales that make up the instrument, suggesting it is a cohesive instrument for assessing functional activity performance and prosthesis use in children with limb deficiency. Initial construct validity of the instrument has been established through empiric strategies. The CAPP-FSI distinguishes between children with upper and lower limb deficiency, and scores on the "Does the Activity" scale are correlated with degree of physical impairment.

In summary, the CAPP-FSI may be useful as a clinical outcome measure in addressing third-party payer concerns about costs of prosthetic devices. Although further refinement and validation are necessary, the CAPP-FSI also is promising for future investigations of health outcome following other clinical interventions designed to improve function of children with limb deficiency. The psychometric analysis of a functional status inventory for preschool children with limb deficiency currently is underway.[26] This standardized measure, similar in construction and design to the CAPP-FSI, is designed for children ages 3 to 6 years.

Patient/Parent Satisfaction With Prosthesis and Functional Status

Patient satisfaction continues to gain interest as a major outcome variable in today's health-care market.[27] There is mounting evidence linking patient satisfaction to a variety of health outcome and health-care utilization factors, including adherence to medical regimens,[28,29] understanding and retention of medical information,[30] mental health status,[31] changing providers,[32] withdrawal from prepaid health plans,[33] and malpractice litigation.[34] Because of these relationships, insurers and health policy makers are particularly interested in assessing patient satisfaction and its impact on health-care costs and clinical outcome.

The assessment of specific dimensions of patient satisfaction may be especially relevant for children with limb deficiency and their unique prosthesis requirements. Previous studies have shown relationships between several "satisfaction-like" variables and prosthesis use in children with limb deficiency. For example, prosthesis comfort and complaints about repair needs have been linked to the amount of time that children wear their prostheses.[35,36] Children who avoid wearing their prosthesis due to dissatisfaction with its comfort, performance, or appearance may be less independent than they otherwise would be. In this era of cost containment, prescriptions for prostheses that are not worn obviously are difficult to justify to third-party payers.

The Child Amputee Prosthetics Project Prosthesis Satisfaction Inventory (CAPP-PSI)[37] measures the degree of parents' satisfaction with their child's prescribed prosthetic device in regard to fit, function, appearance, and service. Parents rate 14 items divided into three scales: (1) parent-rated child satisfaction with prosthesis (eg, "Does your child like the way that his/her prosthesis fits?"); (2) parent satisfaction with prosthesis (eg, "Are you happy with the way your child's prosthesis helps him/her perform daily activities?"); and (3) parent satisfaction with service (eg, "Are you satisfied with how long it takes to repair your child's prosthesis?").

Preliminary psychometric studies of the CAPP-PSI have been completed.[37] Evidence for internal consistency reliability is excellent. Cronbach's alpha coefficients are high (range, 0.80 to 0.90) for all three scales,[38,39] suggesting the CAPP-PSI is a reliable instrument for assessing satisfaction with the prosthetic component prescribed for a child with limb deficiency. There also are significant correlations between prosthesis satisfaction and patterns of prosthesis wear and use and of prosthesis appearance as rated on visual analog scales.

The ability to accurately assess prosthesis satisfaction and link it to compliance with prosthesis wear and use patterns has the potential to enhance prosthesis prescribing practices, clinical interventions, and ultimately, clinical outcome for children with limb deficiency. For example, parent input regarding appearance, function, and fit of the prosthesis may be critical for the child's future compliance. Adequate training and assessment sessions to ensure the best match between child and prosthesis in terms of comfort, function, and appearance may be important prior to ordering the child's actual device. The integration of parents into early training sessions may be imperative. Further, prosthesis satisfaction may require ongoing monitoring as children develop and their prosthetic needs change.[40]

Prosthesis Wear and Use

The assessment of prosthesis wear and use patterns also may be important outcomes in the evaluation of health-care services specific to the pediatric limb deficiency population. The amount of time that children wear and use their prostheses likely is related to other important health outcomes, such as functional status, patient satisfaction, quality of life, and other psychosocial variables.

Pruitt and associates[37] describe a measure in which parents are asked to estimate the amount of time during the previous week their child wore the prescribed prosthesis and the amount of time their child used his/her prosthesis for activities across a range of situations including home, school, with friends, and during social occasions. The range is from "all of the time" to "none of the time." Parents also estimate "overall" prosthesis wear and use time. Although this measure has not undergone psychometric study, the frequency of prosthesis wear and use has been related to prosthesis satisfaction scores as measured by the CAPP-PSI. Further reliability and validity studies are needed.

Additional psychometric studies will include test-retest reliability (to ensure stability of the measure across time) and further validation studies. The parent-rated CAPP-FSI, for example, could be compared to children's own reports of their prosthesis use and behavior to establish concurrent validity. Validity also could be established through high correlations between the CAPP-FSI and other, more general measures of functional abilities (eg, Functional Disability Inventory)[41] and low correlations between the CAPP-FSI and instruments designed to measure unrelated child characteristics. Factor analysis eventually could be accomplished with an adequate sample size. Longitudinal designs are needed to establish how reliably the CAPP-FSI and CAPP-PSI predict prosthesis use and participation in everyday activities as well as to establish their sensitivity to change in functional status and satisfaction following other health-care interventions.

Psychosocial Stressors

In a series of studies, Varni and his associates found that children with limb deficiencies who reported higher levels of perceived stress also reported higher levels of depressive symptoms and lower levels of general self-esteem.[17,18,42] The value of these studies has been to demonstrate how certain daily hassles, which we have termed microstressors, affect the occurrence of depressive symptoms and reduction of self-esteem, and to suggest that many of these stressors may be successfully altered.

Resistance Factors

Intrapersonal Factors

Few empirical investigations exist in the published literature concerning the relationship between temperament and the psychological adaptation of chronically ill and handicapped children. In the study by Varni and associates,[43] the theoretical perspective and measurement methodology of Buss and Plomin[44] was used to test the relationship between temperment and adaptation. Essentially, Buss and Plomin define temperament as a set of inherited personality traits that appear early in life. They have selected personality traits that they theorize appear in infancy, provide a foundation for later personality development, and exclude transient individual differences. They include inheritance as part of their definition of temperament and exclude personality traits that originate solely as a result of environmental influences.[44]

Chess and Thomas[45] have postulated that temperament characteristics must be considered within the context of the environment to predict psychological adjustment. Within their model, child temperament and environmental demands, in other words, child temperament characteristics that maximally "fit" or "match" the demands imposed by the child's social environment are expected to result in more favorable adaptation. Although this Goodness-of-Fit theoretical model is intuitively appealing, there has been relatively little research to investigate its validity in children with chronic illness or physical handicaps.

In 1989 we studied the relationship between family function and child temperament relative to the psychological and social adaptation of children with limb deficiencies. Certain aspects of temperament and family psychosocial environment could be used to predict the degree of adaptation in these children.[43] More family cohesion, moral-religious emphasis, and organization, in combination with less family conflict, predicted better psychological and social adaptation, and greater child emotionality predicted greater behavior problems and lower social competence. Moreover, the interaction between family cohesion and child emotionality significantly predicted behavior problems.

Socioecologic Factors

Varni and associates[46] investigated the adaptational correlates of multiple perceived social support domains in children with congenital/acquired limb deficiencies. Higher perceived classmate, friend, parent, and teacher social support correlated significantly with lower depressive symptoms and trait anxiety, and higher general self-esteem. In hierarchic multiple regression analyses, demographic variables were not significant predictors of depressive symptoms, trait anxiety, or general self-esteem. The child's perception of classmate social support was the only variable that predicted all three psychological adjustment factors in this controlled study. The children who perceived high classmate social support had fewer depressive and anxious symptoms and higher self-esteem.

Finally, Varni and his associates tested the integrated model of perceived stress and perceived social support in children with limb deficiencies. Varni and associates[42] investigated the interaction of social support and perceived microstressors and found a direct connection between the two. Next, Varni and associates[17] investigated how general self-esteem affects the relationship between stress and social support. In addition to the direct effects of microstressors and perceived classmate social support on depressive symptoms, a small indirect effect of perceived classmate social support through general self-esteem was also found. The finding, that classmate social support reduces depressive symptoms, confirms the observation that the negative reaction of a peer group to visible physical differences has a strong negative effect on the child with a limb deficiency.[47,48]

A low level of classmate social support represents a vulnerability factor for children with limb deficiencies in that it increases the risk for depressive symptoms and low self-esteem. Although self-esteem may not show an independent effect on depressive symptoms after controlling for social support, it may be instrumental in other aspects of these children's lives, such as their persistence on difficult or challenging tasks, their vocational choices, their tendency to take calculated risks in new situations, and their selection of a primarily cosmetic versus primarily functional prosthetic device. Previous studies have shown that self-esteem is determined not only by social support, but also by self-perceived competence/adequacy in the following domains: physical appearance, social acceptance, scholastic competence, athletic competence, and behavior.[18,49] Finally, whereas 72% of the variance in depressive symptoms was accounted for, additional variables may also play a part. For instance, family functioning and parental adjustment have also been shown to be significant predictors of emotional and behavioral adjustment in children with limb deficiencies.[43,50]

Taken together, the results have implications for intervention strategies designed to promote coping with the social consequences of limb deficiencies. A promising approach recently developed attempts to teach children the social skills needed to handle teasing, name-calling, and other peer social interactions.[1] Social skills selected for intervention may include improving conversation skills and increasing cooperative play, positive peer interactions, peer acceptance and friendship-making, and how to handle teasing and name-calling on the playground.[51] Varni and Setoguchi[1] describe in detail these techniques for handling teasing and name-calling from peers. Research is needed to evaluate the effects of social skills training on the long-term psychological and social function of children with limb deficiencies.

Perceived Physical Appearance

In our society (and perhaps more generally, in our species), physical attractiveness represents a prominent personal characteristic that systematically influences interpersonal interactions, perceptions, and inferences about an individual's ability.[52–54] This "beauty-is-good" prejudice has been found across all age groups.[55,56] Therefore, it might logically be expected that children with visible physical differences would experience discrimination in their social environment (CP Varni, PhD, unpublished data, 1993). During the childhood years, physical appearance and social acceptance are important predictors of adjustment.[56] The social psychology of physical appearance in our culture negatively influences attitudes and behaviors toward persons with physical handicaps.[57] Children with physical differences are hypothesized to be at high risk for these negative social perceptions and behaviors and resultant loss of self-esteem.[18]

Recently, Varni (unpublished data, 1993) proposed that the individual's perception of his or her physical appearance determines psychological adjustment. In more colloquial terms, "beauty is in the eyes of the beholder," whether the beholder is the individual or those in his or her social environment. Within the risk and resistance theoretical framework,[12–14] limb deficiencies are hypothesized as a chronic strain risk factor, more specifically, a disease/disability parameter. Higher perceived physical appearance, however, is hypothesized as a resistance factor, more specifically a dimension of stress processing.

To clarify the relationship between perceived physical appearance and adaptation, which may aid the development of treatment interventions, a model was generated based on the empiric literature with physically healthy children. In Harter's[49] multidimensional model of general self-esteem, perceived physical appearance is the most robust predictor, followed sequently by social acceptance, scholastic competence, and athletic competence. This theoretical framework in which perceived physical appearance predicts general self-esteem and psychological distress is also consistent with the generic literature on body image disturbance.[58,59]

In a study of 51 8- to 13-year-old children with limb deficiencies, Varni and Setoguchi[60] found that higher perceived physical appearance predicted lower depressive and anxious symptoms and higher general self-esteem. In a comparison of children and adolescents with limb deficiencies, Varni and Setoguchi[61] found that adolescents rated their perceived physical appearance considerably lower than did the children. As they grew older, the children showed a trend toward lower perceived physical appearance.

A study by Varni and Setoguchi[16] tested the conceptual model in adolescents with limb deficiencies. Consistent with previous findings, total limb loss was not significantly correlated with perceived physical appearance in adolescents with limb deficiencies. Age and gender also were not significantly correlated with perceived physical appearance. These findings suggest that the adolescent's perception of his or her physical appearance is relatively independent of the objective rating of total limb loss. Higher perceived physical appearance correlated significantly with lower depressive symptoms, lower trait anxiety, and higher general self-esteem. Path analysis findings indicate that the effect of perceived physical appearance on psychological distress was mediated by general self-esteem. Therefore, the effects of perceived physical appearance on depressive and anxious symptoms may be attenuated by interventions designed to enhance self-esteem.[62]

In addition to perceived physical appearance, perceptions of scholastic competence, athletic competence, social acceptance, and close friendship were also found to increase self-esteem. Because these domains may in fact be modifiable, interventions targeted toward promoting competence/adequacy may enhance general self-esteem.[62]

Varni and Corwin[62] have described a number of skills that can enhance self-esteem, including decision-making and problem-solving, social skills, expressing feelings, and positive self-talk. These cognitive-behavior therapy techniques have been widely used with physically healthy adolescents, and their systematic application to pediatric chronic physical disorders is only at the beginning stages of experimental validation. Alternatively, albeit perhaps more difficult, a focus on ameliorating body dissatisfaction, modeled after research in eating disorders,[63–65] might be modified to address the perceived physical appearance concerns of adolescents with limb deficiencies. By drawing from cognitive-behavior therapy interventions with adolescents and young adults without physical disorders, a rational and logical clinical plan can be developed for those adolescents with physical differences who may be experiencing socioemotional distress.

Cultural Factors in Children's Adjustment to Limb Deficiency

The Wallander/Varni disability-stress-coping model[13] proposes that adjustment is a function of risk factors (condition parameters, functional independence, and stress) and resistance factors (intrapersonal, socioecologic, and stress processing) that have direct and indirect effects on a child's adjustment to a chronic illness or disability. One aspect of this model is the role that cultural factors play in a child's adjustment to limb deficiency. In terms of the Wallander/Varni model, cultural factors belong to the category of socioecologic factors and can influence a child's adjustment in two ways: (1) indirectly, through the child's or family's appraisals of the disability, their experiences with the health-services system in general and the child's prosthesis specifically, and/or expectations of proper behavior by the child or those around him; and (2) directly, via utilitarian resources and parental familiarity and comfort with the health-services system.

Indirect Effects

Appraisals of Illness and Disability

Cultural factors may influence stress processing and thus adjustment by shaping the child's appraisal of his or her limb deficiency. It is hardly a new idea to state that there is a distinction between disease and illness.[66] Whereas disease has come to mean the physiologic process or "deviation from clinical norms, an organic pathology or abnormality,"[67] illness is the individual's interpretation or appraisal of that disease. The partial dependence of the subjective perception of illness on the person's interpretation of the disease is illustrated by research on why and when individuals decide to seek medical treatment. The correlation between disease and medical help-seeking is not perfect. Rather, "the likelihood of seeking care for a minor symptom increases when a person is in a bad mood, has a negative event happen in everyday life, lacks social support, or has no one to talk to."[68] Findings of individual differences in health appraisals are complemented by cultural variations in illness appraisal. In rural Greece, for example, measles, mumps, whooping cough, and chicken pox are not considered diseases but are thought to be a normal part of the process of growing up. Thus, illness is a "cultural category that an individual uses to interpret his or her experiences."[69] In certain cultures, disability is seen as a punishment from God, whereas in other cultures, for example traditional Mexican-Americans, a certain amount of bad luck is expected in this world.[70]

Expectations and Appraisals of Health Care

Cultural factors also shape expectations and appraisals of the health-care system and the child's and family's experience and satisfaction with the prosthesis. Medical anthropologists have written of the "crisis of rising expectations" seen in Anglo-Americans' dealings with the health-care system.[71] This group is thought to have such high expectations that anything less than perfect service and perfect health is seen as unacceptable. Other groups, for example traditional Mexican-Americans, who view health professionals with great respect, are more likely to accept actions and statements of health professionals at face value.

Appropriate 'Sick' Behavior

Cultural factors could influence adjustment by shaping the child's interpretation of the limb deficiency as well as the child's understanding of the socially acceptable role of an ill person.[72] Cultural variations exist in the way people respond to pain and disability. Zboworski's[73] classic study of pain expression in Jewish-American, Italian-American, and Anglo-American patients laid the foundation for research examining the impact of culture on the social expression of illness. In fact, the construct of disability is highly culturally and socially determined.[74] Moreover, the way in which someone with an illness or disability is expected to act, as well as the way in which people in their environment are expected to act towards that person varies across culture.[69] In some cultures, stoicism is valued while in others, people are expected to express their distress.[75] In German-American families, family members express little emotion and make few concessions when caring for a sick relative, while in Mexican-American families, it is customary for family members to pamper a sick relative.[75]

Direct Effects

Cultural factors also can affect a child's adjustment to limb deficiency. Socioeconomic and cultural variations entail variations in utilitarian resources and knowledge of and access to health services. Families with more means can arrange and pay for ancillary or supportive services for their child as well as tutors, after-school help, and so forth. Inability to speak English will make it more difficult to access the health-care system and to make the child's needs understood.

Using the Wallander/Varni model, we examined some of the indirect and direct effects of cultural background. We compared Spanish- and English-speaking parents of 4- to 16-year-old children with limb deficiencies in their responses to questionnaires regarding satisfaction with their child's prosthesis and the prosthesis service (CAPP-PSI),[37] perceptions of their child's functional status CAPP-FSI,[25] CAPP-FSI-Y,[26] and perceptions of their child's social and psychological functioning (the Child Behavior Checklist–Parent Report Form (CBCL).[76] We used language as a proxy measure for culture, assuming that Spanish-speakers in Los Angeles were less acculturated to the dominant Anglophone culture than were self-identified Anglophone Hispanics. We did not examine intraethnic differences (for example, distinguishing between Mexican-Americans and Puerto-Rican-Americans).

In this sample, both English- and Spanish-speaking children experienced similar (re)habilitation as a result of the prosthesis. Despite this similarity in the more 'objective' measure of adjustment, there were differences in how parents from the different cultures perceived their child's prosthesis and their child's social and psychological functioning.

Indirect Effects

Although we did not assess children's appraisals of their limb deficiency, we were able to gather data on parents' appraisals of the health-care system as well as their child's "sick" behavior. Spanish-speaking parents rated themselves more satisfied with their child's prosthesis and with the prosthesis service. If the proposition is correct that, by and large, less acculturated Mexican-Americans are more likely to have greater respect for health-care professionals and to expect some degree of misfortune in their lives, it could be that this higher satisfaction is, to some degree, culturally based.

Mexican-American patients are thought to be more expressive of their suffering than are Anglo-Americans, and Mexican-American families are said to be more indulgent and tolerant of a sick person's behavior than are Anglo-Americans.[75] Thus, we should expect Spanish-speaking parents to rate their children as having more psychological and social difficulties than English-speakers. Although all parents rated their children as essentially similar to a community sample, Spanish-speaking parents rated their children as higher in internalizing and externalizing behavior problems, as engaging less often in social activities, and as less socially competent.

Although these results may be a result of Spanish-speaking children's difficulty in adapting to the prosthesis, parental ratings of their own and their child's satisfaction and of the child's functional status, indicate that this is unlikely. It may be that these problems existed before the prosthesis. Epidemiologic studies have shown that Puerto Rican children have worse scores on the CBCL than do mainland US children.[75] However, Mexican-American children are epidemiologically similar to Anglo-American children in indicators of developmental and functional status.[77]

Direct Effects

Another explanation for these ratings of social and psychological functioning is that cultural factors directly affect child adjustment. That is, the Spanish-speaking families have fewer resources and experience more racism and marginalization than do English-speakers, and this translates directly into poorer child adjustment. In fact, the correlations within each group between socioeconomic status and ratings of social and psychological functioning are significant. Within the English- and Spanish-speaking groups lower socioeconomic status is related to worse scores on the CBCL.

Clearly, more research on this subject is needed, and the above interpretations should be considered within the context of this lack of research. An important starting point is to define and operationalize culture. While early definitions reflected culture as static and comprising a distinct set of beliefs, values, and morals, more recent anthropological writing has viewed culture as dynamic and changing–influenced by social transformations, social conflicts, power relationships, and migrations.[74] Future research should also take care to include the child's appraisals of his or her limb deficiency. Ultimately, researchers and practitioners will benefit by appreciating that adjustment to limb deficiency is many-faceted and multidetermined. Just as there are likely to be individual differences in adjustment, the child's cultural background should be considered as well.

Summary

The measurement and predictive pathways of HRQOL in pediatric limb deficiency have in recent years been the target of programmatic research efforts. These data have clarified the assessment and prediction of health and adaptational outcomes in pediatric limb deficiency. Empirically identifying the potentially modifiable risk and protective factors linked to health outcomes, in combination with state-of-the-art measurement technology, provides the infrastructure for enhanced clinical services for children and adolescents with limb deficiencies now and into the future.

References

1. Varni JW, Setoguchi Y: Psychosocial factors in the management of children with limb deficiencies. *Phys Med Rehabil Clin North Am* 1991;2:395–404.

2. Setoguchi Y, Rosenfelder R (eds): *The Limb Deficient Child.* Springfield, IL, CC Thomas, 1982.

3. Mariner WK: Outcomes assessment in health care reform: Promise and limitations. *Am J Law Med* 1994;20:37–57.

4. Mulley AG Jr, Eagle KA: What is inappropriate care? *JAMA* 1988;260:540–541.

5. Donabedian A: The quality of care: How can it be assessed? *JAMA* 1988;260:1743–1748.

6. Patton JG, Shida-Tokeshi J, Setoguchi Y: Prosthetic components for children. *Am J Phys Med Rehabil* 1991;5:245–264.

7. Varni JW, Katz ER, Seid M, Quiggins DJ, Friedman-Bender A: The Pediatric Cancer Quality of Life Inventory-32 (PCQL-32): I. Reliability and validity. *Cancer,* in press.

8. Varni JW, Katz ER, Seid M, Quiggins DJL, Friedman-Bender A, Castro CM: The Pediatric Cancer Quality of Life Inventory (PCQL): I. Instrument Development, Descriptive Statistics, and Cross-Informant Variance. *J Behav Med,* in press.

9. Varni JW, Setoguchi Y: Screening for behavioral and emotional problems in children and adolescents with congenital or acquired limb deficiencies. *Am J Dis Child* 1992;146:103–107.

10. Seid M, Sadler BL, Peddecord KM, Kurtin PS: *Accountability: Protecting The Well-Being of America's Children and Those Who Care for Them.* Alexandria, VA, National Association of Children's Hospitals and Related Institutions, 1997.

11. Wilson IB, Clearly PD: Linking clinical variables with health-related quality of life: A conceptual model of patient outcomes. *JAMA* 1995;273:59–65.

12. Varni JW, Wallander JL: Pediatric chronic disabilities: Hemophilia and spina bifida as examples, in Routh EK (ed): *Handbook of Pediatric Psychology.* New York, NY, Guilford Press, 1988, pp 190–221.

13. Wallander JL, Varni JW: Adjustment in children with chronic physical disorders: Programmatic research on a disability-stress-coping model, in La Greca AM, Siegel LJ, Wallander LJ, Walker CE (eds): *Stress and Coping in Child Health.* New York, NY, Guilford Press, 1992, pp 279–298.

14. Wallander JL, Varni JW: Appraisal, coping, and adjustment in adolescents with a physical disability, in Wallander JL, Siegel LJ (eds): *Adolescent Health Problems: Behavioral Perspectives.* New York, NY, Guilford Press, 1995, pp 209–231.

15. Pearlin LI, Lieberman MA, Menaghan EG, Mullan JT: The stress process. *J Health Soc Behav* 1981;22:337–356.

16. Varni JW, Setoguchi Y: Perceived physical appearance and adjustment of adolescents with congenital/acquired limb deficiencies: A path-analytic model. *J Clin Child Psychol* 1996;25:201–208.

17. Varni JW, Setoguchi Y, Rappaport LR, Talbot D: Effects of stress, social support, and self-esteem on depression in children with limb deficiencies. *Arch Phys Med Rehabil* 1991;72:1053–1058.

18. Varni JW, Rubenfeld LA, Talbot D, Setoguchi Y: Determinants of self-esteem in children with congenital/acquired limb deficiencies. *J Dev Behav Pediatr* 1989;10:13–16.

19. Greenfield S, Solomon NE, Brook RH, Davies-Avery A: Development of outcome criteria and standards to assess the quality of care for patients with osteoarthrosis. *J Chronic Dis* 1978;31:375–388.

20. Kantz ME, Harris WJ, Levitsky K, Ware JE Jr, Davies AR: Methods for assessing condition-specific and generic functional status outcomes after total knee replacement. *Med Care* 1992;30(suppl 5):MS240–MS252.

21. Lembcke PA: Measuring the quality of medical care through vital statistics based on hospital service areas: I. Comparative study of appendectomy rates. *Am J Public Health* 1952;42:276–286.

22. Mendez MA: Evaluation of a myoelectric hand prosthesis for children with a below-elbow absence. *Prosthet Orthot Int* 1985;9:137–140.

23. Stein RB, Walley M: Functional comparison of upper extremity amputees using myoelectric and conventional prostheses. *Arch Phys Med Rehabil* 1983;64:243–248.

24. Weaver SA, Lange LR, Vogts VM: Comparison of myoelectric and conventional prostheses for adolescent amputees. *Am J Occup Ther* 1988;42:87–91.

25. Pruitt SD, Varni JW, Setoguchi Y: Functional status in children with limb deficiency: Development and initial validation of an outcome measure. *Arch Phys Med Rehabil* 1996;77:1233–1238.

26. Pruitt SD, Varni JW, Seid M, Setoguchi Y: Functional status in limb deficiency: Development of an outcome measure for preschool children. *Arch Phys Med Rehabil*, in press.

27. Abramowitz S, Cote AA, Berry E: Analyzing patient satisfaction: A multianalytic approach. *Quality Rev Bull* 1987;13:122–130.

28. Korsch BM, Gozzi EK, Francis V: Gaps in doctor-patient communication: 1. Doctor-patient interaction and patient satisfaction. *Pediatrics* 1968;42:855–871.

29. Sherbourne CD, Hays RD, Ordway L, DiMatteo MR, Kravitz RL: Antecedents of adherence to medical recommendations: Results from the Medical Outcomes Study. *J Behav Med* 1992;15:447–468.

30. Ley P: Patients' understanding and recall in clinical communication failure, in Pendleton D, Hasler J (eds): *Doctor-Patient Communication.* London, England, Academic Press, 1983, pp 89–107.

31. Marshall GN, Hayes RD, Mazel R: Health status and satisfaction with health care: Results from the Medical Outcomes Study. *J Consult Clin Psychol* 1996;64:380–390.

32. Marquis MS, Davies AR, Ware JE Jr: Patient satisfaction and change in medical care provider: A longitudinal study. *Med Care* 1983;21:821–829.

33. Ware JE Jr, Davies AR: Behavioral consequences of consumer dissatisfaction with medical care. *Eval Prog Plan* 1983;6:291–297.

34. Penchansky R, Macnee C: Initiation of medical malpractice suits: A conceptualization and test. *Med Care* 1994;32:813–831.

35. Boyle M, Tebbi CK, Mindell ER, Mettlin CJ: Adolescent adjustment to amputation. *Med Pediatr Oncol* 1982;10:301–312.

36. Tebbi CK, Petrilli AS, Richards ME: Adjustment to amputation among adolescent oncology patients. *Am J Pediatr Hematol Oncol* 1989;11:276–280.

37. Pruitt SD, Varni JW, Seid M, Setoguchi Y: Prosthesis satisfaction outcome measurement in pediatric limb deficiency. *Arch Phys Med Rehabil* 1997;78:750–754.

38. Cronbach LJ: Coefficient alpha and the internal structure of tests. *Psychometrika* 1951;16:297–334.

39. Helmstadter GC (ed): *Principles of Psychological Measurement*. New York, NY, Appleton-Century-Crofts, 1964.

40. Jain S: Rehabilitation in limb deficiency: 2. The pediatric amputee. *Arch Phys Med Rehabil* 1996;77(suppl 3):S9–S13.

41. Walter LS, Greene JW: The functional disability inventory: Measuring a neglected dimension of child health status. *J Pediatr Psychol* 1991;16:39–58.

42. Varni JW, Rubenfeld LA, Talbot D, Setoguchi Y: Stress, social support, and depressive symptomatology in children with congenital/acquired limb deficiencies. *J Pediatr Psychol* 1989;14:515–530.

43. Varni JW, Rubenfeld LA, Talbot D, Setoguchi Y: Family functioning, temperament, and psychological adaptation in children with congenital or acquired limb deficiencies. *Pediatrics* 1989;84:323–330.

44. Buss AH, Plomin R (eds): *Temperament: Early Developing Personality Traits*. Hillsdale, NJ, L Erlbaum Associates, 1984.

45. Chess S, Thomas A (eds): *Temperament in Clinical Practice*. New York, NY, Guilford Press, 1986.

46. Varni JW, Setoguchi Y, Rappaport LR, Talbot D: Psychological adjustment and perceived social support in children with congenital/acquired limb deficiencies. *J Behav Med* 1992;15:31–44.

47. Harper DC, Wacker DP, Cobb LS: Children's social preferences toward peers with visible physical differences. *J Pediatr Psychol* 1986;11:323–342.

48. Richardson SA: Age and sex differences in values toward physical handicaps. *J Health Soc Behav* 1970;11:207–214.

49. Harter S: The determinants and mediational role of global self-worth in children, in Eisenberg N (ed): *Contemporary Topics in Developmental Psychology*. New York, NY, Wiley, 1987, pp 219–242.

50. Varni JW, Steoguchi Y: Effects of parental adjustment on the adaptation of children with congenital or acquired limb deficiencies. *J Dev Behav Pediatr* 1993;14:13–20.

51. Varni JW, Katz ER, Colegrove R Jr, Dolgin M: The impact of social skills training on the adjustment of children with newly diagnosed cancer. *J Pediatr Psychol* 1993;18:751–767.

52. Adams GR: Physical attractiveness research: Toward a developmental social psychology of beauty. *Hum Dev* 1977;20:217–239.

53. Benson PL, Karabenick SA, Lerner RM: Pretty pleases: The effects of physical attractiveness, race, and sex on receiving help. *J Exp Soc Psychol* 1976;12:409–415.

54. Dion KK: Children's physical attractiveness and sex as determinants of adult punitiveness. *Dev Psychol* 1974;10:772–778.

55. Jones RM, Adams GR: Assessing the importance of physical attractiveness across the life-span. *J Soc Psychol* 1982;118:131–132.

56. Lerner RM, Lerner JV: Effects of age, sex, and physical attractiveness on child-peer relations, academic performance, and elementary school adjustment. *Dev Psychol* 1977;13:585–590.

57. Richardson SA: Attitudes and behavior toward the physically handicapped. *Birth Defects* 1976;12:15–34.

58. Cash TF, Pruzinsky T (eds): *Body Images: Development, Deviance, and Change.* New York, NY, Guilford Press, 1990.

59. Thompson JK (ed): *Body Image Disturbance: Assessment and Treatment.* Elmsford, NY, Pergamon Press, 1990.

60. Varni JW, Setoguchi Y: Correlates of perceived physical appearance in children with congenital/acquired limb deficiencies. *J Dev Behav Pediatr* 1991;12: 171–176.

61. Varni JW, Setoguchi Y: Self-perceived physical appearance in children and adolescents with congenital/acquired limb deficiencies. *J Assoc Child Prosthet Orth Clin* 1991;26:56–60.

62. Varni JW, Corwin DG (eds): *Growing Up Great: Positive Solutions to Raising Confident, Self-Assured Children.* New York, NY, Berkley Books, 1993.

63. Butters JW, Cash TF: Cognitive-behavioral treatment of women's body-image dissatisfaction. *J Consult Clin Psychol* 1987;55:889–897.

64. Rosen JC, Cado S, Silberg NT, Srebnik D, Wendt S: Cognitive behavior therapy with and without size perception training for women with body image disturbance. *Behav Ther* 1990;21:481–498.

65. Wilfley DE, Agras WS, Telch CF, et al: Group cognitive-behavioral therapy and group interpersonal psychotherapy for the nonpurging bulimic individual: A controlled comparison. *J Consult Clin Psychol* 1993;61:296–305.

66. Cassell EJ (ed): *The Healer's Art: A New Approach to the Doctor-Patient Relationship.* New York, NY, JB Lippincott, 1976.

67. McElroy A, Townsend PK (eds): *Medical Anthropology in Ecological Perspective,* ed 2. Boulder, CO, Westview Press, 1989.

68. Lynch WD, Edington DW, Johnson A: Predicting the demand for healthcare. *Healthcare Forum Journal* 1996;39:20–24.

69. Hutchinson JF: Quality of life in ethnic groups, in Spilker B (ed): *Quality of Life and Pharmacoeconomics in Clinical Trials,* ed 2. Philadelphia, PA, Lippincott-Raven, 1996, pp 587–593.

70. Lassiter SM (ed): *Multicultural Clients: A Professional Handbook for Healthcare Providers and Social Workers.* Westport, CT, Greenwood Press, 1995.

71. Vener AM, Krupka LR, Climo JJ: Drug usage and health characteristics in non-institutionalized Mexican-American elderly. *J Drug Educ* 1980;10:343–353.

72. Helman C (ed): *Culture, Health, and Illness: An Introduction for Health Professionals,* ed 2. London, England, Wright, 1990.

73. Zborowski M: Cultural components in responses to pain. *J Social Issues* 1952;8:16–30.

74. Guarnaccia PJ: Anthropological perspectives: The importance of culture in the assessment of quality of life, in Spilker B (ed): *Quality of Life and Pharmacoeconomics in Clinical Trials,* ed 2. Philadelphia, PA, Lippincott-Raven, 1996, pp 523–528.

75. Galanti GA (ed): *Caring for Patients From Different Cultures: Case Studies From American Hospitals.* Philadelphia, PA, University of Pennsylvania Press, 1991.

76. Achenbach TM, Edelbrock CS (eds): *Manual for the Child Behavior Checklist and Revised Child Behavior Profile.* Burlington, VT, TM Achenbach, 1983.

77. Arcia E, Keyes L, Gallagher JJ: Indicators of developmental and functional status of Mexican-American and Puerto Rican children. *J Dev Behav Pediatr* 1994;15:27–33.

Index

Page numbers in italic refer to figures or figure legends.